THEY CALLED IT SHELL SHOCK

THEY CALLED IT SHELL SHOCK

Combat Stress in the First World War

Wolverhampton Military Studies No.24

Stefanie Linden

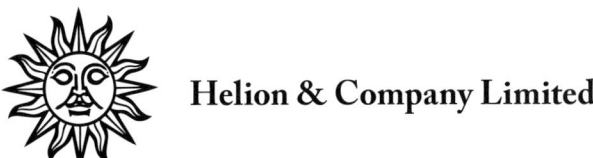

Helion & Company Limited

Helion & Company Limited
26 Willow Road
Solihull
West Midlands
B91 1UE
England
Tel. 0121 705 3393
Fax 0121 711 4075
Email: info@helion.co.uk
Website: www.helion.co.uk
Twitter: @helionbooks
Visit our blog at http://blog.helion.co.uk/

Published by Helion & Company 2016
Designed and typeset by Mach 3 Solutions Ltd (www.mach3solutions.co.uk)
Cover designed by Paul Hewitt, Battlefield Design (www.battlefield-design.co.uk)
Printed by Short Run Press Limited, Exeter, Devon

Text © Stefanie Linden 2016
Images © as individually credited
Maps drawn by George Anderson © Helion & Company 2016

Every reasonable effort has been made to trace copyright holders and to obtain their permission for the use of copyright material. The author and publisher apologize for any errors or omissions in this work, and would be grateful if notified of any corrections that should be incorporated in future reprints or editions of this book.

Cover: 'Blown up, mad' by William Orpen, (Imperial War Museum, London, ART 2376)

ISBN 978-1-911096-35-1

British Library Cataloguing-in-Publication Data.
A catalogue record for this book is available from the British Library.

All rights reserved. No part of this publication may be reproduced, stored in a retrieval system, or transmitted, in any form, or by any means, electronic, mechanical, photocopying, recording or otherwise, without the express written consent of Helion & Company Limited.

For details of other military history titles published by Helion & Company Limited, contact the above address, or visit our website: http://www.helion.co.uk

We always welcome receiving book proposals from prospective authors.

Contents

List of Illustrations	vi
List of Maps	xi
Foreword	xii
Series Preface	xv
Author's Preface and Acknowledgements	xvii
1. A Red-Letter Day for Professor Charcot	19
2. Shell Shock on Both Sides of the Trenches	34
3. From the Fields of Flanders to the Temple of Neurology	41
4. What Major Mott made of Shell Shock	71
5. Neuve Chapelle and Hill 60	83
6. 20 May 1917: One Day on the Shell Shock Ward	105
7. The Mental World of Terror	120
8. Dream Worlds	136
9. The Ultimate Way Out: Suicide in the Trenches	146
10. Desertion	158
11. Madness on the Streets of London and Berlin	177
12. Believe Me, He Will Be Cured	191
13. The Obsession with the Shell	217
14. Shell Shock and PTSD: The Debates Go On	232
Bibliography	250
Index	261

List of Illustrations

A portrait of J.-M. Charcot – head and shoulders in profile; photograph circa 1875. (Wellcome Library, London)   19

Jean-Martin Charcot demonstrating hysteria in a patient at the Salpêtrière; lithograph after P.A.A. Brouillet, 1887. (Wellcome Library, London)   21

From *Études cliniques sur l'hystéro-épilepsie ou grande hystérie* by Paul Marie Louis Pierre Richer; published: Delahaye et Lecrosnier, Paris, 1881; second period: clownism, Plate III. (Wellcome Library, London)   23

From *Études cliniques sur l'hystéro-épilepsie ou grande hystérie* by Paul Marie Louis Pierre Richer; published: Delahaye et Lecrosnier, Paris, 1881; third period: *attitudes passionnelles*, Plate IV. (Wellcome Library, London)   24

A photograph of Private Albert W. of the 5th Dragoon Guards, 1915. (Queen Square Archives, London)   29

Troops supposedly 'going over the top' at the start of the Battle of the Somme in 1916, photographed by Canadian official photographer Ivor Castle. This photograph was widely (and misleadingly) published as a portrayal of an actual British attack; however, it was actually taken during a training exercise behind the lines. The breech cover, which is clearly visible on the rifle of the soldier in the foreground, was edited out in contemporary publications of the photograph; Canadian First World War Official Exchange Collection, 1916, CO 874. (Imperial War Museum, London)   35

James S., a machine gunner from the 9th Royal Fusiliers, who was blind, deaf and mute after spending six hours in a dugout with his dead comrades; written communication between James and his doctor, 1917. (Queen Square Archives, London)   36

Two patients in the hospital, April 1915; photograph, Queen Square Reports. (Queen Square Archives, London)   42

The chapel at Claybury Asylum, Woodford, Essex; photograph by the London & County Photographic Co., Bromley, Kent [1893?]. (Wellcome Library, London)   45

List of Illustrations   vii

Claybury Asylum, Woodford, Essex; photographs by the London & County Photographic Co., Bromley, Kent [1893?]. Top: the recreation hall; bottom: a nurses' day room. (Wellcome Library, London)   46
The Royal Victoria Hospital, Netley; postcard. (Author's own archive)   48
The National Hospital for the Paralysed and Epileptic, circa 1914. (Queen Square Archives, London)   50
Victor Horsley in his operating theatre at Queen Square; photograph; QSA/1518. (Queen Square Archives, London)   50
Paul Ehrlich and Sahachiro Hata working on Salvarsan; public domain. (Wikipedia: https://de.wikipedia.org/wiki/Paul_Ehrlich#/media/File:Paul_Ehrlich_and_Sahachiro_Hata)   51
Minutes from the Board of Management meeting, 10 November 1914, National Hospital for the Paralysed and Epileptic, London; appended to the minutes is an article by Lord Knutsford: 'To the editor of the Daily Mail' (exact date unknown) (Queen Square Archives, London).   53
The letter by Rachel F. Alexander, 10 November 1915; letter preserved in case record Adolf S., Dr Tooth, 1915, male L-Z. (Queen Square Archives, London)   55
Consultants at Queen Square, 1904; QSA/15391. (Queen Square Archives, London)   57
Surgery at the Hotel Claridge ('*Hôpital Anglo- Belge*'): Flora Murray is giving the anaesthetic, Hazel Cuthbert is the surgeon to the left of the picture and Majorie Blandy is to the right; photograph. (Imperial War Museum, London)   59
A view of one of the ANZAC landing places. (From *The Times History and Encyclopaedia of the War*, part 64, Vol 5, Nov 9, 1915, p.450)   61
Sir Victor Horsley in uniform, 1915; QSA/14049. (Queen Square Archives, London)   62
The Dardanelles: a dressing station; an operation in progress. (From *The Times History and Encyclopaedia of the War*, Science and the Health of Armies, part 67, Vol 6, Nov 30, 1915, p.47)   64
In memory of Colonel Sir Victor Horsley, who died on service at Amara, 16.7.16; Sir Victor Horsley's grave, Amara, photograph; QSA/1808. (Queen Square Archives, London)   66
Private Henry M. from the 18th Hussars; photograph attached to case record. (Queen Square Archives, London)   68
Munition workers in a shell warehouse at the National Shell Filling Factory, Chilwell, Nottinghamshire, Q_30018. (Imperial War Museum, London)   72
An examination of the skull and brain – a method of removing the brain after it is severed from the body. (Wellcome Library, London)   74
A photograph of Frederick Walker Mott. (Wellcome Library, London)   75

German soldiers surrender, as Canadian support waves advance across Vimy Ridge at the beginning of the Battle of Arras, 9 April 1917; CO 001155. (Imperial War Museum, London) 79

Neuve Chapelle – fighting in the village; photograph taken by an officer of the Worcester Regiment, Lt. M.A. Hamilton-Cox. (Mercian Regiment Museum, Worcester) 84

The churchyard, Neuve Chapelle; photograph taken during the battle, 10 March 1915. Note the crucifix standing after the heavy bombardment; Q 56178. (Imperial War Museum, London) 92

Officers of 'C' Company, 1st Battalion, Cameronians (Scottish Rifles) taking a tea break in the trenches at Grande Flamengrie Farm – on the Bois Grenier sector of the line – in May 1915; Q 51632. (Imperial War Museum, London) 95

A German battery of chlorine gas cylinders being prepared for an attack, and awaiting the right weather conditions to prevent blowback, similar to the arrangement at Hill 60 in May 1915; open domain. (Private collection) 99

'A Whiff of the Kaiser's Gas' – *Western Mail*, 13 July 1915: '… it was the use of gas by the Germans in the Second Battle of Ypres, which began on 22 April 1915 that caused the greatest condemnation. It went against the 1907 Hague Convention on Land Warfare, which prohibited the use of "poison or poisoned weapons"'; cartoon by Joseph Morewood Staniforth, Cartooning the First World War Project. (Cardiff University) 100

British casualties of the gas attack on Hill 60 receiving treatment at No.8 Casualty Clearing Station, Bailleul; Q 114867. (Imperial War Museum, London) 102

A Zeppelin bomb damage display, with a cabinet containing evidence of bomb damage in Queen Square from a Zeppelin raid in September 1915. It includes a note describing the event, photos, part of a garden railing and a fragment of the bomb; QSA/15424. (Queen Square Archives, London) 106

The National Hospital on 8 September 1915 after the Zeppelin raid; photograph, QSA/15429. (Queen Square Archives, London) 106

Frederick Kempster – the world's tallest man – occupying two hospital beds; QSA/12389. (Queen Square Archives, London) 109

Frederick Kempster – a photograph in the hospital yard at Queen Square. (Queen Square Archives, London) 109

The Reverend John Back, vicar of St George the Martyr and the National Hospital; QSA/1814. (Queen Square Archives, London) 110

John Back ward, National Hospital; QSA/1328. (Queen Square Archives, London) 112

Blown up, mad. William Orpen; ART 2376. (Imperial War Museum, London) 121

Karl Kleist, during a lecture at Frankfurt University, demonstrating a catatonic state; photograph taken by one of his students circa 1939. (Author's own archive)   122

Shell-shocked soldier; Pte E., severe hyperadrenalism and hyperthyroidism with exophthalmos, resulting from prolonged terror; Fig. II, 1; Hurst, Arthur, *Medical Diseases of the War.* (London: Edward Arnold, 1918)   123

'Shining Angels throw a protective curtain around men from the Lincolnshire Regiment at Mons'; Alfred Pearse, published in *The Chariots of God* by a churchwoman in 1915. (London: AH Stockwell, 1916)   137

'Gott in Himmel! I am shocked!' – *Western Mail*, 1 September 1914: 'In this cartoon, a German soldier recoils with shock and surprise, as he touches the "live wire" of British resistance at the Battle of Mons. The battle itself has gained a mythic status as victory against overwhelming odds, and this is perpetuated by the reported sighting by soldiers of the Angels of Mons. In this cartoon, an elderly German soldier is clearly dismayed, as he confronts the steady gaze of a youthful British Tommy. The shock has caused him to fall backwards – losing his rifle, helmet, ammunition and a string of sausages.' Cartoon by Joseph Morewood Staniforth, Cartooning the First World War Project. (Cardiff University)   138

A collection of German spies, cartoon; from Hirschfeld, M. and Gaspar, A., *Sittengeschichte des ersten Weltkrieges* (Hanau: Müller & Kiepenheuer, 1929; re-print of the 2nd revised edition, 1980), p.399.   139

Welsh people during a revival meeting on a field in Anglesey. (Anglesey Archives, Llangefni)   145

Otto Dix, '*Toter Sappenposten*' ('Dead Sentry'), from 'Der Krieg'; etching, 1924. (British Museum, Artists' Rights Society)   147

A visit of the Kaiser to the Citadel in Belgrade – the first German Emperor to do so since Friedrich Barbarossa (12th century), 19 January 1916; photograph, Q 27202. (Imperial War Museum, London)   148

Methods used by Americans to mark stragglers and deserters; photograph, Q 70742. (Imperial War Museum, London)   159

German and Dutch guards at a frontier post on the border between both countries, Q 88209. (Imperial War Museum, London)   160

Two German deserters being questioned by an intelligence staff officer at First Army Headquarters, Ranchicourt, 5 March 1918; Q 10715. (Imperial War Museum, London)   163

Familien-Freibad Wannsee/Berlin; postcard, 1916. (Author's own archive)   168

'John Bull: "What extraordinary creatures! And to think that they are British, too!"' – *Western Mail*, 21 January 1916; cartoon by Joseph Morewood Staniforth, Cartooning the First World War Project. (Cardiff University)   172

A photograph of an RFC pilot, which was taken by Lieutenant William
George Dundas – a reconnaissance photographer of the 82nd Squadron,
Royal Flying Corps; photograph kindly contributed by Louisa Cantwell.
(The Great War Archive, University of Oxford) 178

Results of an aerial collision: the aircraft to the far right appears to be a Bristol
F2b; that to the far left, a de Havilland DH4, which were introduced
respectively in March and April 1917; photograph taken by Lieutenant
William George Dundas – image kindly contributed by Louisa Cantwell.
(The Great War Archive, University of Oxford) 179

Flourmills after the Silvertown explosion; the grain silos and warehouses of
the flourmills were amongst the 17 acres that the Port of London Authority
estimated were damaged. John H. Avery photographed the wreckage
immediately after and throughout the reconstruction, which was completed
in 1921; photograph taken on 25 January 1917 – image ID: 141272.
(Museum of London Picture Library) 182

Cartoon, R. Pallier, 'Le Rire rouge', 1917; from Hirschfeld, M. and Gaspar,
A., *Sittengeschichte des ersten Weltkrieges* (Hanau: Müller & Kiepenheuer,
1929; re-print of the 2nd revised edition, 1980), p.116. 184

Berlin Alexanderplatz, 1915; postcard. (Author's own archive) 186

'Cheer up, sweetheart, you will be back at the front in a week's time'; from
Hirschfeld, M. and Gaspar, A., *Sittengeschichte des ersten Weltkrieges* (Hanau:
Müller & Kiepenheuer, 1929; re-print of the 2nd revised edition, 1980), p.131. 192

Discharge against medical advice: Dr Yealland's handwriting, patient's
signature; Queen Square Records, Dr Taylor, 1917, male L-Z: case record
James T. (Queen Square Archives, London) 193

A graduation photograph of Lewis Ralph Yealland, 1912. (With kind
permission of Dr Susan Yealland, family archive) 196

'Kaufmann method' caricature; from Hirschfeld, M. and Gaspar, A.,
Sittengeschichte des ersten Weltkrieges (Hanau: Müller & Kiepenheuer, 1929;
re-print of the 2nd revised edition, 1980), p.360. 200

Christmas in a soldiers' ward, 1916; QSA/15491. (Queen Square Archives,
London) 203

A referral letter for Private Harry T., which was written by S. Farquhar
Buzzard, consultant at Queen Square. (Queen Square Archives, London) 204

Wounded soldiers in invalid chairs being taken around the grounds of No.4
London General Hospital, Q 27814. (Imperial War Museum, London) 210

The basket-making class at Lonsdale House; photograph, QSA/15492.
(Queen Square Archives, London) 211

Getting fit to return to the trenches: German wounded undergoing scientific
treatment in a Berlin hospital. (From *The Times History and Encyclopaedia of
the War*, part 57, Vol 5, Sept 21, 1915, p.197) 212

Florence Stoney (centre) with her sister, Edith – a physics lecturer at the London (Royal Free) School of Medicine for Women – in 1899, and their father, G. Johnstone Stoney (the Irish physicist, who coined the word 'electron'). During the war years, Edith left her teaching career to work in field hospitals, in order to provide X-ray and electrotherapy services to wounded soldiers and civilians with the Scottish Women's Hospitals (SWH); PH/10/4 Chrystal album no.2 (Newnham College Archives, Cambridge) 225

Angst der Londoner vor den Zeppelinen ('Londoners in fear of Zeppelin raids'), postcard. (Author's own archive) 228

The church of St Bartholomew the Great and the surrounding area (Bartholomew Close) after the Zeppelin air raid on 8 September 1915; photograph, V0029993. (Wellcome Library, London) 229

The world's first electric tram – the Groß-Lichterfelde Tramway – began operation in 1881 in the Lichterfelde neighbourhood of Berlin, Germany and was produced by Werner von Siemens; a direct current was supplied through the rails. (Photograph in public domain) 237

'On the cemetery in Ypres: "Remind me, why did we actually kill each other?"'; from Hirschfeld, M. and Gaspar, A., Sittengeschichte des ersten Weltkrieges. (Hanau: Müller & Kiepenheuer, 1929; reprint of the 2nd revised edition, 1980, p.569) 245

List of Maps

1 The Gallipoli Peninsula and the Dardanelles. (Map by George Anderson) 65
2 Neuve Chapelle. (Map drawn by George Anderson) 85
3 'The Battle of Neuve Chapelle, March 10–12, 1915, trench line before and after the battle' (Map drawn by George Anderson) 93
4 The Western Front and the Dutch/Belgian/German border area; remarkably, Musketeer Wilhelm B. moved relatively freely back and forth between the three countries [Coblenz reserve base; Venlo, where Wilhelm lived in a big community of German deserters; Dinant, where Wilhelm was arrested by German military police; Neuss (parents' house), on the west bank of the Rhine; München-Gladbach (modern Mönchengladbach), where Wilhelm met his friend, is located west of the Rhine – halfway between Düsseldorf and the Dutch border]. (Map drawn by George Anderson) 161

Foreword

On 4 October 1916, during the Battle of the Somme, James S. – a machine gunner from the 9th Royal Fusiliers – was buried together with 11 of his comrades after a shell exploded in a dugout in which they were sheltering. He alone survived, surrounded by their mutilated bodies. When pulled out six hours later he was blind, deaf, dumb and paralysed. Meanwhile, not far away 39-year-old German Pioneer Franz B. was not doing well either. Overcome by terror and continuous nightmares, he started to develop fits and loss of consciousness. Both would end up in hospitals largely given over to dealing with the new kind of injuries that had turned into an epidemic, Franz to the Charité in Berlin and James went to the National Hospital for the Paralysed and Epileptic in London.

In 1989 I went to work at the hospital that had treated James, now called The National Hospital for Neurology and Neurosurgery or simply "Queen Square". I was one of the small number of psychiatrists working in this neurological Holy of Holies. Every Thursday afternoon I was permitted to see my patients in what was called Consulting Room B. It was a vast room, its four walls covered with large book cases from floor to ceiling. Each shelf was filled with large case books, their spines embossed with the name of the giants of Queen Square – Gowers, Hughlings Jackson, Buzzard, Holmes, Ferrier and so on. I was only allowed to use this shrine because Thursday afternoon was when all the neurologists attended the "Gowers Round", during which reputations were made and unmade. Whenever one of my patients decided not to turn up, I would open the casebooks at random and read the stories they contained. I was captivated by the accounts of neurasthenic maids, neuralgic office workers, and finally shell shocked soldiers, although I don't recall James S.

22 years later psychiatrist and medical historian Stefanie Linden was introduced to the same material, no longer in such a spectacular setting as Room B, but now safely in the Queen Square archives, albeit still uncatalogued. She soon located James S. and many others. A few were already well known – scholars such as Elaine Showalter had drawn on Lewis Yealland's accounts in "Hysterical Disorders of Warfare", and novelists such as Pat Barker had done likewise. But Linden now shows how Barker embellished Yealland's account, which in turn was an embellishment of the original case record. As with so much else surrounding the story of psychiatry in the Great War, Barker's fictional caricature in the Regeneration trilogy is still the version most likely to endure, as it is both a school set text and a Hollywood film. It would be

wonderful to think that the book you are about to read receives both accolades – but in the meantime I hope that students and members of the public do take Linden's work to heart as much as they have done Pat Barker's.

One of Linden's many strengths is to give equal weight to not just James S. and his comrades, but also Franz B. and his, avoiding some of the Anglocentric focus of earlier scholarship.[1] She shows not just the similarities, but also the differences in the experiences of shell shock either side of the trenches. Her observations on the increased prevalence for example of pseudo neurological presentations in German rather than British service personnel emphasises the importance of cultural factors in how these disorders manifest themselves. This can sometimes be overlooked in the contemporary explosion of research activity to find a universal explanation for the phenomena across time and space, and hence a single test or biomarker, let alone treatment.

Shell shock only had a brief medical and military life in Britain. First used in 1915 in Myers's famous Lancet paper, it was over by 1917, banned by the Adjutant General, and disappeared from medical discourse shortly after. It only appears in modern psychiatry textbooks in the ritual first chapter on history, where it is usually, and erroneously, described as an early manifestation of what we now call post-traumatic stress disorder. Sometimes this is accompanied by some words to the effect that back then psychological trauma was misunderstood, poorly recognised, and that the person afflicted was more likely to be executed than treated. It takes its place in a Whiggish narrative in which we move from ignorance to our contemporary enlightenment, another questionable assumption.

And yet just as shell shock was being eclipsed in medicine and the military, it shifted into literature and culture. Well before "All Quiet", Rebecca West, A.P. Herbert, Dorothy Sayers and Virginia Woolf had all used it. In "Mrs Dalloway" Woolf introduces us to the shell shocked soldier Septimus Smith, his initials those of Siegfried Sassoon, described as a sensitive poet from Stroud, and thus beginning the linkage between shell shock, the officer class and poetic sensibility. And from literature it moved into the vernacular. Google will confirm that not a day passes without some troubled politician, defeated sports manager or distraught celebrity being described as "shell shocked", and as I write the most troubling computer virus currently doing the rounds is labelled "shell shock".

It was therefore no surprise to see how shell shock took a central place in the extraordinary range of commemorative activities across the United Kingdom marking the centenary of the Great War. This has occurred on a scale not seen in any of the other countries that had participated in the conflict. This is probably because the First World War was the defining event of our century. It was not only the most costly war we have ever fought, but also the most significant event in our modern social and political history. For the United States the story of the First World War was

---

1 Wessely S. Essay Review: Hysterical Men: War, Psychiatry and the Politics of Trauma. History of Psychiatry 2004:15:489-494.

overshadowed in every respect by the Second. Amongst the European participants only in this country has it not been overshadowed by the many and terrible consequences that would follow 1914-1918 – defeat, revolution, occupation, collaboration, totalitarianism or genocide. So the 2014 commemoration and remembrance events in the United Kingdom focussed largely on the cultural memory of futility, slaughter and suffering – and at the heart was our contemporary reading of shell shock. As part of the anniversary most TV channels broadcast a steady stream of dramas and drama documentaries concerned with the war. I can only remember one that did not include shell shock as an important and in some cases dominant theme (the exception was a production focussed exclusively on the events of the July Crisis). Many also linked this with the endlessly powerful imagery of military executions. Much the same was true of the numerous smaller scale creative films commissioned by the Imperial War Museum, or new theatre dramas launched across the country. Quite what Sassoon or Owen would have made of "Shell Shock- the Musical" which had a brief nationwide tour will remain one of the "what ifs" of history.

We should not be surprised that shell shock so comprehensively outlived its military and medical obituaries. The word retains its power - it is not just a description of a particular syndrome, restricted in time and place – it is now the metaphor for the British experience of the Great War. It defies translation – try using French or German translation software for it and you will see what I mean. It captures the impact of the shell on the body, on the mind, and on society and culture. Myers himself agreed that his diagnostic category had outlived its purpose, but could not have anticipated that what he had created would move from a discarded diagnosis to becoming the most potent symbol of the suffering, futility despair, meaninglessness and misery that has come to symbolise the Great War.

Shell shock has been well served by the historians, and Dr Linden draws from and pays tribute to many in the course of this book. But it is her inspired usage of the new and detailed clinical descriptions she has uncovered principally at Queen Square and the Charité that brings a new fresh perspective on the experience and nature of shell shock. Her command of clinical knowledge, historical scholarship and her engaging style has resulted in what will become a classic. If only it could be a film as well.

Professor Sir Simon Wessely
Regius Professor of Psychiatry, Institute of Psychiatry,
Psychology and Neurology; King's College London
President, Royal College of Psychiatrists.

The Wolverhampton Military Studies Series
Series Editor's Preface

As series editor, it is my great pleasure to introduce the *Wolverhampton Military Studies Series* to you. Our intention is that in this series of books you will find military history that is new and innovative, and academically rigorous with a strong basis in fact and in analytical research, but also is the kind of military history that is for all readers, whatever their particular interests, or their level of interest in the subject. To paraphrase an old aphorism: a military history book is not less important just because it is popular, and it is not more scholarly just because it is dull. With every one of our publications we want to bring you the kind of military history that you will want to read simply because it is a good and well-written book, as well as bringing new light, new perspectives, and new factual evidence to its subject.

In devising the *Wolverhampton Military Studies Series*, we gave much thought to the series title: this is a *military* series. We take the view that history is everything except the things that have not happened yet, and even then a good book about the military aspects of the future would find its way into this series. We are not bound to any particular time period or cut-off date. Writing military history often divides quite sharply into eras, from the modern through the early modern to the mediaeval and ancient; and into regions or continents, with a division between western military history and the military history of other countries and cultures being particularly marked. Inevitably, we have had to start somewhere, and the first books of the series deal with British military topics and events of the twentieth century and later nineteenth century. But this series is open to any book that challenges received and accepted ideas about any aspect of military history, and does so in a way that encourages its readers to enjoy the discovery.

In the same way, this series is not limited to being about wars, or about grand strategy, or wider defence matters, or the sociology of armed forces as institutions, or civilian society and culture at war. None of these are specifically excluded, and in some cases they play an important part in the books that comprise our series. But there are already many books in existence, some of them of the highest scholarly standards, which cater to these particular approaches. The main theme of the *Wolverhampton Military Studies Series* is the military aspects of wars, the preparation for wars or their prevention, and their aftermath. This includes some books whose main theme is the technical details of how armed forces have worked, some books on wars and battles, and some books that re-examine the evidence about the existing stories, to show in a different light what everyone thought they already knew and understood.

As series editor, together with my fellow editorial board members, and our publisher Duncan Rogers of Helion, I have found that we have known immediately and almost by instinct the kind of books that fit within this series. They are very much the kind of well-written and challenging books that my students at the University of Wolverhampton would want to read. They are books which enhance knowledge, and offer new perspectives. Also, they are books for anyone with an interest in military history and events, from expert scholars to occasional readers. One of the great benefits of the study of military history is that it includes a large and often committed section of the wider population, who want to read the best military history that they can find; our aim for this series is to provide it.

Stephen Badsey
University of Wolverhampton

Author's Preface and Acknowledgements

In my journeys through the patient records of shell shock hospitals in Britain and Germany, I often encountered soldiers who were traumatised in the same battle – just on different sides of the front line. On 4 October 1916, during the Battle of the Somme, James S. – a machine gunner from the 9th Royal Fusiliers – had just gone over the top when heavy bombardment forced him to retreat to a German dugout; a heavy shell explosion buried him and 11 of his comrades inside. Smothered in debris, burnt soil and mud, James found himself to be the sole survivor. He had to remain in the dugout with his dead comrades for six hours – praying for help until he was finally rescued. James was blind, deaf and dumb; his legs were paralysed. His vision returned soon, but the other problems remained.

While James was buried in the German dugout, German Pioneer Franz B. was in a state of panic: the continuous shooting and air raids terrified him and kept him awake at night. Images of death and destruction flashed up in front of his eyes during the day and haunted him in his nightmares. Franz suddenly felt dizzy, made a moaning sound and fell to the ground. His arms and legs started jerking violently; it took two hours for him to regain consciousness.

James was sent to the National Hospital at Queen Square, whereas Franz's odyssey through the German military hospital system ended at the Charité in Berlin. Both of them had witnessed immeasurable suffering, and had been psychologically scarred. They were victims of the epidemic of trauma that, at some point, threatened to overshadow all other medical problems of the war. The stories of James and Franz reveal the human condition: the basic human reactions to fear and loss that transcend all political and ideological differences.

Reading and comparing the hospital records from London, Berlin and another great German neuropsychiatric institution – the War Hospital in Jena – has been a fascinating experience, and I hope to convey this fascination in this book. Its aim is to link micro- with macro-history – making connections between the fates of individual soldiers and the workings of a hospital, and the vicissitudes of this world-changing conflict and the developments of medicine and science.

I first became interested in the history of medicine when I worked on the marvellously preserved records of the North Wales Asylum in Denbigh, under the guidance of psychiatrist Professor David Healy and historian Margaret Harris, during my psychiatric training. Although my work on post-partum psychosis and the religious revival movement was concerned with different kinds of trauma and emotional upheaval, it taught me how strongly culture can shape psychiatric diseases. I was impressed by the many cases of previously healthy farmers, labourers and housewives who developed a transient psychosis after attending spiritual meetings in the chapels of Snowdonia. Clearly, intense emotions – even positive ones – could trigger mental illness. I turned my interest to the collective trauma of the era: the Great War. How would soldiers react to the experience of combat – the constant shelling, the threat of gas attacks and the unimaginable horror of life in the trenches? Would the war produce an increase in mental illness – and if so, of already familiar diseases, or completely new presentations? And what exactly was meant by the ambiguous term 'shell shock', which is so often used, but seldom properly defined?

I gratefully acknowledge the support of the Wellcome Trust, which funded my PhD on the traumatic reactions to combat stress in the First World War at the Centre for Humanities and Health at King's College London; I am particularly grateful to my supervisor, Professor Edgar Jones, who was always available to discuss any matters relating to the history of war and psychiatry; I greatly benefited from meetings with Dr Bonnie Evans, Professor Andrew Lees and Dr James Hawes on matters of medical and cultural history; I am also grateful for the opportunity to discuss my evolving work with the students and fellows at the centre's stimulating research meetings.

This work crucially relied on the generosity of the institutions holding the medical case records and other archival material from the Great War: I am grateful to the Queen Square Archives Committee and the late librarian Louise Shepherd for access to the substantial historical collections of the National Hospital; I also wish to thank the Queen Square Library and Archives staff – Sarah Lawson, Kate Brunskill, Jackie Cheshire, George Kaim and Rossana Rizzo – for all their support and enthusiasm over the past five years. I am indebted to Jonathan Evans, Trust Archivist at the Royal London Hospital Museum and Archives for alerting me to the Queen Square records. Professor Volker Hess generously provided access to the historical collections of the Charité; my work in Jena was made possible by the kind support of Professor Heinrich Sauer – one of Binswanger's successors as head of the psychiatry department – and Professor Joachim Bauer of the State Archive of Thuringia.

The following institutions and individuals kindly provided permissions to reproduce illustrations or archival material: Dr Susan Yealland, Louisa Cantwell, the British Newspaper Archive, the Museum of London, The Great War Archive/University of Oxford, the Wellcome Library, the Mercian Regiment Museum in Worcester, the Queen Square Library and Archives, Cardiff University, the British Museum, the Anglesey Archives, the Newnham College Archives/University of Cambridge, the Library and Archives Canada, and the Imperial War Museum Collections.

I am very pleased that this book appears in a series that is dedicated to military history because I am convinced that medical and military historians can learn a great deal from each other; I certainly benefited greatly from the encouragement of my publisher, Duncan Rogers, and commissioning editor, Dr Michael LoCicero.

I hope that this history of shell shock will help us remember the soldiers and those who cared for them in the year of the centenary of the Battle of the Somme.

1

A Red-Letter Day for Professor Charcot

The drama of hysteria

Paris, 14 December 1888: the next generation – having experienced unimaginable trauma – would look back in disbelieving wistfulness at the capital of the 19th century in the Belle Époque. Here, in the cultural heart of the mighty continent which ruled the world, in the broad and gorgeous boulevards laid down by Haussmann to resurrect Paris from the disasters of 1871, progress and rationality themselves seemed enshrined – and all that was most rational and progressive in Paris was headed that day (where else?) to the legendary Salpêtrière Hospital to experience one of the famous demonstrations of Jean-Martin Charcot, the professor of neurology, at this foremost hospital of the French capital. Charcot had started his memorable series of lectures and clinical conferences in 1862; in 1881, he was appointed to the first chair of 'Diseases of the Nervous System'.

A whole generation of neurologists built on his pioneering work on neuropathology and neurological disorders, such as *sclérose en plaques* (multiple sclerosis), amyotrophic lateral sclerosis (the progressive loss of nerve cells of the motor system that disabled American baseball legend Lou Gehrig – leading to its alternative name 'Lou Gehrig's Disease') and Parkinson's disease (which he named

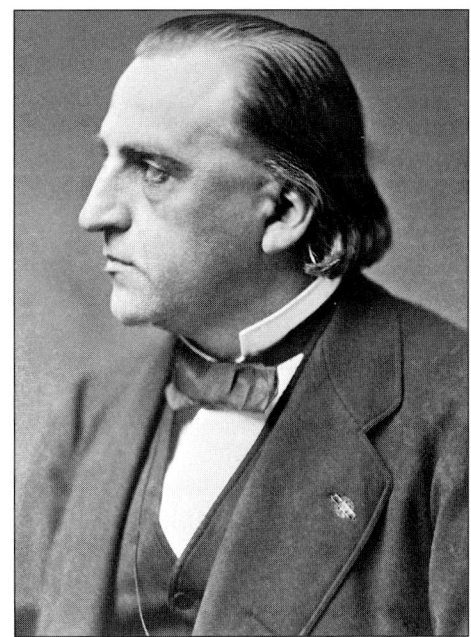

A portrait of J.-M. Charcot – head and shoulders in profile; photograph circa 1875. (Wellcome Library, London)

after the English apothecary who had first described it); however, Charcot's professional reputation was founded on his public demonstrations of hysterical fits and their treatment with hypnosis.

Charcot was an international celebrity, whose death in 1893 would be covered in newspapers worldwide:

> Charcot married a rich wife and lived in a splendid mansion in the Boulevard St Germain. The house is full of fine old tapestries, and profusely decorated with enamels, inlaid ivories, painted tiles, and repoussé metal, the work of his wife and daughters. [...] Although patients went from all parts of the world to consult the Professor, he reserved three days a week for study and research. Many of his students have attained high positions in their profession.[1]

In the 1870s and 1880s, Charcot's theatrical demonstrations, which generally involved the hypnotism of young and attractive female patients, were the talk of Paris and attracted great audiences – ranging from ladies of the high society to visiting doctors from all the medical centres of the world. In his lecture theatre, the well-heeled *habitués* of Parisian salon life rubbed shoulders with the most ambitious trainee doctors of Europe – men like the young Sigmund Freud, who had visited Paris three years before, especially to study with Charcot. Their medical training would not be complete without a visit to the Salpêtrière – the greatest scientific centre in France for the study of the pathology, diagnosis and treatment of nervous diseases. Paris had been the medical lecture theatre of the world since the golden age of the learned societies in the 18th century, and collective demonstrations and cures of strange ailments were popular ever since the German physician Franz Mesmer had arrived to promote the therapeutic use of magnetism.

On this unseasonably mild day in 1888, hundreds of spectators pour into the spacious lecture theatre, which had been the scene of Charcot's conferences for many years. It is crowded to excess not only by the students of Paris, but by physicians from every part of the world.

One of them is Ernest Abraham Hart – the renowned British ophthalmic surgeon and well-known medical journalist – who after his return to Britain would eagerly draft a report for the *British Medical Journal* (the central organ of British medicine):

> The walls are adorned with a fine picture of Pinel, one of the great celebrities of the Salpetriere, striking off the chains of the lunatics – from which he was the first to free them – in one of the courtyards of the Salpetriere. At the further end is a platform, from which the Professor, surrounded by the patients selected for the purpose, delivers his clinical lectures.[2]

1 'Social scraps' – *Hull Daily Mail*, 18 August 1893, p.2.
2 Hart, Ernest, 'Medical Paris of today. Notes made in December, 1888' – *British Medical Journal*, 9 February 1889, pp.322-324.

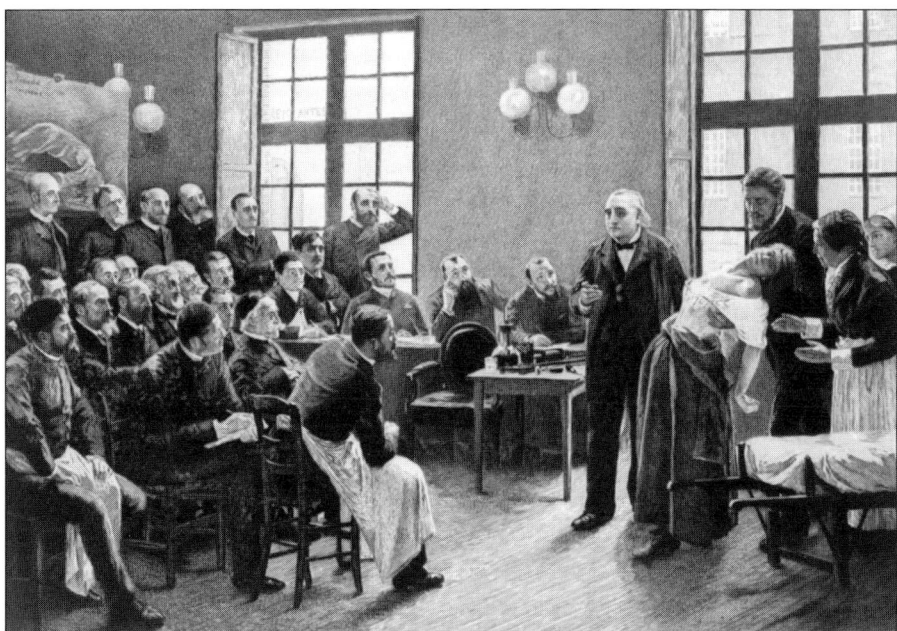

Jean-Martin Charcot demonstrating hysteria in a patient at the Salpêtrière; lithograph after P.A.A. Brouillet, 1887. (Wellcome Library, London)

When Charcot enters the theatre for his weekly Friday lecture, the curious spectators are instantly captivated by his imposing character – 'resembling the first Napoleon, and having also a likeness to the medallions of Dante'. The British doctor-journalist would observe 'that Charcot, sober in manner, clear in diction, picturesque in illustration, original in conception [and] indefatigable in research, […] spares neither time, thought, labour, nor wealth in using all the methods of clinical illustration, artistic, histological, chemical, and pathological'.[3] The patients for these presentations are carefully chosen: they travel to Paris from all parts of the world to consult the celebrity doctor.

Today's case would be a textbook example of the *arc de cercle* typical of hysterical fits:

> After auscultation of the lungs increased breathing rate, walks slowly to the sofa, lies down, then moves quickly with the whole body, shouts several times, then loses consciousness; when the physician says: 'now the patient has a seizure' answers: 'no, this is not yet the real one', trembles with the whole body, then

---

3 Hart, Ernest, 'Special Correspondence: Medical Paris of today. Letter from Mr. Ernest Hart' – *British Medical Journal*, 2 February 1889, pp.266-268.

screams again, bends the head backwards while forming an arch with the spine, then see-saws with the whole body, moves up and breathes heavily.[4]

Dramatic displays of convulsing bodies were typical of the very public medical culture of the *fin de siècle* and fed the widespread belief in the degeneracy of the human race. Hysteria was a very popular diagnosis in the 19th century: the affected patients – almost all of them female – suffered from a wide range of mental, neurological and physical symptoms. The term 'hysteria' referred to theories of Hippocrates and other doctors from ancient Greece. Although the enlightened doctors of the 19th century had long abandoned the notion that a wandering uterus [Greek: *hystere*] caused nervous weakness, the term 'hysteria' remained popular in medical terminology. Its medical use continued well into the 20th century, and it is still used to describe a tendency to emote in front of others in popular language. Long before Charcot, doctors had recognised that it was more fruitful to search for the causes of hysteria in the patient's mental condition and social circumstances than in their lower abdomen. They also realised that if there was an organic, physical explanation for the varied bodily symptoms, it had to be based on an understanding of the brain rather than the uterus. One generation before Charcot, Paul Briquet, who had diligently studied 430 patients with hysteria in Paris hospitals, concluded that hysteria was a disease of the brain – specifically of that part 'where affective functions are located'.[5]

Charcot had seen the various faces of hysteria: he 'tamed and catalogued' hysteria as he had done with such success in other areas of neurology.[6] Charcot concluded that 'all the varieties of hysterical attack [were] only derivative abortive forms of the major variety, and that its phenomena, far from being abandoned to the caprices of chance, [were] under the influence of laws which seem at least as rigorous as those which regulate the organic affections of the nervous system'.[7] Seizures lay at the core of this *grande hystérie*, which Charcot divided into four stages: in the *epileptiform* stage, the patient exhibited fits – typically tensing the whole body before starting rapid jerking movements; the second stage was characterised by dramatic physical displays – often culminating in an *arc-de-cercle* position, where the back was arched and the body only rested on the back of the head and the heels; this stage could be followed by *attitudes passionelles*: patients posed as if being crucified, or in the throes of erotic ecstasy; in the final stage, patients resembled the classical inmates of the asylum of the time – wandering about aimlessly under the influence of some inner voice, or driven by inscrutable mental images.[8]

---

4   Historisches Psychiatriearchiv Charité M8906/1918: Krankenakten.
5   Shorter, Edward, *From Paralysis to Fatigue: A History of Psychosomatic Illness in the Modern Era* (New York: The Free Press, 1992), p.212.
6   Shorvon, Simon, 'Fashion and cult in neuroscience – the case of hysteria' – *Brain*, 130:12 (2007), pp.3,342-3,348.
7   Hart, 'Special Correspondence', p.267.
8   Scull, Andrew, *Hysteria* (Oxford: Oxford University Press, 2009), p.115.

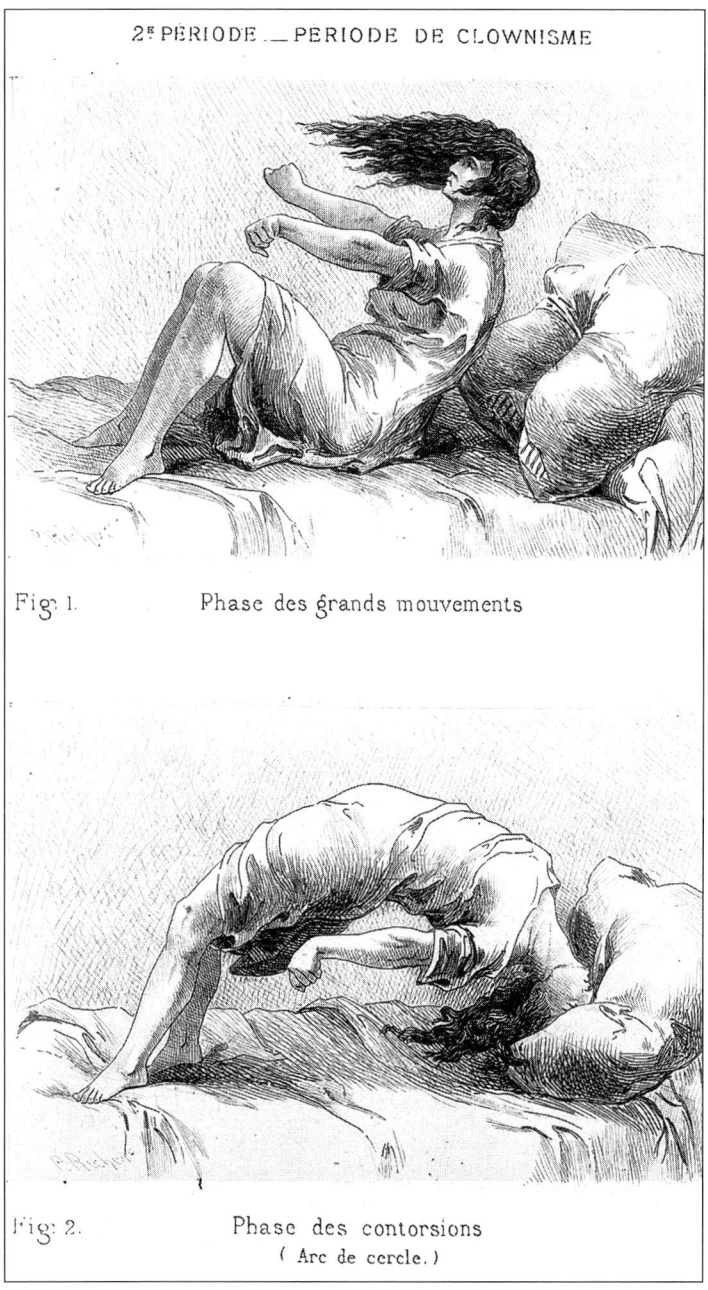

From *Études cliniques sur l'hystéro-épilepsie ou grande hystérie* by Paul Marie Louis Pierre Richer; published: Delahaye et Lecrosnier, Paris, 1881; second period: clownism, Plate III. (Wellcome Library, London)

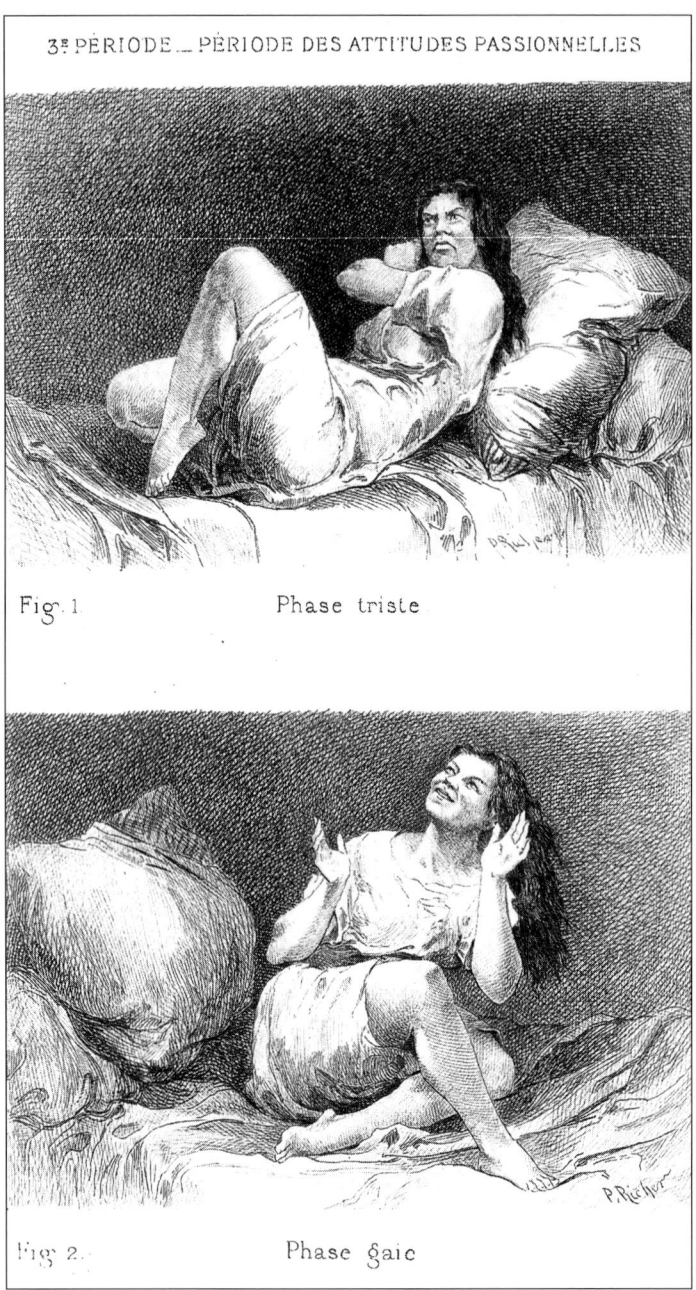

From *Études cliniques sur l'hystéro-épilepsie ou grande hystérie* by Paul Marie Louis Pierre Richer; published: Delahaye et Lecrosnier, Paris, 1881; third period: *attitudes passionnelles*, Plate IV. (Wellcome Library, London)

Charcot mainly presented young, female patients at his educational sessions – yet, could men be affected by hysteria as well? This possibility deeply challenged the gender stereotypes of the 19th and early 20th century: men were supposed to be in control of their emotions and bodies; however, as his clinical experience increased, Charcot found it harder and harder to deny that men could be affected by hysteria as well, and finally opened a ward for male hysterics at the Salpêtrière in 1882.[9] Ethnic and racial stereotypes played a role as well: German visiting scholars looked at Charcot's procession of hysterical men in disbelief and malicious joy; surely, this had to be a specifically French phenomenon.[10] However, Charcot rejected the claim that male hysteria was more common in France than elsewhere in Europe.[11] He believed that these disorders occurred in every army and amongst the working men of every country 'if only they were intelligently looked for'; however, he remarked that 'it would be a red-letter day for him when he should meet with the condition in a Prussian cuirassier'. Strict military discipline and self-control did not go well with conventional conceptions of hysteria.

Had he lived to see the First World War, Charcot would have had his red-letter day – pretty much on a daily basis. Indeed, hysterical seizures raged among the German forces and compromised discipline and order – and the vignette from the beginning of this chapter, a typical example of *grande hystérie*, was not actually taken from Charcot's stage performances, but from the medical records of a German hospital for traumatised soldiers of the Great War. The patient who 'bends the head backwards while forming an arch with the spine, then see-saws with the whole body, moves up and breathes heavily' is not a troubled young woman from *fin de siècle Paris*, but 39-year-old German Pioneer Franz B. – a joiner in civilian life. Franz had been drafted into a railway regiment on 29 June 1915 and was soon sent to the Eastern Front; in June 1916, he was transferred to Sedan in Northern France. Although Franz had never been involved in frontline fighting, he became increasingly anxious and could not bear the shooting and air raids. On 4 October 1916, he had his first fit. Numerous attacks followed – increasing in frequency and severity – so that an admission to the psychiatric department of the Charité University Hospital in Berlin seemed inevitable. The Charité doctors had to concede that Franz was a clear-cut case of male hysteria; however, many doctors – particularly in Britain – were still reluctant (or even refused) to believe in its existence in able-bodied men.

---

9   Scull, *Hysteria*, p.125.
10 Nonne, Max, *Anfang und Ziel meines Lebens. Erinnerungen* (Hamburg: Hans Christians Verlag, 1971), pp.177-178.
11 'REVIEWS AND NOTICES. Leçons du Mardi à la Salpêtrière. Par Professeur Charcot' – *British Medical Journal*, 2:1015 (1890), pp.1,015-1,016.

Male hysteria in Britain?

'Is Male hysteria Non-existent or only Unrecognised in Great Britain?' This was the title of the article by Ernest Hart, published in the *British Medical Journal* on 2 February 1889, in which he described the Napoleonic features of Charcot.[12] At that time, hystero-epilepsy was seen as 'a nervous disease of women of great rarity, affecting them especially during the child-bearing period of life; sometimes, though rarely, occurring before the actual commencement of menstruation, and continuing after its cessation'.[13] Charcot's female patients were chronic cases; they had usually suffered from these hysteric attacks for many years. Some of them also seemed to have fallen under Charcot's spell: sometimes, the only way to break this spell and escape Charcot's dominant personality was the discharge from the Salpêtrière, while others had to wait until the death of the grand master of hysteria for their symptoms to disappear; however, Ernest Hart also reported about 'cases of *male* hysterics of the most striking, various, and complex varieties' at the Salpêtrière. This colourful array of male inpatients – among them agricultural and town workers – exhibited all the features of hysteria that were commonly associated with female patients. To the British physician, this came as a surprise and substantially challenged his medical knowledge and experience. Hart's brief encounter with male hysteria in Paris left a lasting impression and prompted him to review his clinical assessments and diagnostic judgements. Although his practice was mainly confined to patients with eye and ear diseases, and hardly ever brought him into contact with nervous disorders, he was now able to identify hitherto unrecognised cases of major hysteria in three of his male patients: two of these 'cases of the gravest character' had previously been misdiagnosed as 'epilepsy' and 'insanity' respectively. According to Hart, all three men were cured by isolation and moral treatment – a predecessor of psychotherapy. Hart's visits to Paris had revolutionised his medical thinking and, as he noted in his 1889 publication, had estranged him from many of his English colleagues, who believed that male hysteria was a French disease which did not exist in England at all. Conversely, Hart concluded that 'a considerable number of cases [of male hysteria] exist, in this country [England] and in all parts of Europe, which are not recognised, and which are subject to a good deal of maltreatment for grave organic disease, whereas they belong to the class of partial or complete hysteric affections'.[14] The ophthalmic surgeon here displays remarkable insight into the dangers of 'maltreatment' arising from over-reliance on organic diagnoses – and things have not changed much in the last 125 years. In the modern medical world, many patients with functional neurological syndromes

---

12   Hart, 'Special Correspondence', p.266.
13   Gamgee, Arthur, 'An account of a demonstration on the phenomena of hystero-epilepsy and on the modification they undergo under the influence of magnets and solenoids; given by Professor Charcot at the Salpêtrière' – *British Medical Journal*, 2:928 (1878), pp.545-548.
14   Hart, 'Special Correspondence', p.268.

undergo multiple diagnostic procedures in the desperate search for a physical cause, and each futile diagnostic test only serves to entrench the organic model more deeply – making it increasingly difficult to tackle the root of the underlying psychological problems.

A quarter of a century later, when Europe plunged its entire manhood into an abyss of mutual destruction, the medical profession finally had to recognise that men could indeed develop hysteria. British medical experts reluctantly admitted that hysterical fits were more common in soldiers than in the civilian male population, where they were believed to be extremely rare events; however, they categorically denied that major hysterical seizures, with displays of bizarre behaviour and gross emotional outbursts, could be part of the male behaviour repertoire. Arthur Hurst, a shell shock specialist who did describe a hysterical fit with 'opisthotonus' [*arc de cercle* movement] in a soldier in his standard textbook on *Medical Diseases of the War*, was obviously repelled by this display of strange effeminate behaviour. His only way out was to identify the soldier as a 'malingerer' and an 'unwilling conscript'.[15] The British regarded hysterical fits in soldiers with utmost suspicion, as the following case from the National Hospital at Queen Square in London clearly demonstrates.

'Like a boor trying to stifle a guffaw'

Hysterical seizures could take various forms: although Charcot's classical *grande hystérie* was characterised by a particular sequence of events, seizures in soldiers could be manifold and even vary considerably in one individual. Twenty-one-year-old Private Albert W. of the 5th Dragoon Guards – 'a sturdily built youth of peculiar facial appearance and sullen expression' – was treated at the National Hospital between 4 July and 9 August 1915.[16] Albert, the oldest of six children and the son of a company sergeant major of the 10th Sussex Regiment, had been in the army for one and a half years when he was sent to France in August 1914. While in France, 'he was perfectly well, and although he was shaken by severe shell fire at times, he thinks that this was not more the case with him than with others. He was always able to sleep soundly and uninterruptedly and to eat well'. After four months in the trenches, he was invalided home with a shrapnel wound of the hand, which soon healed. When sufficiently recovered, he was sent on home duty to Aldershot – waiting to be sent across to France with a draft. In early June 1915, he woke up one night in a start and found himself in an attack in which he did not lose consciousness, but screamed, kicked violently with his legs and pulled off his bedclothes. Although fully aware of his surroundings, he was not able to answer questions during the attack. From then on, he suffered from

---

15 Hurst, Arthur F., *Medical Diseases of the War* (London: Edward Arnold, 1918), pp.97-98.
16 Queen Square Archives (QSA), Queen Square Records, Dr Tooth, 1915, male L-Z: case record Private Albert W.; all subsequent quotations referring to this case are taken from this record.

these nocturnal attacks on a daily basis – up to 10 times a night. Soon, Albert started having attacks during the day as well; however, these were slightly different from the ones occurring at night. Albert described a 'queer feeling like something crawling up his legs, going up his back and into his head and causing giddiness'. During the days, Albert managed to suppress full-blown seizures by pressing his hands to his eyes. Albert was initially admitted to the Maudsley Hospital – a recently established psychiatric hospital in South London; however, Albert continued to have seizures – and they seemed to become more dramatic over time. On the night of his admission to the National Hospital, Albert rose from his sleep and 'at once the left face was drawn up in a spasm, quite slowly, he bellowed in a low tone, but loudly, sat up in bed kicking his legs'.

His neurologist, Dr Francis Walshe, wrote in the notes:

> On my attempting to remove all the bedclothes from him he clutched them and resisted my doing so in a well coordinated manner. The kicking was but of moderate violence and did not move his whole body at all. It quieted down in a few seconds and he sat still in bed. On asking him if he had finished he nodded and said 'yes'. He then lay down and went to sleep.

Another attack occurred when Albert was physically examined in his bed:

> Suddenly with a low moaning sound the left face was drawn into a grimace, resembling a particularly stupid laugh in which the right side of face was relatively little involved. He at once placed his hand over the mouth, and then bore a striking resemblance to a boor trying to stifle a guffaw. The head was slightly raised from the pillow and all during the attack he seemed quite conscious and fixed the observer very definitely with his gaze, which never wandered. During the few seconds – circa 15 – that this condition lasted there was an up and down movement of the legs of small amplitude. When it ceased his head fell back on the pillow, he sighed and wiped his forehead with the right hand. He was at once able to discuss the attack, of which he had been fully aware in all its details. There had clearly been no obscuration of consciousness.

Albert had numerous seizures, with changing patterns of behaviour. He often stopped in the middle of a fit (for example, to put a plate off the bed to a place of safety) – resuming the attack afterwards. The doctors had no doubts about the hysterical nature of these attacks: first, the typical signs and symptoms of epileptic 'grand mal' seizures (such as incontinence of urine, loss of consciousness and changes in pupillary reactions) were missing; Albert never bit his tongue during a seizure, or injured himself in any other way. There was no family history of epilepsy, and Albert had not suffered from seizures before his military training. Other facts also pointed towards a diagnosis of non-epileptic, or 'functional' fits. The Queen Square doctors brought to light that Albert had had attacks of screaming when seven years old, which his

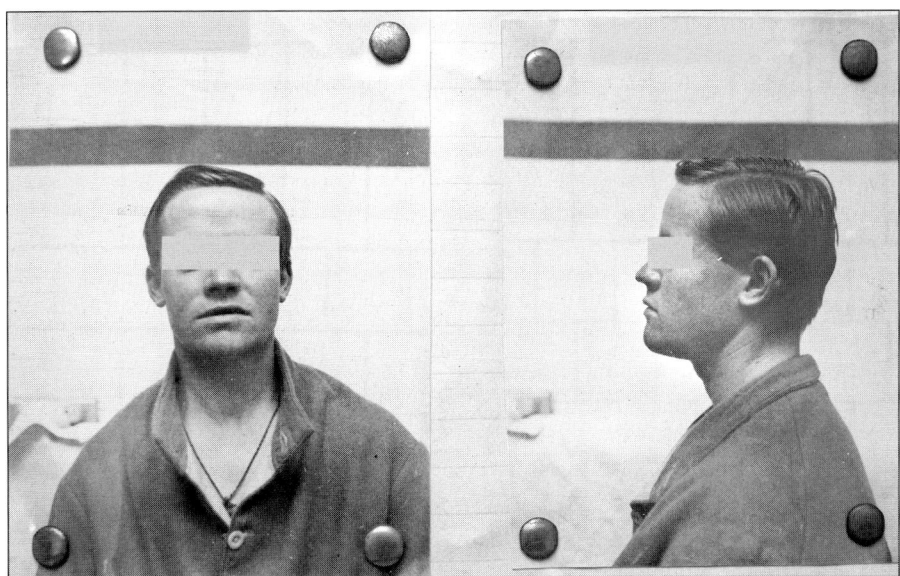

A photograph of Private Albert W. of the 5th Dragoon Guards, 1915.
(Queen Square Archives, London)

mother described as 'hysterical'. Furthermore, Albert admitted that he had suffered from 'other bouts of attacks like those now present when 12 and 16 years old'. With his 'somewhat sullen demeanour', he gave the impression 'of not being quite a frank witness concerning his condition'. The doctors documented in the notes: 'There is some reason to suppose from his history that at the time the present attacks appeared, he was expecting to be sent shortly to France again'. The seizures clearly had a purpose, and as this possibility became more remote, his seizures decreased 'in numbers and severity'. The Queen Square doctors realised that he would never be able to face military service again. Albert was discharged as 'unlikely to be of further military value'.

Hysterical seizures occurred in about seven percent of all soldiers without confirmed organic brain disease admitted to Queen Square during the war years. Queen Square doctors frowned upon these patients, because they were difficult to treat and proved to be highly 'contagious', as illustrated in the case record of 29-year-old ex-soldier William Charles L., who was admitted to the Queen Square Annex on 31 July 1919.

William had had his first fit five months previously when he

> ... saw a discharged soldier in a fit while in [the] street, and went to his aid. When the man recovered [the] patient himself had one (his first) which he was told lasted about ½ hour. Remembers nothing as to an aura or condition during fit – was told he was quite unconscious and was talking and swearing about the Germans. He was able to walk home after but as in subsequent fits felt rather

giddy and sick. Next fit occurred a week later while at a music hall at which reference to Germans was being made. Lasted over an hour but could walk home slowly after it. Since then they have become more frequent sometimes having as many as 3 or 4 a day.[17]

This patient continued to have fits during his hospital stay – sometimes lasting between four and five hours; they left him physically and mentally exhausted. William's fits were characterised by struggling and 'talking nonsense, normally about Germans'; he was finally discharged 'in status quo'. The Queen Square doctors had given up on Albert and William. Men of their disposition were of no further use for the military.

The hysteria of the Prussian cuirassier

The British deniers of male hysteria were correct in one respect: Charcot's *grande hystérie* – the dramatic display of functional seizures – was relatively uncommon amongst British servicemen. The most striking difference between clinical presentations at Queen Square and Berlin was indeed the much higher proportion of functional seizures among German soldiers.[18] One of these German soldiers with 'violent nervous attacks' was 21-year-old Musketeer Gustav B., who had originally been seen in the ENT outpatient clinics. Gustav had been in the trenches in France between June 1915 and June 1916, and involved in heavy fighting. In June 1916, he was buried after a shell explosion, lost consciousness and had to be dug out by his comrades. One month later, he was in the trenches again and suffered a minor head injury. He became deaf in his right ear, developed severe tic-like movements in his right eyelid and right hand, and also started having seizures. He was sent to several military hospitals at the base and at home, where he was treated with electricity and hypnosis. The seizures were triggered by strong emotions or unexpected loud noises. When the Charité psychiatrists enquire about his seizures, Gustav

> … suddenly falls off the chair, in fact slowly slides off the chair, then lies still for about 2 minutes on his back with crossed, clenched fists, breathing heavily. All the sudden starts lashing about, throwing his body about, makes arc of cercle movements with his back. Does not react to call. […] Hitting the table and chairs with his head and body in quite a reckless manner. […] Duration of the whole attack 5 minutes.[19]

---

17 QSA: Queen Square Records, Dr Tooth, 1919, male L-Z: case record William Charles L.
18 Linden, Stefanie C., Hess, Volker and Jones, Edgar, 'The Neurological Manifestations of Trauma: Lessons from World War I' – *European Archives of Psychiatry and Clinical Neuroscience*, 262: 3 (2012), pp.253-264.
19 Historisches Psychiatriearchiv Charité M7286/1917: Krankenakten.

Other soldiers suffered seizures that lasted for hours; they maintained bizarre postures or exhibited repetitive movements for long periods of time. One of them was 20-year-old Grenadier Eugen B. of the Kaiser Franz Regiment, who started having seizures during his military training. The slightest noise or unexpected movements or vibrations caused violent attacks of jerking, with Eugen rhythmically drumming on his mattress with his arms and legs and making noises as if he was in pain.[20]

Another soldier who was treated at the Charité was 30-year-old Territorial Richard N. – a waiter in civilian life, who had first developed seizures during his regular military service in the years before the war. In a courageous act, he had dived into the Rhine to pull two drowning civilians out of the water. Afterwards, he fainted and from then on was 'haunted' by the image of one man he had rescued from the river. He was discharged from military service, and the images disappeared for 10 years until he was drafted again on 14 September 1916. From that day onwards, the image of the man who had nearly drowned in front of his eyes emerged again. Along with the tenacious images came the seizures, which could be triggered by any kind of arousal and upset. During such a seizure, Richard typically fell to the ground before his arms and legs started jerking; he shouted out loud and clenched his fists. With froth around his mouth, he shouted phrases like 'give me my rifle' while gesticulating and grabbing at the air.[21]

Seizure disorders like this hardly ever resolved naturally, but had a tendency to increase in frequency and severity over time. Soldiers with these attacks were commonly referred to a specialist seizure centre like the Charité in order to rule out genuine epilepsy. Numerous publications in German-language journals confirmed the epidemic occurrence of hysterical seizures in the German military.[22] Ernst Jolowicz, for example, reported high numbers of functional seizures among his large cohort of 4,581 patients at a military hospital in Posen [present-day Poznań in Poland – at the time, part of the German Empire]. Particularly young men seemed to be prone to develop seizures: indeed, 25 percent of Jolowicz's military patients below the age of 20 presented with functional seizures. Jolowicz, who published widely on psychotherapy and suggestion after the war (and was later forced to flee Germany because of his anti-Nazi activities), observed that many patients had erroneously been labelled as epileptic when they actually suffered from a functional seizure disorder. He also found that functional seizures mainly occurred in the lower ranks and working-class men, and were more common among Polish (as opposed to German) soldiers fighting in the German Army. With the typical class and ethnic bias of German doctors of this time, Jolowicz concluded that functional seizures represented the most primitive expression of hysteria in the 'simple-minded human being'.

---

20   Historisches Psychiatriearchiv Charité M4717/1915: Krankenakten.
21   Historisches Psychiatriearchiv Charité M6603/1916: Krankenakten.
22   For example: Meyer, Semi, 'Die nervösen Krankheitsbilder nach Explosionsschock' – *Zeitschrift für die gesamte Neurologie und Psychiatrie*, 33:1 (1916), pp.353-370; Leva, J., 'Epilepsie im Kriege' – *Archiv für Psychiatrie und Nervenheilkunde*, 65 (1922), pp.386-410.

Another striking observation was that soldiers frequently developed functional seizures without having been exposed to actual fighting, often when they prepared for their first battle; others presented with violent displays of convulsions for the first time during their home leave from the front. Many civilians will have been baffled by the sight of bizarrely-moving soldiers on Berlin's central squares or on public transport, which will be described further in Chapter 11. Less public, but equally concerning, were the series of cases of dramatic fits that spread within army bases.[23] Germany was in danger of becoming victim of an epidemic of hysterical seizures, and this is reflected in many of the discussions in the German medical journals of the time.

Conversely, medical discussions and large-scale epidemiological studies conducted by British doctors did not concentrate on functional seizures, but focused on other functional disorders – particularly those related to the heart or the motor system.[24] Dudley Carmalt-Jones, who was in charge of a specialist treatment centre for shell shock (opened in January 1917 at No.4 Stationary Hospital at Arques), conducted a detailed clinical study on functional disorders of the war. He assessed 1,300 patients admitted under the label 'N.Y.D., N.' (not yet diagnosed, nervous) a few days after the onset of symptoms, but only came across three cases of 'violent hysterical fits'.[25]

Charcot's legacy in the war

How can we explain these cultural differences in the expression of war trauma? Seven years before the outbreak of the First World War, Pierre Janet – one of Charcot's eminent pupils – had already asked: "How is it that with one person, the hysteria bears on the arm, with another on the stomach, and that, with a third, it only reaches a system of ideas?" At the end of this book, the reader will have a better understanding of the mechanisms that shaped the expression of distress and the different approaches towards these striking clinical presentations.

The history of shell shock started in the lecture theatres of Paris – and it was Charcot who had introduced male hysteria into a wider medical community. Among the hundreds of doctors who went on a pilgrimage to Paris to witness Charcot's lessons on hysteria were many who would play a leading part in the treatment of

---

23 Rohde, Max, 'Neurologische Betrachtungen eines Truppenarztes im Felde' – *Zeitschrift für die gesamte Neurologie und Psychiatrie*, 29 (1915), pp.379-415.
24 'Disordered Action of the Heart' (DAH) – for example: Fraser, Francis, Wilson, R.M., 'The sympathetic nervous system and the "irritable heart of soldiers"' – *British Medical Journal*, 2:3002 (1918), pp.27-29; Wells, S. Russell, 'A collective investigation of ten thousand recruits with doubtful heart conditions' – *British Medical Journal*, 2:3010 (1918), pp.248-251; Oppenheimer, B.S., Rothschild, M.A., 'The psychoneurotic factor in the "irritable heart" of soldiers' – *British Medical Journal*, 2:3002 (1918), pp.29-31; sensory-motor system – for example: Johnson, W., 'Hysterical tremor' – *British Medical Journal*, 2:3023 (1918), pp.627-628.
25 Carmalt-Jones, Dudley W., 'War-neurasthenia, acute and chronic' – *Brain* 42:3 (1919), pp.171-213.

shell-shocked soldiers during the Great War. The Hamburg physician Max Nonne had first witnessed the therapeutic application of hypnosis by Jean-Martin Charcot in Paris in 1889. Then 28 years of age – and in the final stages of his neurological training – Nonne was truly impressed by Charcot's stage performances. During the First World War, Nonne himself would enter the stage to tame whole companies of hysterical soldiers with hypnotic suggestion. Nonne's lifelong mission to cure hysteria had been spawned in the lecture theatre of the Salpêtrière; the images of Charcot's vivid demonstrations stayed with him all his life.

Half a century after his memorable visit to the French capital, when he was in his late seventies and writing down his memoirs, his encounter with Charcot re-emerged in its original splendour:

> The crowded assembly of doctors from all countries was deeply impressed by the appearance of the genteel professor, meticulously dressed in a black morning suit and sporting the shining red ribbon of the legion of honour. His highly arched brow, his bold aquiline nose, the clean-shaven, forceful, broad, yet graceful chin, the thin lips, the pale complexion, the large, dreamy, steel-grey eyes, the well-formed ears, the fine and noble hands betrayed the old-school aristocrat of letters. His presentations were elegant, unpretentious and calmly determined, and he was always warm and open-hearted towards his patients who regarded it as a kind of privilege to come to the attention of this man, to become the objects of his interest and careful scrutiny. Nevertheless I got the impression that the lectures Charcot gave towards the end of his life were not so much training lessons for aspiring physicians but rather performances on a theatre stage.[26]

Nonne was not the only physician to disseminate Charcot's doctrine: through his numerous disciples, Charcot's ideas were spread throughout Europe and influenced the approach to shell shock. Major Arthur Hurst, who during the First World War would be in charge of the shell shock cases at the Royal Victoria Hospital in Netley (the British Army's principal treatment facility since 1863), was another leading neurologist who eagerly embraced Charcot's ideas on hysteria and suggestion. Aged 28 – like Nonne during his memorable visit – and supported by a prestigious Radcliffe Fellowship, he made his way to Paris to attend outpatient clinics of Joseph Babinski and Joseph Jules Dejerine (both pupils of Charcot). Like Nonne, Hurst would also dedicate great parts of his professional life to the treatment of hysteria. During the war, the two pupils of Charcot – whose paths never crossed – were to take leading parts in the endeavour to conquer the epidemic of shell shock in Britain and in Germany.[27]

---

26 Nonne, *Anfang und Ziel meines Lebens*, p.76.
27 Jones, Edgar, 'War Neuroses and Arthur Hurst: A Pioneering Medical Film about the Treatment of Psychiatric Battle Casualties' – *Journal of the History of Medicine and Allied Sciences*, 67:3 (2012), pp.345-373.

2

Shell Shock on Both Sides of the Trenches

The history of shell shock thus started in the lecture theatres of *fin de siècle* Paris. Here, hysteria was groomed and celebrated; it entertained spoilt audiences, brought fame to physicians and meaning to patients. The battlefields of Flanders seemed a less nourishing ground for the ailments of the civilised world – and still, hysteria flourished in this most unlikely setting, amidst the relentless firing of the shells; in the damp and draughty trenches and on blood-drenched battlefields.

Two individual stories will introduce the reader to this no man's land of disease – and both stories take us to the battlefields of the Somme, on 4 October 1916: James S., a machine gunner from the 9th Royal Fusiliers, has just gone over the top.[1] To escape the heavy bombardment, he and 11 of his comrades retreat to a German dugout, when suddenly a shell explodes and buries everyone inside. Smothered in debris, burned soil and mud, James finds himself to be the sole survivor. He remains in the dugout with his dead comrades for six hours – praying for help – until he is finally rescued and taken to the next base hospital at Camiers. James is blind, deaf and dumb; his legs are paralysed. His vision returns soon, but the other problems remain.

While James is buried in the German dugout, hoping to be found by his own men rather than the enemy, German Pioneer Franz B. – the Prussian cuirassier of Chapter 1 – is in a state of panic.[2] Although he has been transferred to the back area, the continuous shooting and air raids terrify him and keep him awake at night. Images of death and destruction flash up in front of his eyes during the day and haunt him in his nightmares. Franz suddenly feels dizzy, makes a moaning sound and falls to the ground. His arms and legs start jerking violently; it takes two hours for him to regain consciousness.

---

1   QSA: Queen Square Records, Dr Holmes, 1917, male and female L-Z: Case record Private James S.; all subsequent quotations in this chapter referring to this case are taken from this record.
2   Historisches Psychiatriearchiv Charité M8906/1918: Krankenakten; all subsequent quotations in this chapter referring to this case are taken from this record.

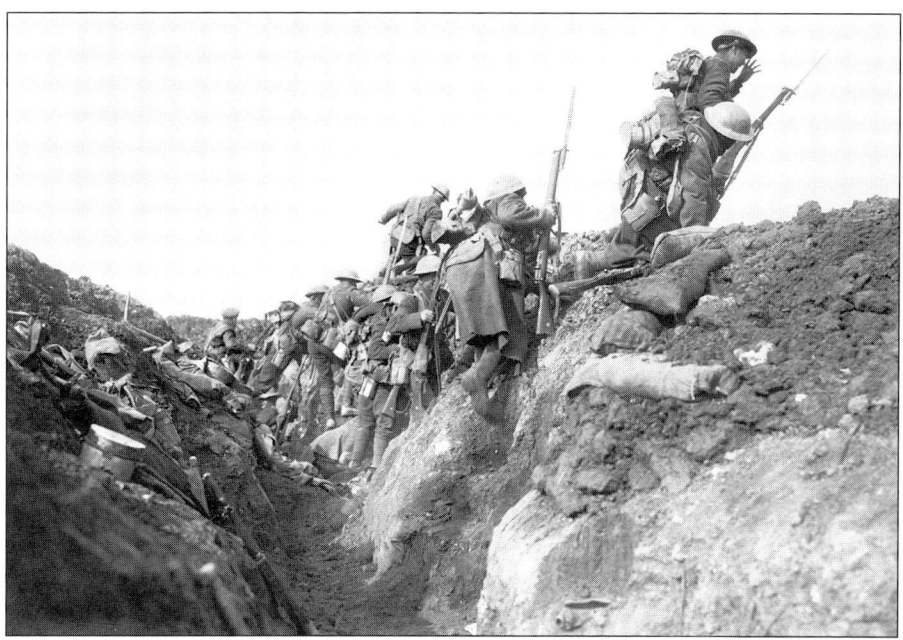

Troops supposedly 'going over the top' at the start of the Battle of the Somme in 1916, photographed by Canadian official photographer Ivor Castle. This photograph was widely (and misleadingly) published as a portrayal of an actual British attack; however, it was actually taken during a training exercise behind the lines. The breech cover, which is clearly visible on the rifle of the soldier in the foreground, was edited out in contemporary publications of the photograph; Canadian First World War Official Exchange Collection, 1916, CO 874. (Imperial War Museum, London)

Clearly, James and Franz were not of much use for the trenches – and as their symptoms did not improve, they were soon sent home for treatment. For both men, this was the beginning of an odyssey through numerous military hospitals in their respective home countries.

Tremblings

James was a 25-year-old well-built Londoner, with blue eyes and brown hair, who had spent his youth in Australia. He had returned from the dominion just in time to enlist in the British Army, together with his four brothers. All brothers went to France and one of them was killed immediately in one of the first battles fought by the British Army in the First World War at Mons; James saw action in several engagements himself. After his burial in the dugout, which miraculously left his body unscathed, he was treated at the Redlands War Hospital at Reading; the 4th London General Hospital at Denmark Hill, which specialised in neurological and psychiatric casualties; the Springfield War Hospital at Tooting, which was housed in the former Surrey

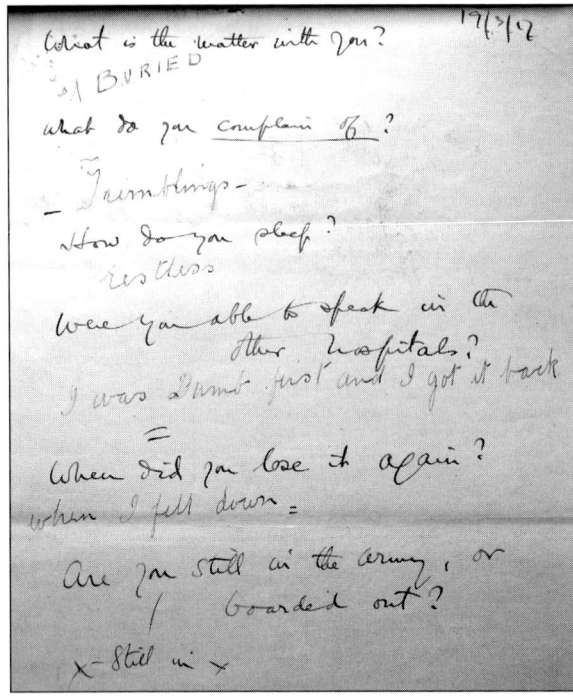

James S., a machine gunner from the 9th Royal Fusiliers, who was blind, deaf and mute after spending six hours in a dugout with his dead comrades; written communication between James and his doctor, 1917. (Queen Square Archives, London)

County Lunatic Asylum; and the Fulham Military Hospital. On 30 March 1917, almost six months after the fateful battle, he was finally admitted to the National Hospital for the Paralysed and Epileptic at Queen Square, London – Britain's foremost neurological institution. According to the admission records, he was still deaf and could not utter a single word forcing him to communicate with his doctor in a written form.

Furthermore, he was unable to walk and could not feel his legs. Whenever he tried to move, his legs went into violent spasms. The doctors found it very difficult to make contact with James, because he turned his head away when anyone spoke to him. He refused to move and resisted all attempts to help him recover his speech and gain control over his legs; he even passed his urine in bed.

By the spring of 1917, the specialists at Queen Square had seen many similar cases and did not waste any time trying to localise the origin of his problems in the brain. They recognised that he was one of the many sufferers of shell shock – the epidemic hysterical disorder of traumatised veterans of the Western – and other – fronts. They immediately diagnosed James with 'functional aphonia and paraplegia' and applied their harsh treatment regime for patients with so-called 'functional disorders' (those without a recognisable organic or physical cause). James's improvement was striking, considering how little progress he had made in the preceding six months. He was treated in strict isolation to calm his nerves and avoid a spread of symptoms to other patients. He was also enrolled in a strict exercise programme; however, the most dramatic part of his treatment was the application of strong (and probably painful) electric currents to his legs. After only a few weeks of treatment at Queen Square, he was able to walk again. His speech returned after persuasion therapy – a form of psychotherapy – and his mood improved considerably. He felt sufficiently recovered to leave the hospital against medical advice on 29 May 1917.

Fits

Franz's odyssey through military hospitals lasted even longer than that of James: it was only in February 1918 that Franz was eventually admitted to the Charité Hospital in Berlin. Similar in standing to the National Hospital in London, the Charité was the German national centre for brain disorders – and doctors there were expected to understand the relationship between psychological war trauma and organic, neurological problems. At the Charité, Franz on numerous occasions was observed to be 'lying on his back, bending his head backwards, forming an arch with his spine, seesawing with his body, and breathing heavily'. This pattern of attack was very familiar to the neurology experts: as we saw in Chapter 1, this *arc de cercle* was indeed Charcot's signature symptom – the ultimate and purest expression of (initially only female) hysteria. The doctors felt uncomfortable seeing a man in such provocative postures; however, there was no way for them to attribute Franz's bizarre postures to epilepsy, or an organic movement disorder. They had to admit to themselves that Franz's attacks were hysteria, pure and simple.

Conversely, the Charité doctors were reluctant to blame wartime hardship and atrocities for his psychological meltdown. They rather wanted to believe in the importance of a 'psychopathic constitution' – an inborn weakness or vulnerability, which predisposed these men to mental breakdown. In this way, doctors could avoid the admission that combat stress could derange soldiers' minds and also – at a more practical level – reduce the number of pension claims that could be made by traumatised soldiers. With their model of constitutional weakness in mind, the Charité doctors dug deep into Franz's history: his foibles, shortcomings and family problems. Franz had worked as a joiner at the piano manufacturer Steinway and Sons in Hamburg, and lost his first wife in 1913 after she had delivered healthy twin boys. He got married a second time in the summer of 1915, which was shortly before he was drafted into the army. According to reports from his family, Franz had always been tender-hearted, highly strung and irritable. Clearly then, his symptoms were not a result of the stresses of war, but an outgrowth of his 'psychopathic predispostion'; yet, although his doctors denied the direct causal link with the war, they still treated him like their other soldier-patients with electrotherapy, which was a mainstay of the treatment at the Charité, like at Queen Square. Franz, too, benefited from it: his attacks soon stopped, but he was still suffering from dizzy spells and felt depressed. This may have been one of the reasons why he was not sent back to the front line, but returned to do construction work in the back area.

These cases from both sides of the trenches demonstrate how the horrific experience of combat in the First World War could paralyse soldiers – both literally and mentally – even if they had not actually suffered any direct injury to their brains. They also show that both acute psychological trauma – in James's case, the loss of 11 comrades to a shell explosion in the dugout – and the enduring stress along and behind the front line could lead to nervous exhaustion and breakdown. The English gunner and the German pioneer both had to spend many months in military hospitals under the care of overstretched army doctors who did not have much to offer them. They finally made it to specialist academic centres in their respective capitals, where they were put under a formalised and relatively harsh treatment regime, which perhaps surprisingly, helped their recovery and rendered them fit enough to support the war effort (if not at the fighting line, then at least at the Home Front).

James was one of the estimated 80,000 British servicemen who suffered severe psychological reactions to combat experience in the First World War. This is a considerable number – amounting to an equivalent of the manpower of four army divisions – and similar estimates have been produced for the German and French Armies; yet, the importance of this epidemic of nervous breakdown amongst servicemen to the military and political leaders becomes even more obvious when we consider that when the first patients started to flood the base hospitals in autumn 1914, it was by no means clear what the ultimate scale of this problem would be.

These traumatised soldiers were also a major source of bewilderment to the medical profession on both sides: the trauma of war produced a great variety of unfamiliar psychological reactions in servicemen of all combatant countries, whether they were involved in active combat or not. Soldiers exposed to similar atrocities developed different symptoms, which could include paralysis, blindness, deafness, constant shaking, frequent fits, aggressive outbursts and severe depression. Initially, the debate circled around the question whether mental and neurological combat reactions were caused by hidden physical effects of shell explosions that might lead to microscopic lesions of the brain or spinal cord. These 'organic' models gave rise to the terms 'shell shock' in Britain and 'traumatic neurosis' in Germany, which remained popular even after the majority of the medical profession had adopted the view that they were caused by psychological, rather than direct, physical trauma. The debate then moved to the question why different individuals who were exposed to similar traumatic experiences reacted in such different ways: this question had captivated physicians since the heyday of female hysteria in the late 19th century.

Military doctors were even more interested in the question why certain patients, but not others, developed these symptoms after exposure to similar atrocities in battle. Was it possible and advisable to identify those that would not withstand the stress of combat and rule them out from military service, or would this just promote a culture of aggravation and malingering? And finally, after some sort of understanding of the presentation and causes of shell shock had been achieved, the next big challenge to the medical system was to come up with effective cures. Although neurologists had gained some experience with treating hysteria and traumatic neurosis since the late

19th century, they were unprepared for the scale and severity of the new epidemic. The scale and importance of the challenge is reflected by the high proportion of articles on shell shock in general medical journals of the time: about one-fifth of papers in *The Lancet* and the *British Medical Journal* – leading sources of information for doctors then, as now – were devoted to the psychological consequences of combat.

Later chronicles of First World War medicine have not been kind to the shell shock doctors. Particularly those who embraced electrotherapy as a therapeutic method have been vilified for their alleged cruelty and lack of empathy by modern historians, political theorists and writers of fiction; Elaine Showalter's *The Female Malady* and Pat Barker's *Regeneration* are just some particularly well-known examples. Both scholarly and popular discussions of shell shock are dogged by myths about the medical response and its consequences – and even the historian Niall Ferguson, otherwise not known for uncritical adoption of received wisdom, perpetuates this simplified view of sadistic doctors who forced shell-shocked soldiers to return to the front line:

> German soldiers evinced similar symptoms and, as in Britain, there was a tendency to punish as much as treat the victims with electric shocks and other equally painful 'remedies'. If there was a German equivalent of Dr William H.R. Rivers, who at least had a human way of getting men back to their work of killing, his deeds have gone unsung.[3]

This book will show that disciplinary measures were only one component of often rather complex treatment programmes, and that very few patients were actually sent back to the front – at least from the specialist treatment units. There is no reason to accuse Rivers – the eminent anthropologist, psychologist and neuroscientist – of being keen on 'getting men back to their work of killing'; in fact, Rivers was rather reluctant to let his officer-patients return to their units and pointed out to them that the psychological defence mechanism – repression – they had carefully built up during his therapy would crumble upon the first contact with military life. Moreover, there were psychoanalytically-minded doctors like Rivers in Germany and Austria-Hungary as well, and proponents of more or less humane treatments could be found on both sides; in fact, it is often difficult to draw clear lines between the more or less ethically acceptable treatments applied by doctors across the theatres of the Great War. Psychoanalysis may seem more humane than electric shock treatment and more likely to cure the root causes, rather than just the symptoms, of war neurosis; however, being cured in this way entailed the risk of having to return to the trenches – and although Rivers himself was not particularly keen on sending his patients back to the front line, German and Austrian psychoanalysts advertised their ability to make traumatised soldiers fit for duty up to the very end of the war.

---

3   Ferguson, Niall, *The Pity of War* (London: Penguin Books, 1999), p.342.

This book draws on a large body of unpublished medical records from several British and German shell shock centres. The reader will enter a world which, since the last veterans of the Great War have passed away, is now inaccessible through living memory. Drawing upon individual histories from two combatant countries – Britain and Germany – this book illustrates the universal suffering of all involved in this conflict and shows how culture can shape individual symptoms. This source material creates a unique opportunity to compare the symptoms and treatments of combat stress in both countries and draw lessons for today – and it also allows us to trace the individual stories of the affected soldiers from their pre-war upbringing through the different stages of their war deployment and hospital treatment, to their adjustment to civilian life after the war. These case histories, and the medical literature of the time, will provide the basis for an analysis of the medical response to shell shock, both in terms of diagnostic models and therapeutic approaches (Chapters 4, 12 and 13). I will analyse the rationale and motivation behind some of the more controversial treatments and try to disentangle the punitive and therapeutic goals. The interaction between doctors and their military patients was certainly more complex than depicted in most fictional accounts, and provides striking insights into British and German culture of the time. In Chapter 3, I will describe the disposal system for psychological casualties and explain why it took some patients so long to arrive at the specialised hospitals. I will also look at those soldiers who developed shell shock symptoms far away from the front line (for example, the surprisingly large number of patients who suffered nervous breakdown while travelling on public transport – see Chapter 11).

During wartime, doctors inevitably find themselves in a conflict of interest between medical and military aims. We will see how doctors on both sides dealt with this conflict and encounter a widespread practice of discharging soldiers as unfit for military duty, which challenges the myth that shell shock doctors considered it their mission to return killing machines to the front line.

3

From the Fields of Flanders to the Temple of Neurology

Shell shock: the new epidemic

Soon after the beginning of the First World War, 'cases of nervous and mental shock' from the battlefields of Flanders began to arrive in England.[1] At first, the medical profession did not pay much attention to these psychological casualties, which were seen as 'the more uncommon clinical products of the present war'.[2] For most of 1914, the British medical press mainly reported single cases: these individual cases of soldiers who suffered 'a complete loss of memory, a total blank', or became blind after a shell explosion,[3] captured the attention of the medical world, but did not cause great alarm; in fact, doctors thought that 'considering the stress of conditions at the front, it is wonderful that there were not more cases of insanity'.[4] Some authors observed a decrease in admissions to mental hospitals and interpreted this as evidence for the invigorating powers of warfare – and one asylum doctor even opined that the monotony of civilian life was much worse for mental health than the catastrophic experiences of wartime:

> It is not the great tragedies of life that sap the forces of the brain and wreck the psychic organism. On the contrary, it is small worries, the deadly monotony of

---

1 Turner, William A., 'Remarks on Cases of Nervous and Mental Shock' – *British Medical Journal*, 1:2837 (1915), pp.833-835.
2 Turner, 'Remarks on Cases of Nervous and Mental Shock', p.833; From a Special Correspondent in Northern France, 'Medical arrangements of the British Expeditionary Force' – *British Medical Journal*, 2:2815 (1914), pp.1,037-1,038.
3 Medical Society of London, 'Surgical experiences of the present war. Functional blindness' – *British Medical Journal*, 2:2813 (1914), pp.938-942; 'Home Hospitals and the War: Brighton, Second Eastern General Hospital: Complete Loss of Memory' *British Medical Journal*, 2:2814 (1914), p.992.
4 By a correspondent, 'Medical Aspects of severe Trauma in War. Insanity and Psychic Trauma' – *British Medical Journal*, 2:2815 (1914), pp.1,038-1,039.

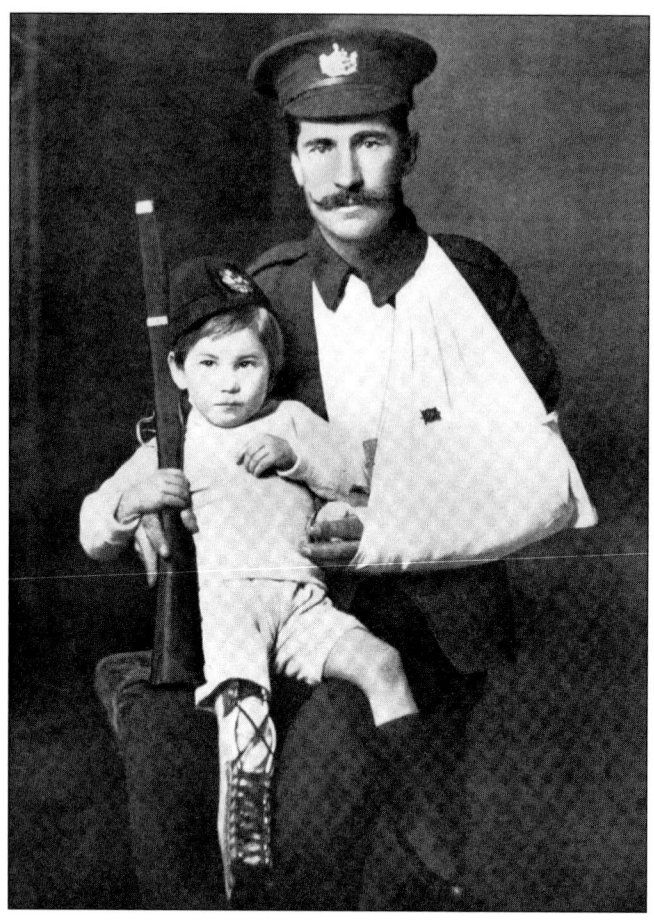

Two patients in the hospital, April 1915; photograph, Queen Square Reports. (Queen Square Archives, London)

a narrow and circumscribed existence, the dull drab of a life without joy and barren of an achievement, the self-centred anaemic consciousness, it is these experiences that weaken and diminish personality and so leave it a prey to inherited predispositions or to the slings and arrows of outrageous fortune.[5]

Yet, advocates of the beneficial effects of war on mental health were soon faced with evidence from the front line that challenged their optimism. On 12 December 1914, the *British Medical Journal* had published an article by T.R. Elliott on a surprising number of paralyses in soldiers without obvious head injury. Elliott, a consultant

5   'Insanity and the War' – *The Lancet*, 186:4801 (1915): pp.553-554; author cites *85th Annual Report of the Belfast District Lunatic Asylum.*

physician to the British Army in France, acknowledged that these disorders were often difficult to distinguish from those caused by brain lesions. In addition, Elliott observed that these reactions to the constant shelling could assume diverse forms: '… the man may become blind, or deaf, or dumb; he may be seized by a violent and coarse tremor that shakes his body for days; or he may be paralysed with a hemiplegia or paraplegia.'[6] Although these soldiers did not show any obvious physical injuries, doctors thought that their symptoms must be caused by the physical effects of the shell explosion; the alternative (psychological) explanation had not yet crossed their minds. To emphasise the organic nature of the injuries, from the winter of 1914-1915 onwards, these cases were labelled as 'shell shock'.[7]

A revolution in British psychiatry

Some of these shell-shocked soldiers who flooded the home hospitals soon after the outbreak of war even developed symptoms that were commonly seen in the mentally insane – the long-term inhabitants of asylums and workhouses. These confused, troubled souls – men frozen with terror and frantic with fear, who had clearly lost touch with the real world – challenged conventional psychiatric thinking: firstly, they had previously been perfectly sane and suddenly developed symptoms that psychiatrists associated with chronic mental degeneration; secondly, they could recover within a few days or weeks. Their favourable outcomes contradicted the common belief that these symptoms predicted a lifelong debilitating illness, such as 'dementia praecox', as schizophrenia was called a century ago; however, some of these men who had developed psychotic symptoms only in response to the war trauma were confined to mental wards for the chronically insane.

These challenging soldier-patients, with their bizarre ideas, unpredictable tempers and emotional outbursts, encountered a psychiatric profession in disarray. Psychological medicine in Britain before the Great War had a pessimistic outlook on therapy and recovery, and the innovative spirit and scientific vigour of Victorian medicine had not captured this unpopular discipline. Furthermore, doctors working in British asylums were not even formally trained in psychological medicine.

The dismal state of psychiatric training before the war was described by Grafton Elliot Smith, a leading brain anatomist, and the young psychologist Tom Hatherley Pear in their wartime book:

> This university's contribution to [the doctor's] psychological knowledge usually consists in showing him a hand full of comparatively hopeless caricatures of

---

6   Elliott, T.R., 'Transient paraplegia from shell explosions' – *British Medical Journal*, 2:2815 (1914), p.1,006. Paraplegia: loss of function of both legs; hemiplegia: loss of function of limbs on one side of the body.
7   Turner, 'Remarks on Cases of Nervous and Mental Shock', p.833.

mentality in his short series of visits to the asylum. It is as if one tried to teach electrical engineering by a few exhibitions of broken-down dynamos, navigation by half-a-dozen cursory inspections of wrecks, finance by a short series of visits to the bankruptcy courts.[8]

The architectural splendour of the Victorian asylum was, in no way, matched by therapeutic efficacy: up to the war, there was little expectation that psychiatrists could cure anybody, as society mainly expected them to keep their patients safe and away from the more respectable part of the citizenship. British doctors argued that German pre-war psychiatry was more forward-looking and much better prepared for the huge influx of soldiers with temporary psychological reactions. In Germany, university outpatient clinics[9] offered treatment in the early stages of mental illness, with a view of full recovery and reintegration into society. Furthermore, German doctors were particularly trained to distinguish between transient and treatable conditions, and chronic mental disorders.

To their credit, British Government ministers were quick to recognise the new psychiatric challenges that arose with the war: they introduced the Mental Treatment Bill on 20 April 1915, with the intention 'to facilitate the early treatment of mental disorder of recent origin arising from wounds, shock, and other causes', as reported in *The Lancet*. Before this bill, treatment in the asylum had been reserved for those with a recognised mental illness, and admission was often for life. In public perception, patients with mental disorders were often put in the same category as common criminals, but the 1915 Mental Treatment Bill now allowed for traumatised soldiers with psychiatric symptoms such as hallucinations and confusion to be treated in an asylum for short periods of time. Whenever improvement allowed them to return into the care of their families, they could be discharged at short notice. This meant that traumatised soldiers were not stigmatised as insane.[10] To be sure, this does not imply that society became more understanding towards people with mental health problems in general, but rather that it exempted its traumatised soldiers from the general prejudice against psychiatric patients.

War medicine adjusts to shell shock

The medical services of the British Expeditionary Force (BEF) had to deal with more than eight million casualties. It is astounding how quickly authorities on both sides managed to organise a system of field, base and home hospitals – stretcher bearers,

---

8   Smith, Grafton E. and Pear, Tom H., *Shell Shock and its Lessons*, 2nd edn (Manchester: Manchester University Press, 1917), p.100.
9   Smith and Pear particularly mention the outpatient clinic at the psychiatric department of the Charité.
10   'Nerves and War: The Mental Treatment Bill' – *The Lancet*, 185:4783 (1915), pp.919-920.

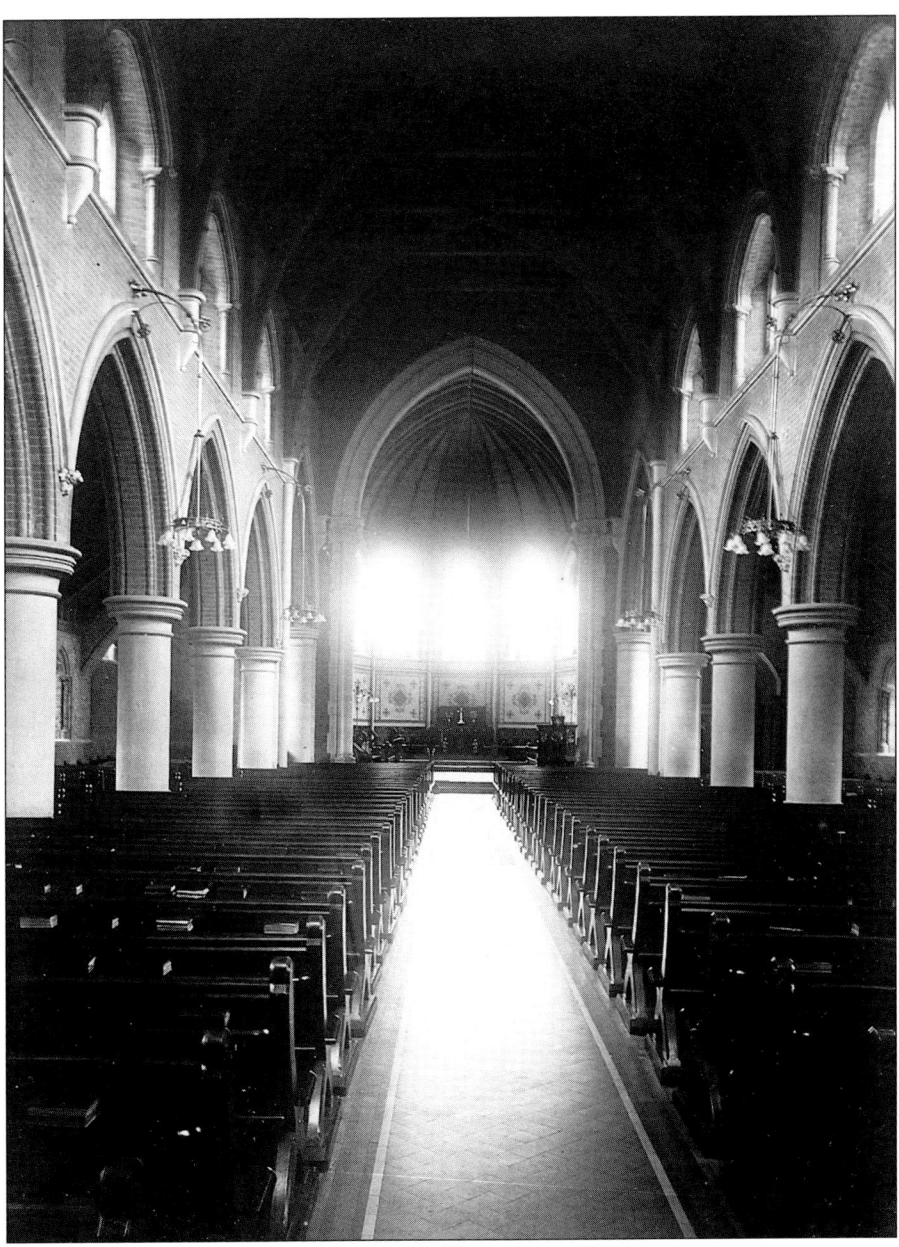

The chapel at Claybury Asylum, Woodford, Essex; photograph by the London & County Photographic Co., Bromley, Kent [1893?]. (Wellcome Library, London)

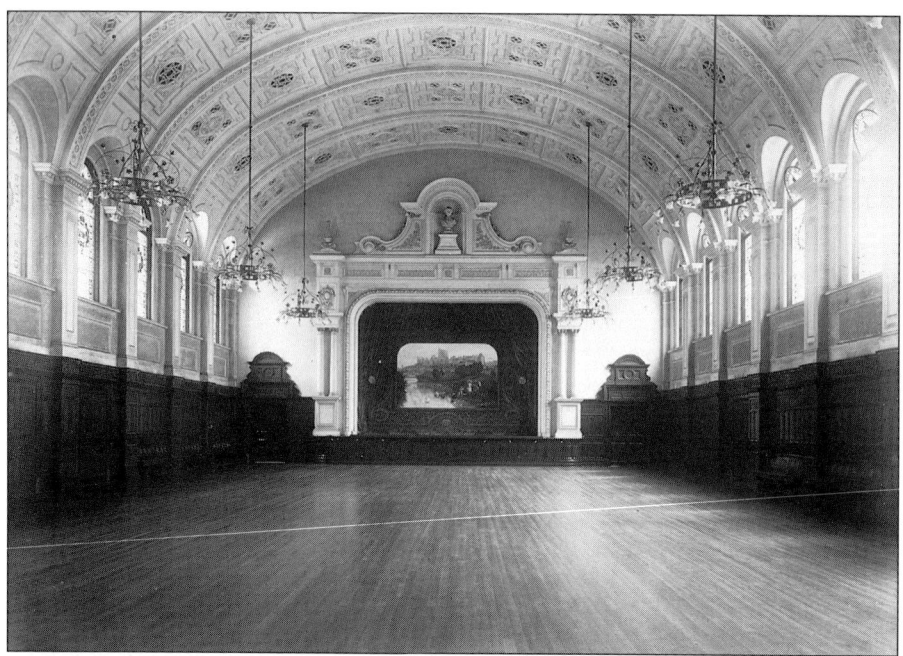

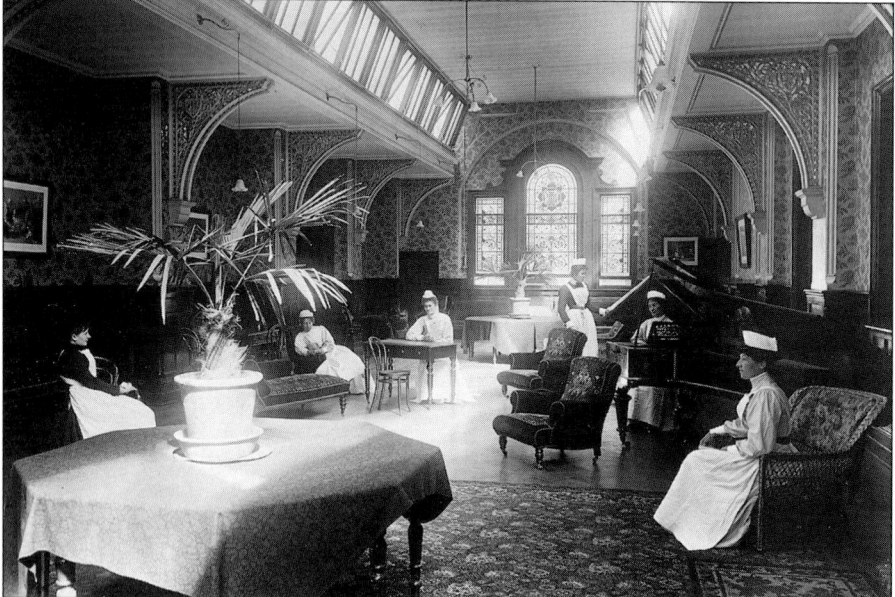

Claybury Asylum, Woodford, Essex; photographs by the London & County Photographic Co., Bromley, Kent [1893?]. Top: the recreation hall; bottom: a nurses' day room. (Wellcome Library, London)

ambulances, clearing stations, hospital trains and ships – to ensure their wounded received medical attention. More than 300,000 hospital beds were set up for military use in the UK, which is twice the number of beds provided by the National Health Service today;[11] the UK organised its war medicine, like its warfare in general, on a truly international scale. We will later encounter a patient who, having been wounded in Mesopotamia, received his first treatment in India before being shipped back to England. Another soldier – from Australia – was wounded in Gallipoli and treated in Alexandria in Egypt, but asked to be transferred to a specialist hospital in London. These cases were no exceptions and illustrate to modern readers just what a logistical achievement the organisation of an effective medical system under the conditions of a worldwide war (and with the limited communication and transport technology of the time) must have been.

Although the scale was unprecedented, at least one could draw on similar experiences and procedures from previous wars. After all, British nurses had set up the first large-scale centres for wounded soldiers during the Crimean War, and had carried on this tradition throughout several colonial wars.[12] Shell shock, however, was, in many respects, the biggest challenge encountered so far. Neither side had prepared a disposal system or treatment facilities for psychologically wounded soldiers, simply because nobody had anticipated (or been prepared to admit) that Prussian grenadiers or Scottish riflemen would fall victim to the effects of combat stress.

At the beginning of the war, British doctors treated their soldier-patients with 'nervous shock' on general wards next to the patients with gunshot wounds. This was clearly inefficient, because the shell shock patients took up beds that were urgently needed for the increasing number of seriously injured servicemen. Moreover, it soon became clear that the atmosphere on a general ward was not conducive to a cure of the nervous symptoms. Specialised treatment facilities were needed – and the British Army set up a sophisticated system for the disposal of these nervous cases from early 1915. At base hospitals in France, patients were labelled as either 'neurological' or 'mental' cases by specially qualified medical officers and separated in designated neurological (or mental) sections. 'Neurological' cases here denoted patients affected by unexplained physical (and sometimes also psychological) symptoms, as opposed to patients suffering from traditional severe forms of mental illness (schizophrenia, manic depressive disorder and general paralysis of the insane, which is a late stage of syphilis): 'By these means cases of functional paralysis, neurasthenia, and the milder psychoses were separated as early as

---

11 <http://www.kingsfund.org.uk/projects/general-election-2010/faqs#beds> accessed 10 December 2015.
12 Rafferty, Anne Marie and Solano, Diana, 'The Rise and Demise of the Colonial Nursing Service: British Nurses in the Colonies, 1896-1966' – *Nursing History Review*, 15:1 (2007), pp.147-154.

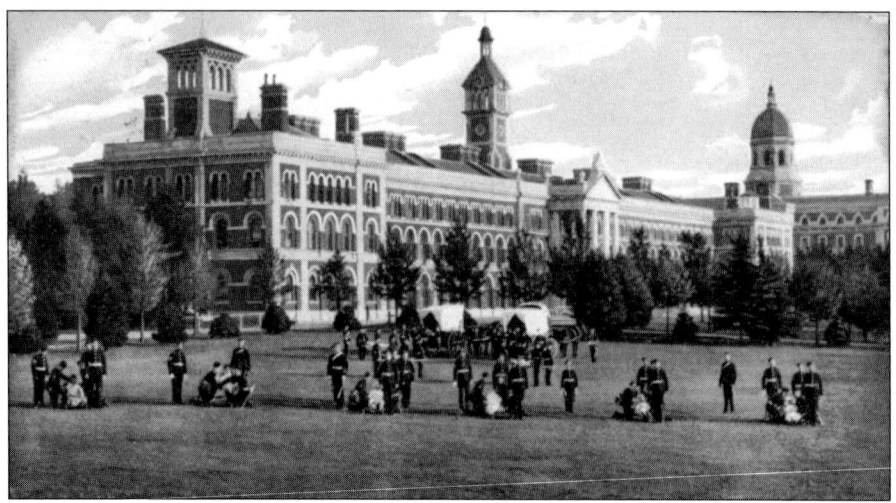

The Royal Victoria Hospital, Netley; postcard. (Author's own archive)

possible from cases of severe mental disorder'.[13] The director-general of the Army Medical Service also established neurological sections in territorial hospitals in the UK, where shell-shocked soldiers were put in the care of physicians who had special experience in diseases of the nervous system.

A limited number of special hospitals were also set up for neurological and psychiatric patients who were not suitable for treatment in general hospitals: from early 1915, two clearing hospitals were in use so that 'all cases should receive a short period of rest and treatment on their return from France before being transferred to the most suitable institutions for final disposal and treatment'. The Neurological Section of the 4th London Territorial General Hospital – which included the Maudsley Hospital, founded in 1916 (and still one of the main specialist centres for clinical psychiatry in the UK today) – took 'all unwounded cases suffering from neurasthenia, the functional paralyses, hysteria and the milder psychoses'. Early in 1918, the Maudsley became independent of the 4th London General and was known as the Neurological Clearing Hospital – a reflection of its size and status. Cases of acute mental disorder, however, were sent to the Royal Victoria Hospital on the South Coast at Netley, Hampshire (which included 'D' Block, which was designed to treat severe mental illness). From the clearing hospitals, some cases could be discharged to furlough and light duty, whereas soldiers with more chronic symptoms were referred to specialist institutions, such as the Red Cross Hospital Maghull in Lancashire (for Northern and Western Commands); the Springfield War Hospital in Tooting, London (for Eastern,

---

13 Turner, William A., 'Nervous and Mental Shock' – *British Medical Journal*, 1:2893 (1916), pp.830-832.

Southern and Aldershot Commands); the Royal Victoria Hospital in Edinburgh (for the Scottish Command); or the King George V Hospital in Dublin (for the Irish Command). Under the direction of Lieutenant Colonel R.G. Rows, a training centre was established in connection with the Maghull Military Hospital, where medical officers were instructed in the basic principles of psychology and psychopathology. Finally, for the most puzzling or treatment-resistant cases of functional neurological symptoms, there was the world's leading neurological hospital, which was situated in Bloomsbury – the cultural and academic heartland of the capital.

In the temple of British neurology

The National Hospital for the Paralysed and Epileptic (today called the National Hospital for Neurology and Neurosurgery) at Queen Square admitted a large number of soldiers with physical injuries, such as serious head trauma; yet, Queen Square also became one of the most important centres for the treatment of shell shock cases.[14] Whereas funding and staff limitations forced many general hospitals to conduct low-cost mass treatments that required minimal input from qualified personnel, the National Hospital had specialist staff, extensive treatment and research facilities and less pressure to discharge patients within short periods of time;[15] it mainly received referrals from military hospitals, such as the Fulham Military Hospital and the First London General Hospital at Camberwell – and some patients were transferred from the two official clearing hospitals ('D' Block Netley and the Maudsley). With only 100 military beds in 1915, Queen Square operated on a much smaller scale than the specialist treatment hospital at Maghull, which had 300 beds – rising to 500 in the second half of the war.[16]

At the beginning of the First World War, the hospital at Queen Square had gained an international reputation for the treatment of neurological disorders and had pioneered neurosurgery in England – and Victor Horsley was the first surgeon in the world who had been appointed to a hospital post as a 'brain surgeon'. By 1900, he had reported a series of 44 operations for gliomas (brain tumours), pituitary operations, procedures on spinal tumours and a process for managing malignant brain swelling.[17]

---

14   Micale, Mark S. and Lerner, Paul F., *Traumatic Pasts: History, Psychiatry, and Trauma in the Modern Age, 1870-1930* (Cambridge: Cambridge University Press, 2001); Jones, Edgar, 'Shell Shock at Maghull and the Maudsley: Models of Psychological Medicine in the UK' – *Journal of the History of Medicine and Allied Sciences*, 65:3 (2010), pp.368-395.
15   Micale and Lerner, *Traumatic Pasts*, pp.213-214.
16   For a detailed account of the treatment at Maghull during the First World War, see Jones, 'Shell Shock at Maghull and the Maudsley'; patient statistics and the number of military beds can be found in *The National Hospital, Report for the year ending 31 December 1914*, Queen Square Archive.
17   Powell, Michael, 'Sir Victor Horsley – an inspiration' – *British Medical Journal*, 333:7582 (2006), pp.1,317-1,319.

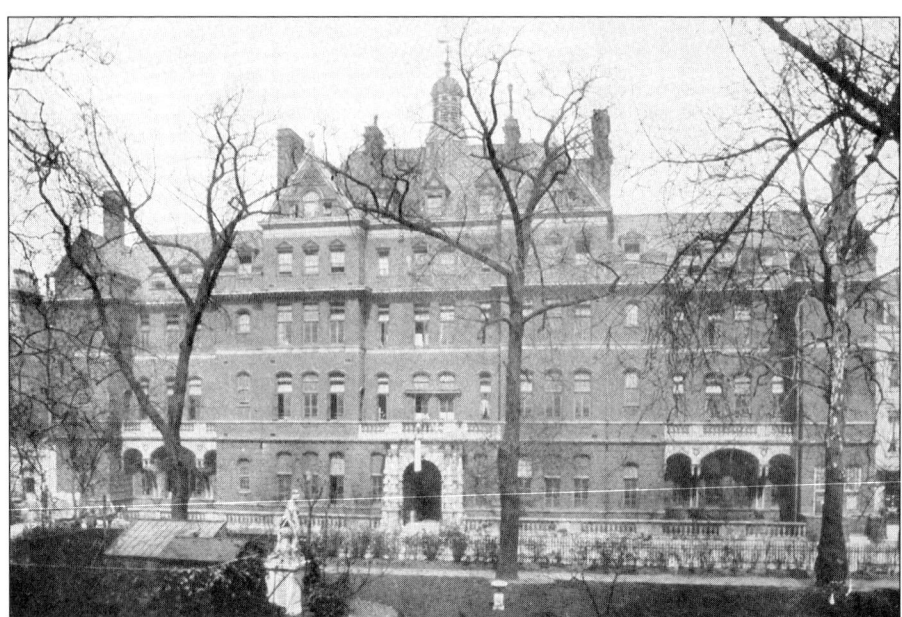

The National Hospital for the Paralysed and Epileptic, circa 1914.
(Queen Square Archives, London)

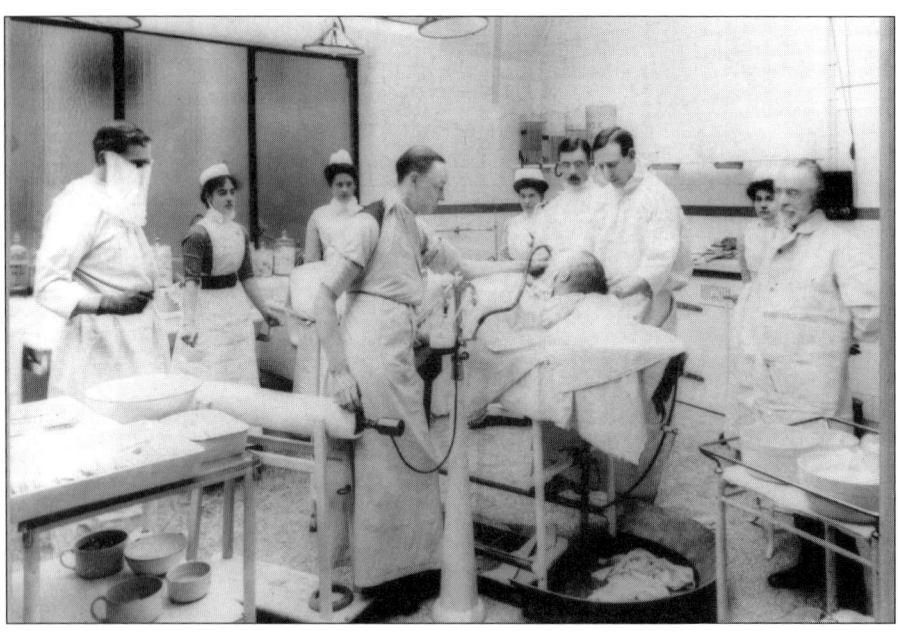

Victor Horsley in his operating theatre at Queen Square; photograph; QSA/1518.
(Queen Square Archives, London)

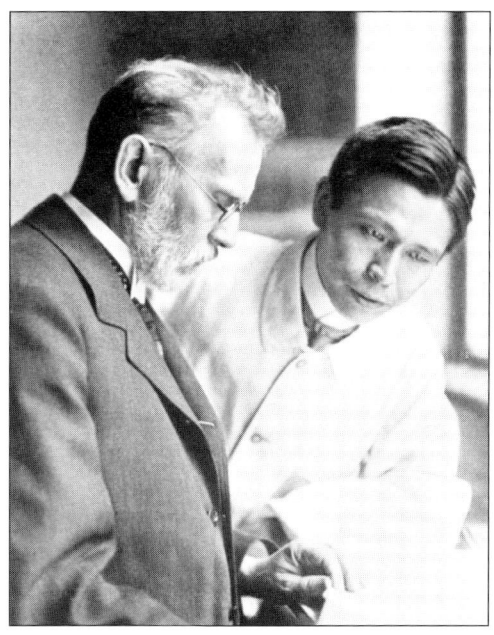

Paul Ehrlich (left) and Sahachiro Hata working on Salvarsan; public domain. (Wikipedia: https://de.wikipedia.org/wiki/Paul_Ehrlich#/media/File:Paul_Ehrlich_and_Sahachiro_Hata)

With his Queen Square colleague, Robert Henry Clarke, he had invented a device for guiding the surgeon to a target within the skull cavity. Similar stereotactic frames are still used in patients whenever pinpoint accuracy is needed, such as for biopsies, brain stimulation and local radiotherapy.

Contemporaries referred to Queen Square as 'the temple of British neurology' and compared its staff to 'a priesthood for the spread of the neurological faith of Britain'.[18] On 6 February 1915, Lord Beauchamp – the president of the National Hospital – announced that the War Office was 'arranging to send soldiers suffering from shock to be treated at the Hospital in wards specially set apart for the purpose';[19] war-related cases continued to be treated at Queen Square until 1926.[20]

The first two British soldiers were admitted to Queen Square in October 1914 – and they were suffering from general paralysis of the insane (GPI). These were the days when syphilis was one of the commonest causes of mental illness, at least in males, and accounted for about 20 percent of all admissions to mental and neurological institutions. The first effective drug for syphilis had been introduced by Sahachiro Hata and Paul Ehrlich in Germany only a few years earlier. Arsphenamine, also known as 'Compound 606', was first marketed by Hoechst in Germany under the trade name Salvarsan in 1910. Salvarsan was a great improvement over the mercury compounds that had been used previously to treat syphilis. The outbreak of the war inevitably affected the supply chain for Salvarsan, but in 1916, 'British-made' Salvarsan and Neosalvarsan (a liquid form of the original powder medication) were produced by the

---

18 Maloney, W.J.M.A., 'Obituary: "The National" and Dr. F.E. Batten' – *Journal of Nervous and Mental Disease*, 49:1 (1919), pp.91-94.
19 *The Times*, 6 February 1915.
20 Holmes, Gordon, *The National Hospital, Queen Square, 1860–1948* (Edinburgh: E. & S. Livingstone, 1954).

Wellcome Chemical Works under the names of Kharsivan and Neokharsivan. GPI was thus not a particular challenge to the Queen Square doctors, although success rates of the new cures remained low.

In early November 1914, the first soldiers with injuries to peripheral nerves and the spinal cord were admitted to Queen Square. These cases, again, were all still very much within the comfort zone of the resident neurologists and surgeons; however, the hospital was soon to be made aware of the problem of 'nervous and mental shock'.

At its meeting on 10 November 1914, the hospital's Board of Management discussed an appeal from Lord Knutsford, the chairman of the London Hospital House Committee, which had been published in the London newspapers:

> There are a certain number of our gallant soldiers for whom no proper provision is at present obtainable but is sorely needed. They are suffering from very severe mental and nervous shock due to exposure, excessive strain, and tension. They can be cured if only they receive proper attention from physicians who have made a specialty of treating such conditions. These men are quite unsuitable patients for general hospitals, as their chance of recovery depends on absolute quiet and on the individual and prolonged attention of the physician. If not cured, these men will drift back to the world as wrecks, and miserable wrecks, for the rest of their lives.[21]

James Collier and William Aldren Turner, two consultant neurologists from the National Hospital, had already offered their support to the War Office. It was decided that Farquhar Buzzard, another consultant neurologist at Queen Square, would draft a letter to Lord Knutsford and the press – pointing out that the National Hospital would accept soldiers with mental and nervous affections – and the War Office was informed that wounded soldiers suffering from any nervous ailment were eligible for admission.[22]

It did not take long for the first shell shock case to arrive at Queen Square: Adolf S., a 22-year-old Belgian soldier who was admitted on 14 November 1914,[23] had lost the use of his legs after a heavy blow to his abdomen with the butt of a rifle on 19 August 1914 during the German capture of Aarschot in Flemish Brabant. After his transfer to England, Adolf was initially admitted to Base Hospital No.1 at Camberwell, London. He suffered from attacks of acute abdominal pain and was still unable to move his legs, which was the reason for his referral to the National Hospital. In the admission records, he was described as a 'highly strung nervous emotional individual',

---

21 Lord Knutsford, 'To the editor of the Daily Mail' – *Daily Mail* (exact date unknown); newspaper cutting appended to the minutes from the Board of Management meeting, 10 November 1914, Queen Square Archives, London.
22 QSA: minutes from the Board of Management meeting; handwritten note, 10 November 1914.
23 QSA: Queen Square Records, Dr Tooth, 1915, male L-Z: case record Adolf S.

Minutes from the Board of Management meeting, 10 November 1914, National Hospital for the Paralysed and Epileptic, London; appended to the minutes is an article by Lord Knutsford: 'To the editor of the Daily Mail' (exact date unknown). (Queen Square Archives, London)

yet 'lively and bright and quick to interpret signs and broken French and German expressions put to him by the examiner'. During his three-month inpatient treatment at Queen Square, which included strict isolation from other patients, he made a slow recovery and was finally discharged to a private convalescent home at Aubrey House in Kensington, West London. The Queen Square experts had not been able to find a medical explanation for his symptoms.

William Cleverly Alexander (1840-1916) – Quaker, city banker and patron of the painter James McNeill Whistler – had purchased Aubrey House, which was a mansion noted for its extensive gardens, in 1873 and moved in with his large family. During the first half of the war, the garden room of Aubrey House accommodated 15 Belgian soldiers who had been discharged from acute treatment at various London hospitals. After the death of the owner, his family offered Aubrey House to the War Office in April 1916 for use as a hospital for officers in conjunction with the neighbouring Moray Lodge, which had become an annexe to the Special Hospital for Officers in Palace Green; they also kept some rooms for Belgian refugees. The hospital operated until April 1920, when the house was reclaimed by Alexander's daughters.

The Alexander family clearly took a personal interest in the fate of their Belgian convalescents: Rachel F. Alexander, the second youngest of William's seven daughters, wrote to Dr Frederick Eustace Batten – a consultant neurologist and specialist in shell shock at the National Hospital – on 10 November 1915 to inform him that Adolf S., 'the little pastry cook', was still in contact with the owners of Aubrey House 10 months after his discharge from the National Hospital and, from time to time, staying at their convalescent unit. According to the letter, Adolf was doing well, walking without problems and staying at a 'big place for reformés Belgian soldiers at Grove House, Ewell' near Epsom, Surrey (about 15 miles south of London). The doctor at Grove House had advised Adolf not to return to work for at least another year because he was still experiencing pain in his abdomen.

During the war years, a total of 13 Belgian soldiers with shell shock, who had fought in Flanders early in the war, were treated at the National Hospital; some of them had escaped German imprisonment and managed to travel to Britain. Communication was often difficult because of the language barrier, but the general attitude of Britons to the almost 250,000 refugees from the largely-occupied Allied country was cordial.

Two further soldiers with unexplained neurological symptoms arrived at Queen Square on 8 December 1914: Walter E., a 23-year-old private from the First Royal Dragoons, suffered from weakness and 'violent trembling' of his legs. On 29 October 1914, he had carried a wounded comrade through severe enemy fire – and the moment he placed him in an ambulance wagon, he lost consciousness and 'knew nothing until he came to himself the next morning at 7-8 am in a Red Cross railway coach in Boulogne'. He never found out how he got there, or what occurred during his period of unconsciousness. He continued his journey and arrived in the base hospital in Camberwell on 6 November. When Walter first came to himself, he 'felt as though he did not have legs'. When he tried to read, the letters ran together and got indistinct; sudden noises caused him to jump.[24]

The other soldier admitted on 8 December was Steward B. – an 18-year-old private of the London Scottish Regiment, who had been sent to the front in mid-October 1914.

The case record provides a harrowing account of this teenager's experience during the first months of the war:

> The life in the trenches was very hard. There was considerable rain. They were not able to get water. The diet consisted of 'bully beef', jam, cheese and bread. The sand would come into the food and this increased the thirst. They had little chance to sleep, the eye-strain was very severe. Patient had a great deal to do with handling wounded and dying soldiers which made a deep impression on him. The first day he was in a trench, he had in his line of vision a pile of corpses one of which had the face turned toward him and appeared to be sleeping – this made such an impression upon him that he cannot free himself of this vision.

24 QSA: Queen Square Records, Dr Batten, 1915, male A-K: case record Private Walter E.

> AUBREY HOUSE,
> KENSINGTON, W.
>
> Nov 10 · 1915
>
> Dear Dr Batten
>
> We ~~~~ still see the little pastry-cook, Adolph ▓▓▓ from time to time — He went to Harrogate, where he got much better, & can now walk quite well — He was very anxious to go back to work, and is now at the big place for reformé's Belgian soldiers at Grove House, Ewell. The doctor there has told him that he mustn't attempt to go to work for about another year. He still has a good deal of pain at times. Lately he came to us for a night or two — I wish I could get him somewhere else, he says the men at Ewell drink a lot, & he is not very happy there — I have heard of a place in London which would I think be nicer for him.
>
> Yours sincerely
> Rachel F. Alexander

The letter by Rachel F. Alexander, 10 November 1915; letter preserved in case record Adolf S., Dr Tooth, 1915, male L-Z. (Queen Square Archives, London)

Just before being sent home, he was five days and six nights in the trenches at a stretch under the above condition. The noises made by shells and the uncertainty of where they would strike caused great uneasiness and strain. Patient's comrades remarked that he did not answer when they spoke to him and appeared not to realize that they were speaking to him. Of this he knew nothing until told later on. He could not hold his weapon properly, nor shoot accurately. He was very shaky. Suffered much from headache. He was sent away from trenches November 14 and arrived at Southampton November 21.[25]

Steward's presentation included almost all the stereotypes that would later form the public image of the shell-shocked soldier. Both Walter and Steward had completely normal physical examinations, and both soldiers showed 'considerable improvement' through massages, exercise and pain medication.

The numbers of soldier-patients admitted to Queen Square increased rapidly after William Aldren Turner (1864-1945), who had recently returned from duty in France, wrote a letter to the chairman of the hospital on 21 December 1914 suggesting that one or two wards be set apart entirely for the treatment of military patients suffering from nervous shock. Turner, a territorial officer in the Royal Army Medical Corps, had been rushed to France in December 1914 as a temporary lieutenant colonel when it became clear that 'nervous and mental shock' casualties were multiplying; he was one of the few doctors at the National Hospital with first-hand experience of casualties in France. As a consultant both at King's College Hospital and the National Hospital, he was responsible for devising a management strategy for shell shock – and in January 1915, was appointed consultant neurologist to the War Office. After the war, he remained adviser on neurology to the War Office and later to the Ministry of Pensions.[26]

While the hospital opened its doors to casualties from France, its capacity to treat patients was initially undermined by the loss of experienced staff like Turner, who had volunteered for military service.[27] Increasingly, however, junior medical posts could be filled by female doctors and retired consultants who returned to take up clinical duties.[28] Later in the war, demands on the clinical staff were intensified by a

---

25 QSA: Queen Square Records, Dr Batten, 1915, male A-K: case record Private Steward B.; the pain medication was 'aspirin'.
26 Holmes, *The National Hospital*, p.64.
27 QSA: minutes from the Board of Management meeting; handwritten note, 10 November 1914. Howard Henry Tooth, consultant neurologist at Queen Square since 1887, informed the Board in writing that he had taken command of a military hospital and would not be able to attend to his duties at the National Hospital for some time; see also QSA: minutes from the Board of Management meeting, 12 January 1915 – absence of W. Aldren Turner: 'A letter was read from Dr. Aldren Turner that he had been called away to France for a period of about two months....'
28 QSA: minutes from the Board of Management meeting; handwritten note, 10 November 1914. Frederick Eustace Batten, dean of the National's Medical School (who had resigned

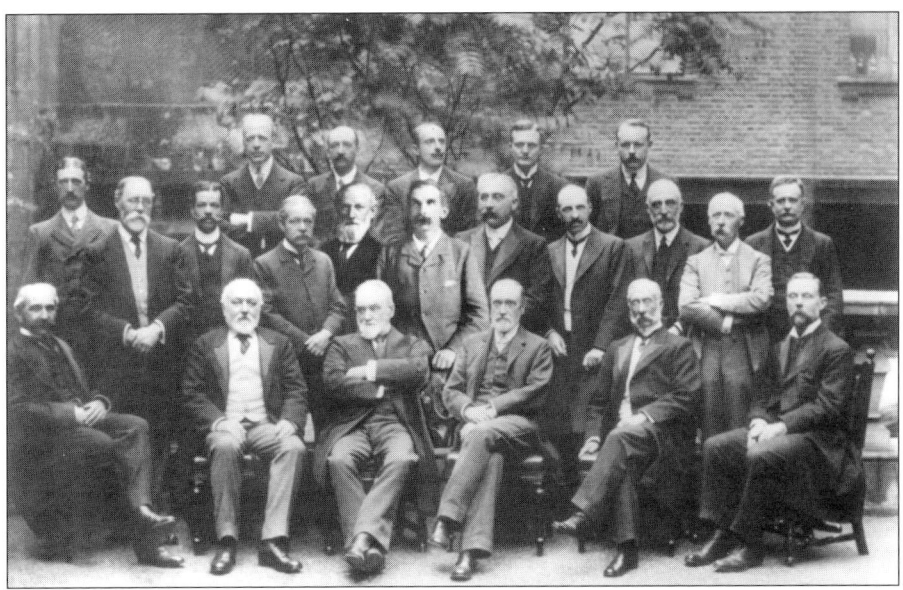

Consultants at Queen Square, 1904; QSA/15391. (Queen Square Archives, London)

request from the Ministry of Pensions to hold special outpatient sessions for wounded servicemen. The high numbers of military casualties led to longer waiting lists for civilian patients and 'complaints by the medical staff that frequently there was no accommodation even for persons who were seriously ill and urgently required indoor treatment'.[29]

The hour of the female doctors

The gaps in medical staffing were gradually filled by women house officers recruited from the only women's medical school of the country: the London School of Medicine for Women (LSMW) at the Royal Free Hospital. The year 1916 had seen the first two female junior doctors at the National Hospital: Drs Violet Turner and Elizabeth Ashby. In 1918, two female doctors – Drs Majorie A. Blandy and Eveleen B. Rivington – would again be responsible for the medical care of all inpatients. Majorie Blandy had already gained considerable experience with surgical cases from the Western Front: newly qualified from the LSMW, she had joined the Women's Hospital Corps (WHC) at the beginning of the war. Under the leadership of the former militant suffragettes Flora Murray and Louisa Garrett Anderson, this remarkable group of female doctors

from his clinical duties in 1909), took responsibility for Tooth's patients in his absence.
29 Holmes, *The National Hospital*, p.59.

successfully ran two military hospitals in France from September 1914 to January 1915. The vast majority of female doctors of the WHC were former students of the LSMW – and because of the strict gender separation of pre-war medicine, none of them would have had experience treating male patients. Although women had been able to qualify as doctors in Britain since the trailblazing efforts of Louisa's mother, Elizabeth Garrett Anderson, in 1865, most hospital appointments remained closed to them. Those who had clinical appointments before the war had been working in women-run hospitals, and several held posts as school medical officers or inspectors; some had built up private practices.

The first French hospital run by the WHC was based in Paris, in the newly-finished Hotel Claridge on the Champs-Élysées , which had been converted into a 100-bed hospital by the French Red Cross. The *'Hôpital Anglo-Belge'* ('Belgian' because there were Belgian refugees on the upper floors), which opened its doors to injured soldiers from the Western Front on 22 September 1914, was self-financed; staff and equipment, including an X-ray machine and two ambulances, came from London. The second hospital run by the WHC opened on 6 November 1914 in the Château Mauricien at Wimereux (on the coast of the Channel). It was officially recognised by the War Office and attached to the RAMC – and by January 1915, the whole Claridge staff had been transferred to Wimereux.

In 1915, the War Office asked the WHC to run a large RAMC hospital in London. Workhouse premises in Endell Street in Covent Garden were rapidly transformed into a 573-bed hospital, which was staffed and administered entirely by women. The Endell Street Military Hospital, run under the direct patronage of the War Office, was the first hospital in the UK established for men by medical women. It remained open from May 1915 to December 1919; in that time, its doctors saw 26,000 patients and performed more than 7,000 major operations.[30]

The wartime shortages of qualified medical staff and the dedication and readiness of gifted women doctors had changed the status of female physicians considerably; however, the successful work of the WHC – in particular, at Endell Street – was not to strengthen the position of female doctors in the years after the war. In fact, the work conditions of female doctors improved very little compared to the pre-war period. Although Marjorie Blandy was one of the first female doctors to work at the National Hospital at Queen Square, she did not advance into a consultant post, unlike most of her male predecessors and successors. In 1922, she married James Purdon Martin – a neurologist who had recently been appointed to the staff and would later rise to the office of dean of Queen Square's Medical School. They had to keep their wedding secret, because women could not keep their jobs once married. Shortly afterwards, Dr Blandy was brave enough to write a letter to the Medical Committee complaining about the insufficient heating in her registrar room, after which she was replaced fairly

---

30 Geddes, Jennian F., 'The Women's Hospital Corps: forgotten surgeons of the First World War' – *Journal of Medical Biography*, 14:2 (2006), pp.109-117.

From the Fields of Flanders to the Temple of Neurology   59

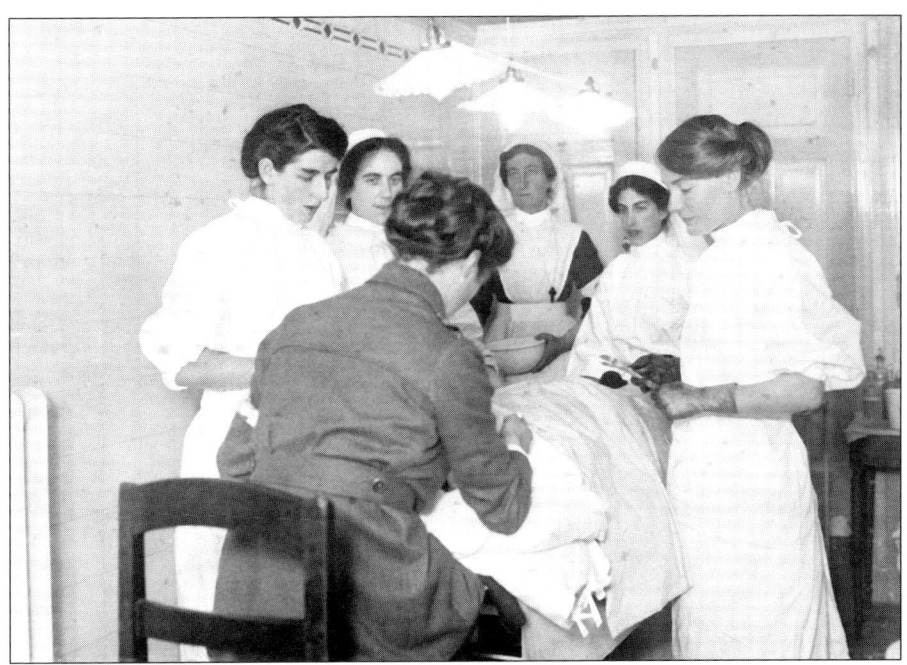

Surgery at the Hotel Claridge ('*Hôpital Anglo-Belge*'): Flora Murray is giving the anaesthetic, Hazel Cuthbert is the surgeon to the left of the picture and Majorie Blandy is to the right; photograph. (Imperial War Museum, London)

quickly. After the war, most WHC doctors married and retired, went into private practice or returned to their former posts at women-run hospitals. None of them went into surgery – the area in which many of them had gained the greatest expertise.[31]

Soldier-patients in the temple of neurology

Between 3 August 1914 and 31 December 1919, 1,212 soldiers and sailors were treated at the National Hospital – accounting for 45 percent of all male admissions. For 462 soldiers (38 percent of all military admissions), doctors could find no identifiable organic pathology. The Queen Square neurologists mainly classified such cases as 'functional disorder', 'hysteria', 'neurasthenia', 'neurosis' and 'shell shock'. The peak of the shell shock epidemic at Queen Square was reached in 1915, when 63 percent of military cases were eventually diagnosed with a psychological disorder.

Who were these patients whom their army doctors considered to be in need of specialist intervention at the most prestigious neurological institution of the empire?

---

31   Geddes, 'The Women's Hospital Corps', p.116.

The vast majority of psychological military casualties were private soldiers; 16 percent were non-commissioned officers, with the ranks of lance corporal, corporal, sergeant and sergeant major. Only four officers with shell shock were admitted to Queen Square during the war years, which is lower than would be expected given their distribution in the army, but can be explained by the existence of dedicated treatment facilities for officers (for example, at Golders Green, North London or Craiglockhart, near Edinburgh). In addition, consultants at Queen Square saw outpatients with war trauma on a private basis (for whom no records survived) – and given the higher ability to pay, there may have been a higher proportion of officers amongst this group.

Most soldiers were British, but there were also Irish, Belgian, Canadian, Australian and South African servicemen. On average, they had developed their symptoms nine months before admission to Queen Square; the mean age on admission was 28 years. The youngest patient was 17, while the oldest was 60 (a solicitor's clerk in civilian life, who was a member of the volunteer reserves). The average length of stay in hospital for soldiers with shell shock was 69 days – exceeding the 53 days of average treatment duration for civilian patients before the war. Four-hundred and thirty-three patients had been involved in frontline service, but 29 soldiers developed functional disorders without even having been exposed to combat.

The international reputation of the hospital was illustrated by the case of George C., a 25-year-old private from the Australian Infantry.[32] George had landed in Gallipoli on the night of 25 April 1915 – and under cover of darkness, but with increasing opposition from the Turkish defenders, he had made his way inland to occupy Pope's Hill (a razor-backed ridge in the heights above ANZAC Cove). In the following months, George was involved in many charges and took part in the disastrous August offensive.

On 7 August 1915 – after three months of fierce fighting – when George's regiment attacked a Turkish trench at sunset, the young Australian broke down. When he regained consciousness, he found himself on a hospital ship that had berthed at the Greek island of Lemnos. From there, he was taken to Alexandria in Egypt, where he arrived on 14 August. George could not remember the circumstances of his breakdown, and he found himself unable to speak, or make any sound at all. George was one of the thousands of wounded soldiers from Gallipoli to be treated at the 21st General Hospital in Alexandria. He was lucky, because conditions at this hospital had substantially improved since the first wounded had arrived from Gallipoli, thanks to a particular link with Queen Square.

The 21st General Hospital, which was located in old barracks adjacent to the Ras-el-Tin Palace, had been in an appalling state: it was infested with flies, enormous cockroaches and rodents, and lacking basic equipment when Victor Horsley took charge in May 1915. The pioneering neurosurgeon from Queen Square had

---

32 QSA: Queen Square Records, Dr Tooth, 1915, male A-K: case record Private George C.

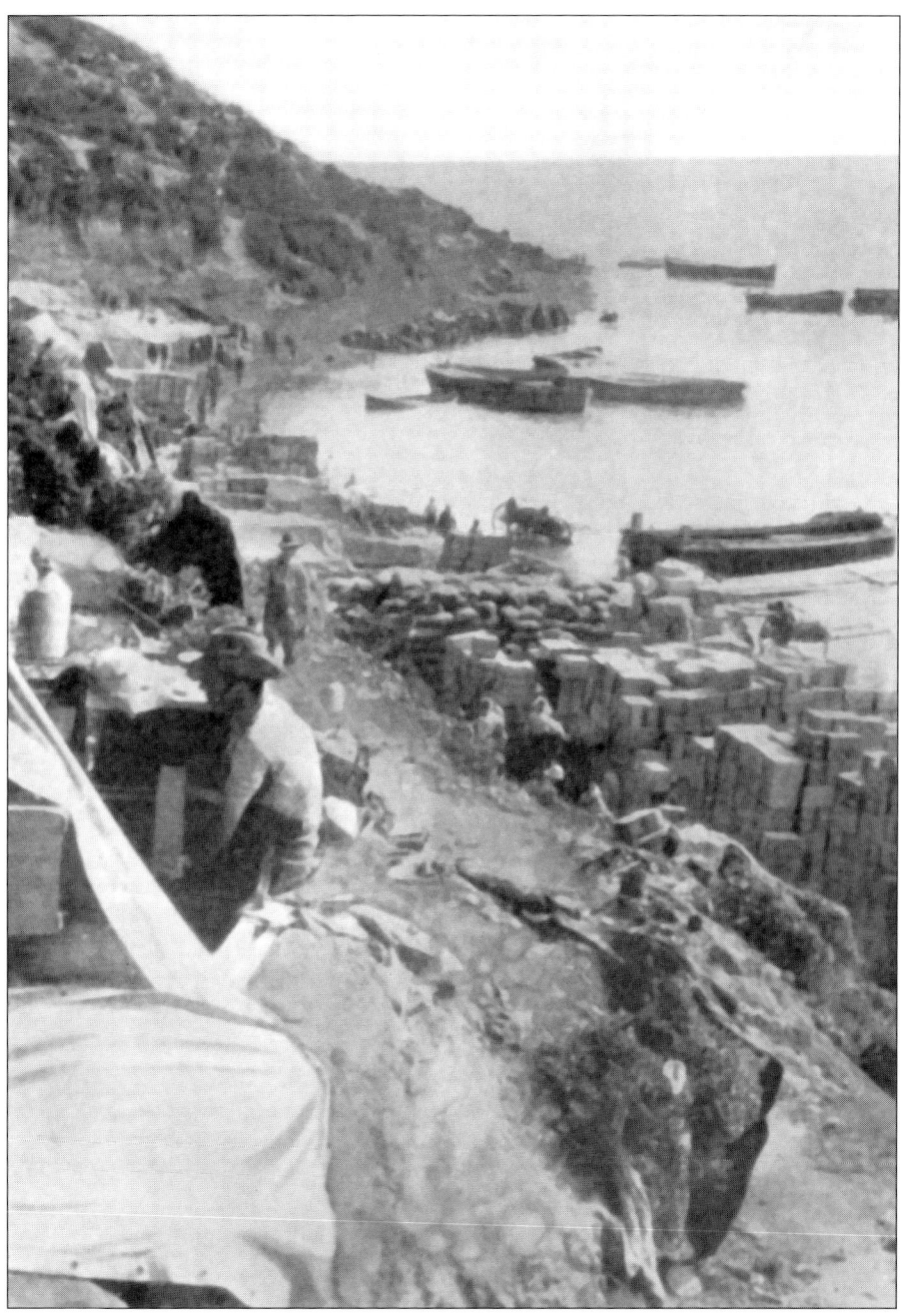

A view of one of the ANZAC landing places. (From *The Times History and Encyclopaedia of the War*, part 64, Vol 5, Nov 9, 1915, p.450)

volunteered for active service in the Middle East soon after the outbreak of the war, and an overhaul of the military hospital in Alexandria was his first major task as a military doctor. Horsley himself took an active part in the dirty work of cleaning and disinfecting the hospital, and ordered modern equipment from England. He acted as surgeon to the 21st General Hospital until on 14 July 1915, he was appointed consultant surgeon to the Mediterranean Expeditionary Force to inspect the surgical facilities throughout the area.

George, who arrived one month later, thus probably never met Victor Horsley in person; however, he would have heard of Horsley's great contributions towards improved treatment facilities for wounded soldiers, and he would have heard of Horsley's home institution: the National Hospital for the Paralysed and Epileptic.

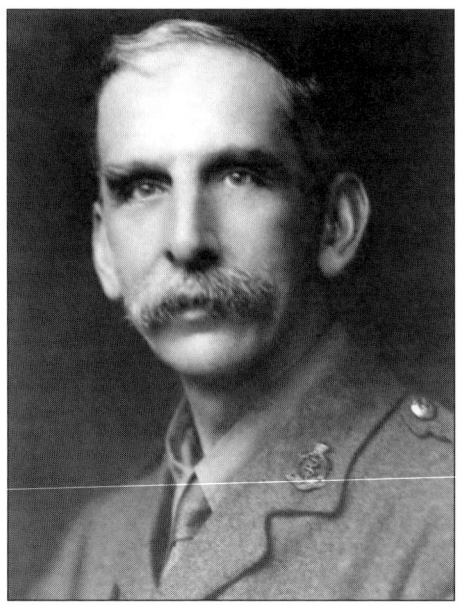

Sir Victor Horsley in uniform, 1915; QSA/14049. (Queen Square Archives, London)

George was convinced that he could only be successfully treated at this world-leading hospital – and although it was difficult, he ultimately managed to obtain his transfer there:

> When in the 21st General Hospital Alexandria Egypt I was ordered home to Australia. … And was told that so many had gone there that they were only sending curable cases there and as mine would be a very long time I would have to go to Australia. But if I wanted to get to England I had to sign to the effect that if I was not cured within three months, I would have to pay my fare back to Australia because I came here on my own decision as the Board had decided to send me to Australia. Anyhow I thought I would give myself a chance as so many had got back their voice in England and I had not been home for 5 years. So I chanced paying my own fare anyhow whatever happening and now I have wrote to Commissioner of Australia Sir George Reid, and he informed me that all would be well with me whatever happened.
>
> I came to England on the Glengorm Castle to Southampton to Camberwell Hospital. I had a coughing for a night or two and since then I have been a bit mixed. I have not spoken a word since I have been in England but one of my mates told me I said three words in Alexandria but over excited myself and the doctor said it would be alright in a few days. By all accounts I could not cough or

whistle but now I do both. And also since I have had a cough I have been able to whisper... I was under treatment by another doctor here somewhere which have seemed done me a little good.[33]

When George was admitted to the National Hospital on 22 October 1915, Victor Horsley was visiting the medical facilities on the Gallipoli Peninsula; lectured to the medical officers in the tented hospital at Sulva Bay on the treatment of head wounds; and visited the field ambulance and casualty clearing stations at ANZAC Cove and Cape Helles.

The young Australian was discharged from the National Hospital as 'cured' on 17 November 1915; his main treatment consisted of breathing exercises and electrotherapy. His firm belief in the effectiveness of the treatment provided at Queen Square may have been a major factor in this positive outcome, and the prospect of having to pay for his return to Australia if treatment failed may have incentivised him further. George never saw active service again, and we do not know if he returned to Australia, or if he built a new life in Britain; however, Victor Horsley – to whose hygienic measures in Alexandria George may have owed his life – never saw his home country again. In April 1916, he moved to Mesopotamia, where his expertise was urgently needed. His indefatigable commitment was taking its toll: on 14 July 1916, he was admitted to the British General Hospital at Amara (on the shores of the Tigris River) with high fever. He died two days later – most likely from heatstroke. He was buried the next day at Amara, with full military honours, in the presence of 80 of his fellow officers.[34]

What was shell shock like?

The symptoms of traumatised soldiers were diverse and could affect every system of the body. British medical journals of the war years were filled with reports of the common shell shock syndromes, such as heart-related problems (called 'disordered action of the heart'), or paralyses of legs or arms. They also recorded less common functional phenomena, such as the 'big belly' (or '*les gros ventres de la guerre*'), which was characterised by an abdomen that was 'excessively prominent, recalling that of a woman seven or eight months pregnant'.[35] 'Miner's nystagmus' – presenting with visual disturbances and rhythmic oscillation of the eyes – was another of the rarer

---

33 QSA: Queen Square Records, Dr Tooth, 1915, male A-K: case record Private George C.; patient's handwritten account attached to case record.
34 Dunnill, Michael S., 'Victor Horsley (1857-1916) in World War I' – *Journal of Medical Biography*, 18:4 (2010), pp.186-193.
35 'An epitome of current medical literature. "Big belly" in soldiers' – *British Medical Journal*, 2:2961 (1917), p.9.

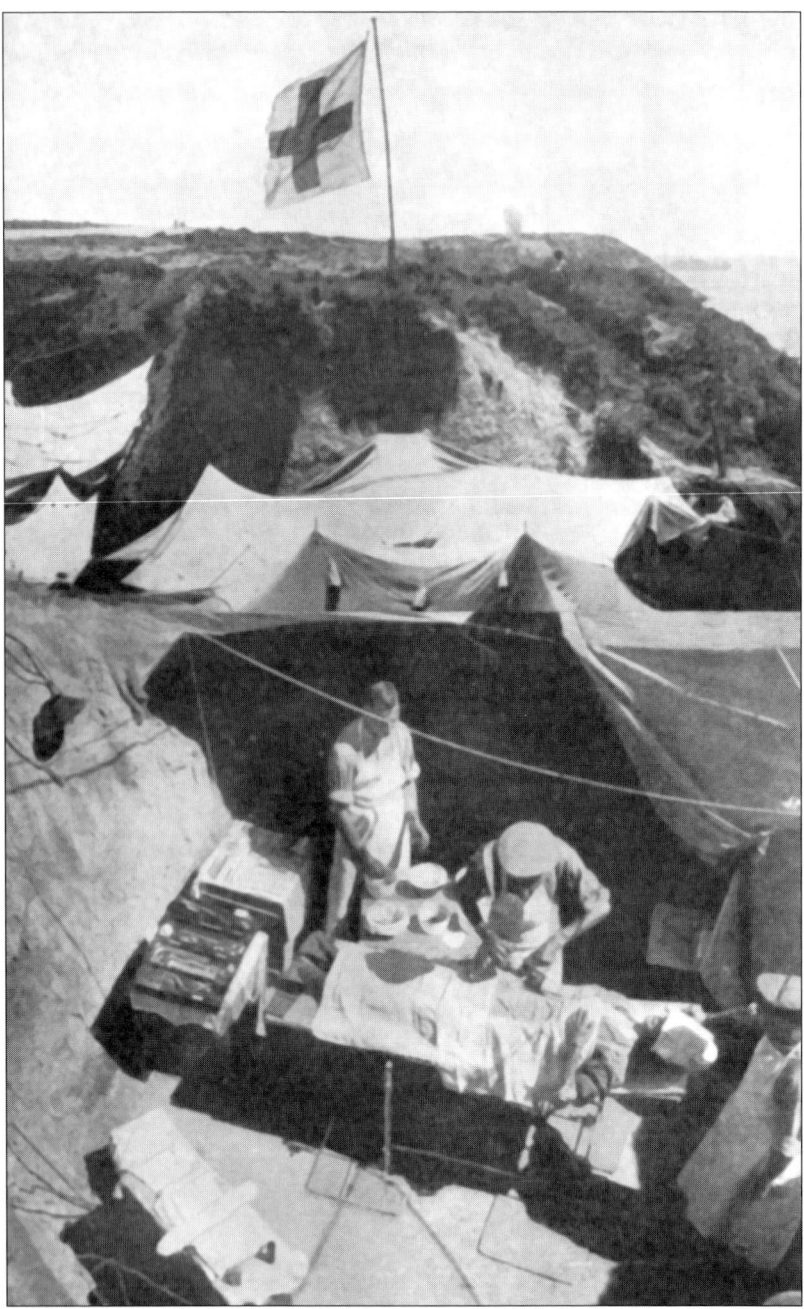

The Dardanelles: a dressing station; an operation in progress. (From *The Times History and Encyclopaedia of the War*, Science and the Health of Armies, part 67, Vol 6, Nov 30, 1915, p.47)

From the Fields of Flanders to the Temple of Neurology 65

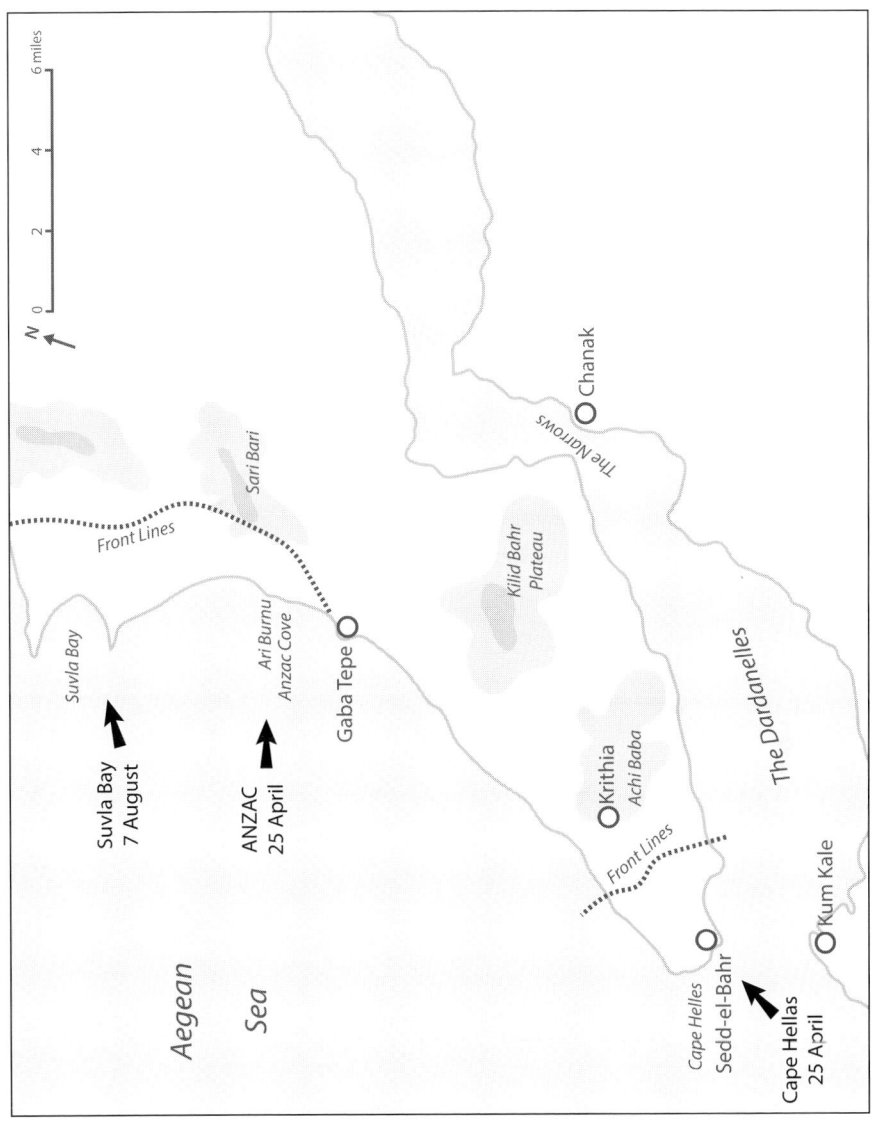

Map 1 The Gallipoli Peninsula and the Dardanelles. (Map by George Anderson)

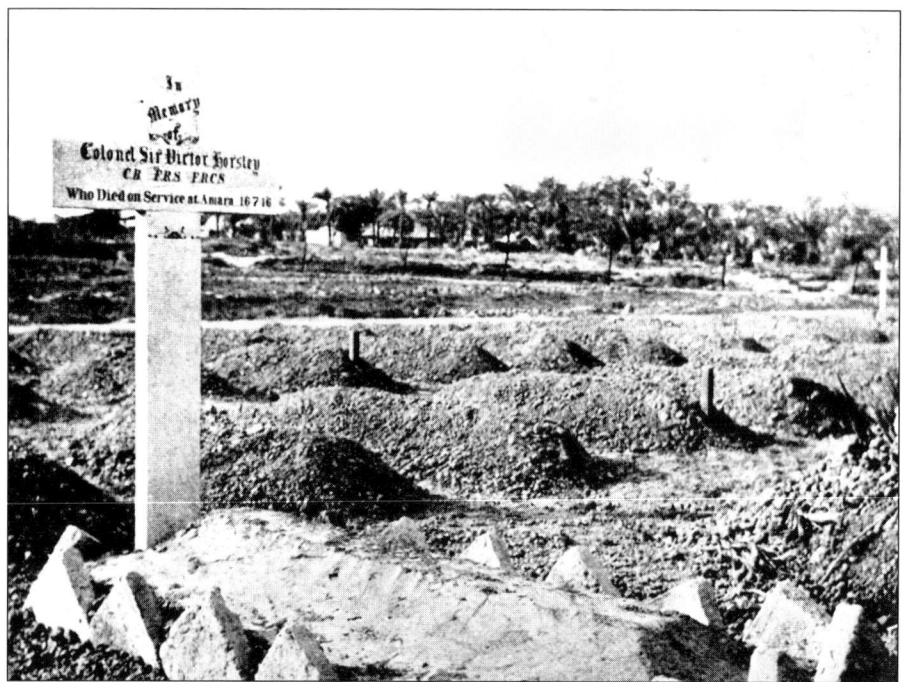

In memory of Colonel Sir Victor Horsley, who died on service at Amara, 16.7.16; Sir Victor Horsley's grave, Amara, photograph; QSA/1808. (Queen Square Archives, London)

conditions; it had been known from peacetime coal miners.[36] This example can serve as a reminder that traumatic neuroses had been recognised throughout the Industrial Revolution, although the scale and intensity with which they occurred during the war was completely unprecedented. Some doctors believed that shell shock symptoms could reflect the nature of the traumatising event in an almost symbolic way: for example, in some patients, a blaze of light across the eyes had led to blindness, or an intolerably intense explosion to deafness.

Queen Square mainly received patients in whom shell shock had affected the control of the limbs. Soldiers suffered unexplained paralyses of their arms or legs, combined with numbness, or an altered sensation in the affected area of the body. The other main group of symptoms included involuntary movements in the form of shaking, tremors or tics, as in the case of 27-year-old Frank D. from the 1st Monmouthshire Regiment. Frank was admitted to Queen Square on 4 May 1915 with a diagnosis of 'functional tremor' and 'neurosis like "dog chorea"'.

36 Harford, Charles F., 'Visual neuroses of miners in their relation to military service' – *British Medical Journal*, 1:2879 (1916), pp.340-342.

The case record reads:

> Patient is a territorial and went out to France in January; he has been quite well up till a week ago, when on April 26th he was buried under a bomb explosion in the trench. He was not unconscious but dazed and all in a tremble, all his limbs were shaking. He was conscious being carried by his comrades out of the trenches to a "dugout". A few hours afterwards he had to cry and he was crying for two days. At the same time his arms began to twitch, very frequently at first. He was transferred to the 12th General Hospital in Rouen and from there here. He has a bad headache since all over the head.[37]

The rifleman showed 'lightening-like synchronous twitching of both arms with contraction of both pectoral muscles, quite involuntary but less frequent if attention is fixed on something else'. After two weeks, he was discharged 'recovered' to a convalescent home.

Another striking example of abnormal motor function was observed in 23-year-old Scottish Private Henry M. from the 18th Hussars, who was admitted to Queen Square on 18 June 1915 with a diagnosis of functional facial spasm:

> On May 13th [1915] patient was struck by several pieces of shrapnel, on the right hand, forearm, shoulder and on the right side of the nose at its base. He was very dazed, but did not lose consciousness. The wounds healed in a month. About a week after being wounded he was operated on in order that a piece of shrapnel might be removed from his face. On recovering from the anaesthetic he found himself unable to move the right side of his face or to open his mouth. This condition, which is quite painless, has persisted since, and he has not eaten solid food or been able to take out his false teeth. He has been fed through a rubber tube inserted between his teeth. In all other respects he feels well. [...] Patient sits up in bed gasping in a highly alarming manner, with his left face in a strong tonic spasm and his jaws tightly set. All efforts to open his mouth are unavailing, so strong is the contraction of his masseters. [...] He declares himself unable to breathe unless sitting up, and when made to lie down, his neck is strongly retracted and set and he breathes violently through his clenched teeth and holds his breath for as long as he can, assuming a purple tinge, which is apt to be disconcerting until one is accustomed to it. By the moral aid given by strong faradism [an electric current applied by the physician] and force applied to the jaw, it was possible to remove a filthy set of false teeth. During this performance he uttered piercing shrieks and foamed and his rigidly held arms shook violently. Tears ran from his eyes, and he sweated profusely from his muscular exertion in resisting the attentions, well intended though they were, of the physician. When

---

37   QSA: Queen Square Records, Dr Tooth, 1915, male A-K: Case record Rifleman Frank D.

asked to close his eyes he was able to do, in fact the left eye is half closed in the spasm. All tests reveal good power in both sides of the face. The facial and jaw spasm would seem to be voluntary and due to frank malingering. In the intervals of this grotesque performance he lies back on the pillow, without any dyspnoea, but he induces an apparent difficulty in breathing at will. Examination reveals no organic disease or injury in either nervous or other systems.[38]

Within four weeks of inpatient treatment, this soldier made a 'practically complete recovery', and he was recommended for home service. This case is noteworthy for several reasons: first, this is a case in which functional symptoms were grafted onto physical injuries. Such cases could be particularly confusing for the medical officers, because it was difficult to tell apart the physical cause and the psychological consequences. As Charles Myers, the psychologist who had originally coined the term 'shell shock' remarked, functional contractures and paralyses often occurred 'after leaving France, often after the removal of a splint following surgical treatment for a wound to the limb received there'. These functional symptoms, which were localised in the same area as the original lesion, could easily be mistaken for the effects of a physical injury.[39] Secondly, this case demonstrates the immense suffering psychologically wounded soldiers experienced and the impact the trauma had on everyday life; thirdly, this is one of the very rare Queen Square cases in which simulation of symptoms was suspected. Even if presentations seemed bizarre or mannered, the genuineness of these conditions was hardly ever doubted by any of the Queen Square doctors, and not a single patient was discharged with a diagnosis of 'malingering' or simulation. Contemporary publications also stressed the rarity of 'pure malingering

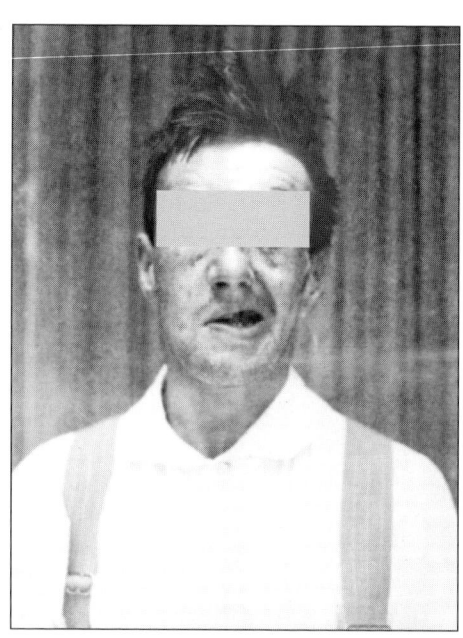

Private Henry M. from the 18th Hussars; photograph attached to case record. (Queen Square Archives, London)

---

38 QSA: Queen Square Records, Dr Tooth, 1915, male L-Z: Case record Private Henry M.
39 Myers, Charles S., *Shell Shock in France, 1914-1918* (Cambridge: Cambridge University Press, 1940), pp.132-133.

[…] in the British and French armies'[40] and the rarity of discussions of malingering in the medical records suggests that this account was not mere propaganda; however, it is also possible that malingerers had been sifted out before reaching Queen Square.

The question of simulation

The hero of the 1954 novel *Confessions of Felix Krull* by German Nobel laureate Thomas Mann suffered a classical functional seizure during his army medical examination. Before, he had provided the military doctors with enough information to conclude that he was suffering from a psychopathic constitution: he had missed his final year of school because he was suffering from psychosomatic complaints, and his father – an alcoholic champagne producer – had committed suicide after his business had collapsed. Almost a typical Charité case, except that Felix Krull had never been to the front line (he obviously did not pass his medical), and his symptoms and history were completely fabricated. Perhaps more conscripts would have attempted simulation if Thomas Mann had published his novel 40 years earlier (it would have been a different novel, because like so many other German intellectuals, Mann was enthusiastic about the war in its early phase), or more doctors would have suspected it. As it was, 'neither military nor medical authorities devoted significant amounts of attention to the simulation issue during the war'. If anything, doctors were concerned that soldiers may have aggravated pre-existing symptoms. Nevertheless, some psychiatrists tried to establish guidelines for the distinction between hysteria and simulation; however, they were at a loss to distinguish these two groups on the basis of clinical symptoms. They concluded that a strong wish to avoid frontline service through illness was dominant both in hysterics and in malingerers: a hysterical origin was considered likely in cases where there was a proven pre-war history of hysterical symptoms – especially in childhood – or evidence of a psychopathic constitution throughout life; conversely, malingering was suspected when symptoms did not vary with the emotional state of the patient, and when no clear triggers could be identified.

Psychological wounds

Cases such as that of Henry M., the Scottish private who could not open his mouth, show that neurological problems (paralyses, involuntary movements, muteness, deafness and blindness) were closely entwined with psychological symptoms. Common symptoms included irritability, difficulty sleeping and increased sensitivity to noise.[41]

---

40   Hurst, Arthur F., *Medical Diseases of the War*, 2nd edn (London: Edward Arnold, 1918), pp.28-29; other physicians who emphasised that cases of malingering were exceptional were Mott and Myers: Mott, Frederick W., *War Neuroses and Shell Shock* (London: Oxford University Press, 1919), p.123; Myers, *Shell Shock in France*, p.40.
41   Hurst, *Medical Diseases of the War*, p.41.

These 'subjective' disturbances, which could be easily overlooked in a cursory examination, could cause considerable suffering and 'make life for some of their victims a veritable hell'.[42] Irritability, sleeping problems and increased sensitivity are all core symptoms of the modern diagnosis of post-traumatic stress disorder (PTSD), which is linked with veterans of the Korean, Vietnam and more recent wars – thus, was shell shock perhaps an early form of PTSD? Or was shell shock a relatively easy way – consciously or subconsciously – to escape frontline duty? These are central questions for the understanding of shell shock, but also for the understanding of the consequences of combat stress across the times and theatres of war; they will be the topic of Chapter 14.

---

42   Smith and Pear, *Shell Shock and its Lessons*, pp.12-13.

4

What Major Mott made of Shell Shock

Paralysis and deafness, twitching and shaking, stuttering and loss of memory – what had happened to all those young healthy men who had eagerly volunteered to fight for their country? Surely, there had to be a simple explanation as to why these men had lost control over their own bodies; why they had become liabilities to the armed forces.

After an initial phase of puzzlement, army doctors on both sides started an intense scientific debate on the causes of these new and perplexing symptoms. The Great War turned into a 'huge psychological experiment' through which the effects of extreme psychological and physical stress on human behaviour could be studied.[1] A central question of the wartime medical debates was whether the symptoms found in soldiers without visible wounds were the result of organic brain damage (produced by shockwaves from explosions), or psychological effects of the traumatic experience. This was not the first time that physical and psychological causes of post-traumatic complaints were pitched against each other: a similar debate had occurred in the second half of the 19th century, when the rapid expansion of rail travel led to numerous railroad accidents – after which passengers (even those without obvious physical injuries) complained about exhaustion, chronic pain and other neurological symptoms. It was clearly beneficial for them to argue that their complaints were caused by the physical impact of the accident rather than the fears and terrors it invoked in the passenger. In this way, they were much more likely to receive compensation from the railway company and avoided the stigma associated with a mental illness. The medical profession failed to solve the conundrum of how these mysterious symptoms – subsumed under the heading of 'railway spine' – evolved. Some neurologists and psychiatrists of the time believed in an organic cause – pointing to physical correlates like microscopic brain lesions or bleedings; many others thought that these presentations looked rather more like a variant of neurasthenia or hysteria – the psychological reactions to trauma

---

1   Fauser, A., 'Kriegspsychiatrische und neurologische Erfahrungen und Betrachtungen' – *Archiv für Psychiatrie und Nervenkrankheiten*, 59:1 (1918), pp.260-280.

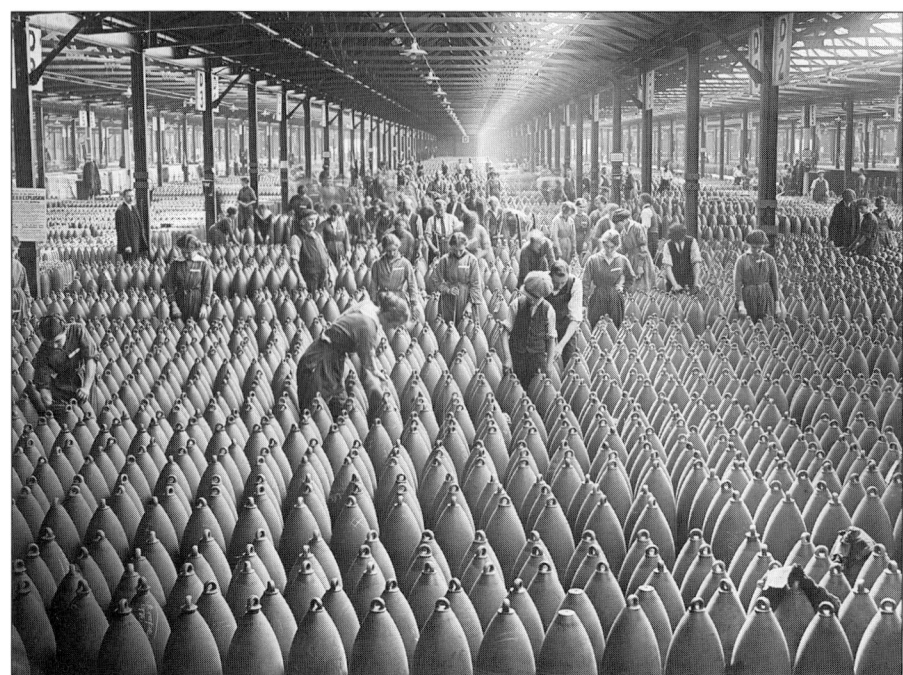

Munition workers in a shell warehouse at the National Shell Filling Factory, Chilwell, Nottinghamshire, Q 30018. (Imperial War Museum, London)

that had initially been studied by Charcot and his pupil, the pioneering psychologist Pierre Janet.

Hermann Oppenheim, a leading German neurologist from Berlin, was one of the foremost advocates of the organic illness model. Following his investigation of injured industrial workers with neurological symptoms before the war, Oppenheim had delineated a distinct disease that he named 'traumatic neurosis'. This term suggested a causal relationship between trauma and symptoms, and implied an organic – yet, at first view, hidden – origin of the disorder. Oppenheim was quick to apply the disease model that he had developed for injured industry workers of pre-war Berlin to shell-shocked soldiers. Here too, he believed that microscopic changes in the brain caused by cerebral concussion were primarily responsible for the strange symptoms – and indeed, the German medical press seemed to provide the evidence for Oppenheim's theories: post-mortem investigations of soldiers exposed to shell explosions revealed cerebral haemorrhages.[2] Similarly, Swiss experiments with rabbits, fish and a rat that

---

2   For example, Harzbecker, O., 'Über die Ätiologie der Granatkontusionsverletzungen' – *Deutsche Medizinische Wochenschrift*, 40:47 (1914), p.1,985.

had been subjected to controlled explosions, but did not have any obvious head injuries, revealed bleeds in the brain[3] – thus, all seemed to be pointing to an organic origin of shell shock.

The early reports from Germany were read eagerly by the British experts who retained a high opinion of the quality – albeit not necessarily morality – of German science throughout the war. A central figure in the British debate, with a position similar to that of Oppenheim in Germany, was Frederick Walker Mott. Mott was one of Britain's leading neuropathologists and had been made a fellow of the Royal Society in 1896 – the highest academic distinction of the empire. During the war, he treated soldiers at the Neurological Section of the 4th London Territorial General Hospital and later at the Maudsley Neurological Clearing Hospital, which was opened as a specialist treatment and research hospital for shell shock in January 1916. Like his German counterparts, Mott embraced the opportunity to study the effects of explosives on the central nervous system.

In 1917, Mott reported on post-mortem examinations of two soldiers who had died at the Western Front after shell explosions without suffering obvious physical injuries.[4] One of them had shown classical symptoms of shell shock: tremors, crying, excitement and paralysis of his legs. After a good night's sleep, induced by morphine and chloroform, he had woken up 'apparently well, and suddenly died'. On the same day, Captain A. Stokes of the Royal Army Medical Corps performed a post-mortem examination in his mobile laboratory: he opened the soldier's skull, but could not detect any major haemorrhage or other lesion on the brain; however, he was surprised to find the cerebrospinal fluid – the liquid surrounding and cushioning the brain and spinal cord – to be blood-tinged. The other soldier, a gunner in the Royal Garrison Artillery, had been sitting in a corrugated iron hut – 50 yards from some boxes of cordite cartridges – when a shell landed and blew up his entire unit. Although he did not have any visible wounds, the soldier lost consciousness, his breathing became stertorous and slow, and he died shortly afterwards. The soldiers' brains were removed, placed in spirit, packaged and dispatched to Major Mott's laboratory in the south of London.

On general inspection, the brains looked as if their blood supply had been cut off. They appeared similar to the brains of animals whose carotid and vertebral arteries – the arteries supplying the brain with blood – had been tied off in an experiment to study the effects of anaemia. On microscopic examination – in particular, of the motor cortex responsible for body movements – Mott found evidence of cell death in the grey matter and small bleeds in the white matter of the dissected brains.[5] He concluded

---

3   Rusca, F., 'Experimentelle Untersuchungen über die traumatische Druckwirkung der Explosionen' – *Deutsche Zeitschrift für Chirurgie*, 132:3-4 (1914), pp.315-374.
4   Mott, Frederick W., 'The microscopic examination of the brains of two men dead of commotio cerebri (shell shock) without visible external injury' – *British Medical Journal*, 2:2967 (1917), pp.612-615.
5   Mott, 'The microscopic examination', pp.612-615.

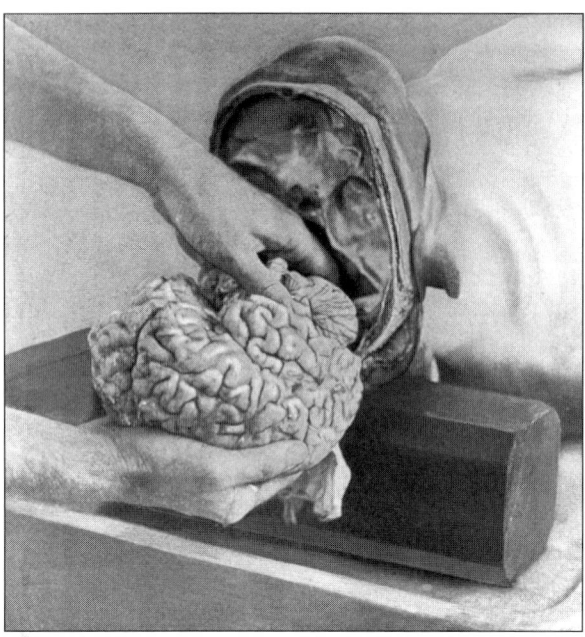

An examination of the skull and brain – a method of removing the brain after it is severed from the body. (Wellcome Library, London)

that these changes must have been caused by the 'enormous forces of compression and decompression generated by the detonation of high-explosives in great shells, aerial torpedoes, and mines'. The blast caused direct damage to the brain and spinal cord, but also triggered 'vibrations' of the bony structures and spinal fluid. Mott opined that these physical effects of the blast led to molecular disturbances in nerve cells – in particular, those responsible for cardio-respiratory function, which could explain the altered breathing pattern in many soldiers. He also tried to explain the anaemic appearance of the soldiers' brains: during the decompression phase, bubbles of gas were released into the bloodstream, which blocked the blood vessels – leading to loss of blood supply. Mott certainly knew about the diving decompression experiments that the Edinburgh- and Jena-trained physiologist John Scott Haldane, who had been admitted to the Royal Society one year after him (1897), had conducted for the Admiralty. In a seminal paper published in 1908, covering more than 100 pages of the *Journal of Hygiene*, Haldane and his colleagues – Boycott and Damant – reported on their use of a pressure chamber to investigate the mechanisms of diving-related injuries in animals and humans. They described how too rapid decompression in goats led to an accumulation of gas bubbles in the spinal cord, tissue death and, ultimately, paralysis.[6]

6   Boycott, A.E., Damant, G.C.C. and Haldane, J.S., 'The Prevention of Compressed-Air Illness' – *Journal of Hygiene*, 8:3 (1908), pp.342-443.

Mott's colleagues, who were based at clearing stations in France, also reported that there was an increased pressure in the cerebrospinal fluid of shell-shocked soldiers, and that it sometimes contained blood or protein (normal cerebrospinal fluid does not contain blood cells and only very little protein); withdrawing fluid by lumbar puncture seemed to relieve acute symptoms.[7] These observations supported Mott's hypothesis about an organic basis of shell shock. Furthermore, Mott noted that not only physical trauma, but also psychological stress, could lead to a sudden fall of blood pressure, lack of blood supply to the brain and consecutive loss of consciousness, amnesia and other symptoms, such as deafness or blindness.[8]

Based on these findings and hypotheses, Mott encouraged his assistant at the Maudsley Hospital, Dr Edith Green – a research scholar of the recently established Medical Research Committee (today's Medical Research Council) – to study the relationship between physiological parameters, such as blood pressure and body surface temperature, and the mental symptoms of shell-shocked soldiers.[9] Green found that psychological recovery – in particular, the disappearance of terrifying dreams – was associated with a gradual rise in blood pressure and body surface temperature. Mott was fascinated by the apparent association between mental and organic processes, which he emphasised in his 3rd Lettsomian Lecture, delivered at the Medical Society of London on 6 March 1916: 'Every state of consciousness which is habitually repeated leaves an organic impression on the brain, by virtue of which that same state may be reproduced more readily at any future time in response to a suggestion fitted to excite it.'[10]

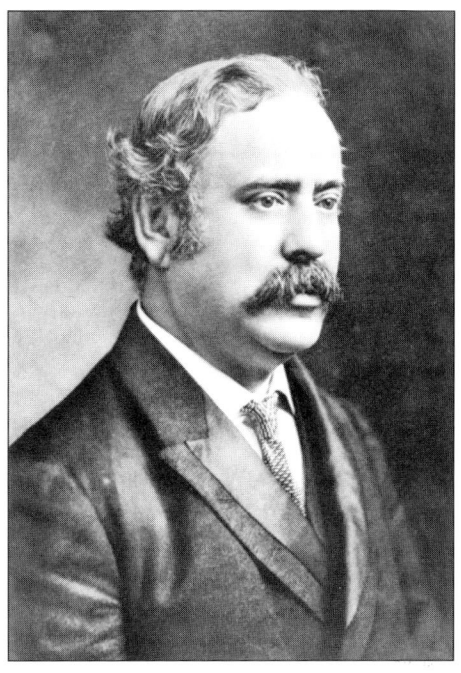

A photograph of Frederick Walker Mott. (Wellcome Library, London)

---

7   Mott, Frederick W., 'The Chadwick Lecture on Mental Hygiene and Shell Shock during and after the War' – *British Medical Journal*, 2:2950 (1917), pp.39-42.
8   Mott, *War Neuroses and Shell Shock*, p.22.
9   Green, Edith M.N., 'Blood pressure and surface temperature in 110 cases of shell shock' – *The Lancet*, 190:4908 (1917), pp.456-457.
10   Frederick W. Mott, 'The Lettsomian Lectures on the effects of high explosives upon the Central Nervous System', delivered before the Medical Society of London. Lecture III, delivered on 6 March – *The Lancet*, 187:4828 (1916), pp.545-553.

Mott was not the only physician of the time who was interested in the 'organic impressions' of psychological states: in fact, the interdependence between psychological and physiological processes was widely recognised at the time, even by psychoanalytically-minded physicians like Charles Myers.[11] In 1884, the founder of American psychology, William James, had proposed that physiological and behavioural responses to environmental stimuli preceded the subjective experience of emotions.[12] James's theory assigned a central role to the autonomic nervous system, which regulates the bodily processes that are not normally under voluntary control, such as heart rate, breathing and digestion; a similar emotion theory had been proposed independently by the Danish physiologist Carl Lange. Both James's and Lange's theories shared the premise that feelings were generated in the body, and Mott was clearly under the influence of this theory; however, some leading British shell shock doctors did not subscribe to James's emotion theory: an alternative model had been developed by Walter Cannon, who had studied with James at Harvard. Cannon believed that emotional stimuli were primarily processed in the brain, which then separately generated both bodily responses and feelings. This theory, which was first presented by Cannon in 1915,[13] found supporters among the more psychologically-minded shell shock doctors, such as Grafton Elliot Smith – anatomist and one of the fathers of brain mapping – and his colleague, Tom Hatherley Pear. Central to Smith and Pear's work on shell shock was the idea that '… one of the greatest sources of break-down under such circumstances [they refer to the war situation] is intense and frequently repeated emotion. …'[14] They developed a model in which bodily reactions were secondary to emotions such as fear, rage or despair, and thus inverted the hierarchy of physical and psychological factors of trauma proposed by Mott.

The fall of the organic model

While Mott was still collecting evidence for physical consequences of shell explosions, the organic model was falling rapidly out of favour within the German medical community. The arguments against an organic origin – put forward in the German medical literature between 1915 and 1917 – had been all too convincing: firstly, the neurological and psychological symptoms of soldiers responded surprisingly well to psychological therapies, such as hypnosis or persuasion – a precursor of modern psychotherapy. If these post-combat disorders were curable through

11 Myers, *Shell Shock in France*, p.13.
12 James, William, 'What is an emotion?', *Mind*, 9:1884, pp.188-205; Friedman, Bruce H., 'Feelings and the body: the Jamesian perspective on autonomic specificity of emotion' – *Biological Psychology*, 84:3 (2010), pp.383-393.
13 Cannon, Walter B., *Bodily Changes in Pain, Hunger, Fear and Rage: An Account of Recent Researches into the Function of Emotional Excitement* (New York, London: Appleton and Company, 1915).
14 Smith and Pear, *Shell Shock and its Lessons*, pp. 6, 8.

psychological interventions,[15] then the underlying mechanisms had to be psychological rather than physiological; secondly, doctors could not find war neurosis in prisoner of war (POW) camps,[16] or soldiers with severe physical injuries.[17] Why did these men, who had been exposed to combat and even suffered severe physical trauma, or the humiliation of imprisonment by the enemy, not develop symptoms of shell shock? There was one plausible explanation: these men – injured or captured by the enemy – were in no real danger of being sent back into battle; they did not have to show bizarre behaviours or debilitating symptoms to escape frontline service. Karl Bonhoeffer, head of the psychiatric department of the Charité in Berlin (and one of the most influential psychiatrists of his time), strongly believed that the wish to escape war and physical threat was the driving force behind most shell shock symptoms. For POWs and severely injured men, this subconscious wish had become true. Because of these and similar arguments, organic theories fell from favour and psychological illness models prevailed. The 1916 congress on war neurosis held by German psychiatrists and neurologists in Munich put an end to the public debate on causal models on the continent, and brought the defeat of Hermann Oppenheim.

Mott followed this debate closely: British medical journals regularly reported about medical practices of the enemy. German journal articles were translated into English and discussed in the British medical press. Yet, not only German psychiatrists, but also Mott's British colleagues revised their illness models. Even Mott, the most passionate promoter of the organic illness model, reconsidered his arguments over the course of the war and moved away from a purely somatic illness model. He no longer considered shell explosions to be the paramount factor, but '… merely the spark which has released long pent up forces of a psychical kind. …'[18] Mott's more integrated causal model took both 'intrinsic' constitutional and 'extrinsic' environmental factors into account. Extrinsic factors included life events, as well as the organic changes caused

---

15 Nonne, Max, 'Über erfolgreiche Suggestivbehandlung der hysteriformen Störungen bei Kriegsneurosen' – *Zeitschrift für die gesamte Neurologie und Psychiatrie*, 37:1 (1917), pp.191-218; Raether, M., 'Neurosen-Heilungen nach der Kaufmann-Methode' – *Deutsche Medizinische Wochenschrift*, 43:11 (1917), pp.321-323.

16 Mörchen, Friedrich, 'Der vorläufige Abschluß der Auseinandersetzung über das Wesen der nervösen Kriegsschädigungen' – *Psychiatrisch-Neurologische Wochenschrift*, 39:40 (1916/1917), pp.301-305.

17 This was a frequent assumption made by contemporary German physicians; yet, both modern (for example, Jones, Edgar and Wessely, Simon, 'British prisoners-of-war: from resilience to psychological vulnerability: reality or perception' – *Twentieth Century British History*, 21:2 (2010), pp.163-183) and contemporaneous (Liebermeister, G. and Siegerist, 'Über eine Neurosenepidemie in einem Kriegsgefangenenlager' – *Zeitschrift für die gesamte Neurologie und Psychiatrie*, 37:1 (1917), pp.350-355) research has shown that POWs, too, developed stress disorders.

18 MacCurdy, John T., *War Neuroses* (Cambridge: Cambridge University Press, 1918); introduction by W.H.R. Rivers.

by shell explosions and exposure to noxious gases; intrinsic (or constitutional) factors made the soldier's central nervous system vulnerable to stress in the widest sense and rendered him susceptible to mental breakdown. The interplay between psychological and physical trauma, and the individual's constitution, determined if they developed symptoms of shell shock. Mott ultimately acknowledged that most cases of shell shock '… did not owe their condition to any pathological changes which would have been recognisable in the central nervous system by any known methods of microscopic investigation… .'[19] Shell shock was not primarily an organic disorder, but a psychological reaction to stress.

Mott moved even further away from his original organic illness model when he emphasised the symbolic meaning of functional symptoms: in his terminology, the patient was 'paralysed by fear', or 'dumb with fear'. The freezing after an emotional trauma could lead to stuporous states or paralysis, and the shock-induced speechlessness to functional mutism. Similarly, tics – involuntary body movements – were sometimes described as repeated 'startling and dodging reflexes' or 'gesture movements of horror'.[20] Mott also believed that hysterical paralyses and contractures (fixed muscle contractions leading to abnormal limb posture) could be remnants of the instinctive immobilisation of an injured limb.

For Mott, these symptoms not only had a symbolic meaning: they also tended to manifest in those parts of the body which had been affected by illness or weakness before;[21] for example, a patient who had fractured his ankle in his childhood was prone to develop a restriction of movement or pain in this part of the body. Similarly, a soldier who had previously suffered from trench fever with malaise and bodily weakness could develop a chronic state of physical and mental exhaustion. In Chapter 11, we will encounter Devitt O., a daredevil pilot who was paralysed and incontinent after a plane crash. Although Devitt's symptoms disappeared, they subconsciously persisted in his mind; it only needed a minor trigger for the symptoms to return.

Following the shock of a trauma, soldiers were in a state of increased suggestibility. They were susceptible to adopt a wide variety of symptoms: these symptoms could mimic a previous illness – as in Devitt's case – or they could be an 'unconscious imitation' of another person's sufferings. An impressive example of the latter phenomenon was cited by psychoanalyst Montague David Eder: a shell-shocked soldier had developed a 'twitch' of the lower jaw. 'This was rather slowly depressed and the mouth opened with a sigh as if about to yawn or take a deep breath'. These spasms occurred frequently – two or three times in a minute at irregular intervals. There was a plausible explanation for these unusual symptoms: not long before the symptoms started, this soldier had witnessed his officer – to whom he had been deeply devoted – die in the

---

19 Mott, *War Neuroses and Shell Shock*, p.5.
20 Mott, *War Neuroses and Shell Shock*, pp.159, 121.
21 Mott, *War Neuroses and Shell Shock*, pp.131-133.

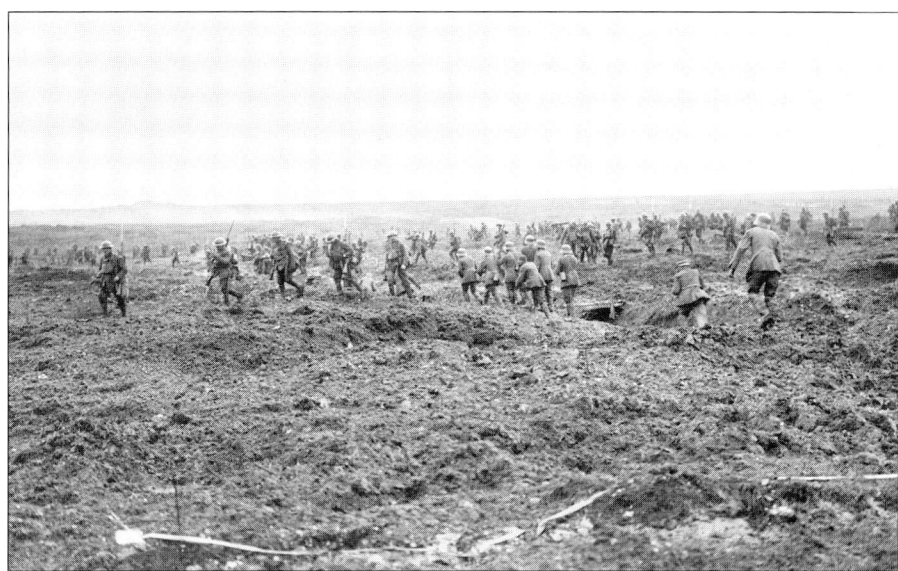

German soldiers surrender, as Canadian support waves advance across Vimy Ridge at the beginning of the Battle of Arras, 9 April 1917; CO 001155. (Imperial War Museum, London)

trenches. The corporal had been gasping for breath in agony, and the traumatised soldier had obviously mimicked this death spasm.[22]

The Queen Square Records illustrate the symbolic character of many functional symptoms – and one striking example is 29-year-old Lance Corporal Patrick R. of the 2nd Leinsters:[23] Patrick, an Irish quarryman who had just got married, enlisted in August 1914 and was sent to France in March 1915. On 20 April 1917, five months before his admission to the National Hospital, his unit had been fighting at Vimy Ridge in Northern France, supported by Canadian troops. At 5:00 p.m., when he had reached the 3rd Line of German trenches, Patrick was hit in the back by a piece of shrapnel. His Lewis automatic machine gun fell out of his hand, but he had a revolver attached to a lanyard, which was suspended from his neck. He tried to find his way back to his own lines, but got lost. When 'he saw two unarmed Germans coming out of a sap, he thought they were making for their rifles and he shot them'. From then on, his right arm was completely paralysed.

Patrick was taken to the nearest casualty clearing station, where a piece of shrapnel was removed from above his right clavicle; then to the General Hospital in Boulogne

22 Eder, Montague D., *War-Shock, the Psycho-Neuroses in War* (London: William Heinemann, 1917), p.39.
23 QSA: Queen Square Records, Dr Wilson, 1917, male and female L-Z: case record Lance Corporal Patrick R.

and, finally on 25 April 1917, to England. Between April and September, he was an inpatient in a psychiatric hospital – the Napsbury Asylum, which was located about 20 miles north of Central London – before he was transferred to Queen Square. When he arrived there on 10 September 1917, Patrick was still unable to move his right arm, which felt numb and lifeless. When doctors attempted to move his arm passively, the muscles went into violent spasms. This phenomenon was called 'negativism', because the affected limb did not do what it was supposed to do, but moved in the opposite direction. It was noted in the case records that Patrick had a 'rather depressed gloomy appearance'. His head was tilted downwards and could not be voluntarily raised. Lewis Yealland, the junior doctor in charge, used faradism and suggestion to restore motor function in Patrick's arm – 'sufficient for him to use it to eat and write'; Patrick was also made to hold his head up. Although Patrick's body functions slowly recovered, the Queen Square doctors decided that Patrick was of no further use for the British Army.

This case impressively demonstrates how the body sometimes expressed psychological scars: Patrick had shot two German soldiers and, as a consequence, the fingers that pulled the trigger stopped working and the whole arm ceased to exist in Patrick's mind. The mental representation of the arm was dissociated from the rest of his body – possibly in an attempt to suppress the memory of the traumatic experience. The spasmodic contractions of the arm – and its tendency to move in the wrong direction – were symbolic of Patrick's inner conflict and ambivalence when he was faced with the enemy. Patrick's dropped head represented his shame and self-abandonment; however, the Queen Square doctors did not spend much time on such psychological explanations. Their approach was much more pragmatic: instead of trying to interpret Patrick's symptoms, Yealland was determined to treat them.

Why had Patrick's right arm ceased to exist in his mind? Before the First World War, French neurologist Joseph Jules Dejerine had already used the term 'psychic forgetfulness' – indicating that patients with a functional paralysis had lost 'the mental representations' corresponding to the non-functioning part of the body: 'The paraplegic hysteric has forgotten in some fashion that he ever had limbs. He no longer seems to be aware that he has any. In fact, he acts as if he never had had any, and as if he had never known what it was to walk'.[24]

Arthur Hurst described the same mechanism: the belief that a particular body part or sensory organ did not work or exist led to a permanent shift of attention – and therefore, consolidation of symptoms:

> Hearing necessitates listening; inattention during a dull sermon results in total deafness to the sermon. In hysterical deafness the patient is so convinced that he cannot hear that he does not listen. Although the sound vibrations reach the

---

24 Dejerine, J. Jules and Gauckler, Ernest, *The Psychoneuroses and Their Treatment by Psychotherapy* (Philadelphia and London: J.B. Lippincott Company, 1913), p.265.

ear in the normal way, they do not give rise to the slightest auditory sensation because of this inattention. […] Just as one must listen in order to hear, so one must look in order to see, and a man who for any reason is convinced that he is blind fails to see because he does not look.[25]

The cases of functional blindness were rare and gained much attention among shell shock doctors: among 462 shell-shocked soldiers treated at the National Hospital, only four suffered from functional blindness – and one of them was 22-year-old Private Philip P. from the Machine Gun Battalion.[26] He was one of the cases that Lewis Ralph Yealland – junior doctor and, by that time, one of the most eminent shell shock specialists – discussed in his famous wartime monograph *Hysterical Disorders of Warfare*.[27] Philip, a farm labourer in civilian life, was 'blown up' and hit by a piece of shrapnel in the left side of his face when fighting in Mesopotamia on 11 January 1917; he was unconscious for several days. When he regained consciousness, he was mute and completely blind. In an operation on 18 January, shrapnel was removed from his eye and left jaw, which was splintered. He was not able to open his mouth for two months – and therefore, could not eat solid food. Philip was sent to Victoria Hospital in Bombay and another operation was performed in March, when a piece of bone was removed from his face. At that time, his voice came back; his sight, however, did not improve. Philip was sent on to England – and on 27 August 1917, he was admitted to St Mary's Hospital in London Paddington. After one week, he was transferred to the National Hospital for treatment. The 'small, well-nourished man with blue eyes, fair hair' and a 'rather fat, round face' was disfigured by a large 'ugly' scar on the left side of his face and a weakness of the muscles of the jaw. When touching his face, he experienced sharp, 'knife-like' pains; he was completely blind in his left eye. Because of marked blepharospasm (an uncontrolled contraction of the eyelid), it was initially impossible to examine Philip's eyes. On the day of his admission, electric currents were applied over Philip's closed eye – and at regular intervals, he was asked to read a vision chart to monitor his progress. Within half an hour, he could see perfectly well with both eyes, and the blepharospasm had subsided. After only two days of inpatient treatment, Philip was discharged from the National Hospital. The observation that even the most disabling shell shock symptoms could sometimes be cured within a matter of days provided the final blow to the organic disease model.

The question of the disease model was very relevant for the choice of treatment; the wartime imperative of returning invalid soldiers to productive roles ran counter to the lack of interest in therapeutic innovation that characterised university psychiatry

---

25 Hurst, *Medical Diseases of the War*, p.118.
26 QSA: Queen Square Records, Dr Turner, 1917, male L-Z: case record Private Philip P.
27 Yealland, Lewis R., *Hysterical Disorders of Warfare* (London: MacMillan and Co., 1918).

of the late 19th and early 20th century.[28] In 1917, Max Nonne, who became known for his successful treatment of war neurosis with suggestion under hypnosis, stated that 'war has taught us to be [...] less fatalistic towards the treatment of functional nervous disorders';[29] the Hamburg-based physician was convinced that war neurosis was curable. The increasing influence of psychological disease models was accompanied by the development and implementation of a vast array of largely psychological interventions for war trauma, which will be discussed in Chapter 12.

---

28 Porter, Roy, *The Greatest Benefit to Mankind: A Medical History of Humanity from Antiquity to the Present* (London: Fontana Press, 1999); Shorter, Edward, *A History of Psychiatry: From the Era of the Asylum to the Age of Prozac* (New York: Wiley, 1997); Neuner, Stephanie, *Politik und Psychiatrie: Die Staatliche Versorgung Psychisch Kriegsbeschädigter in Deutschland 1920-1939* (Göttingen: Vandenhoeck & Ruprecht, 2011), p.55.
29 Nonne, 'Über erfolgreiche Suggestivbehandlung', pp.216-217.

5

Neuve Chapelle and Hill 60

The Western Front in 1915 saw two events that accelerated the intensity and cruelty of trench warfare: the Battle of Neuve Chapelle in March – a partial success for the BEF – and the German gas attacks at Ypres in May. Both of these resulted in numerous medical casualties, but also added considerably to the toll of shell shock victims. Several of these psychological casualties ultimately made it to Queen Square, and the hospital records provide a unique vista on these gruelling battles from the point of view of mentally traumatised soldiers.

The Battle of Neuve Chapelle: four days in March 1915

Neuve Chapelle: a small farming community in Northern France, about nine miles south-west of Armentières, that had already been the scene of bitter fighting in October 1914. The fights were not so much about the village, but about the access to the city of Lille – the industrial powerhouse of Northern France and an important railway junction. Wresting Lille from German control would substantially shift the balance of power in favour of the Allied forces, but before, they would have to seize control of Aubers Ridge – an elevation of 35 metres extending across six miles of the agricultural plain to the east of the village. As long as the Germans held Aubers Ridge, they could oversee British defences and had much drier entrenchment. Aubers Ridge, thus, was a prime target for the BEF's advance into German-held French territory, but the British first had to cross a salient that was under enemy control as well. The plan was to deliver a short, but very forceful, artillery bombardment, followed by an infantry assault; the date set for the attack was 10 March 1915. It seemed the perfect time for an offensive, because the Germans were withdrawing troops to reinforce their armies at the Eastern Front.

The night before the attack was wet, with light snow, which turned to damp mist in the early hours of the first day of battle. Many young men had been waiting for this day in febrile anticipation. Some of them were experienced soldiers, while others were expecting to see action for the first time. Nine of the British soldiers, of very different ranks and backgrounds, later ended up at the capital's shell shock treatment centre at Queen Square.

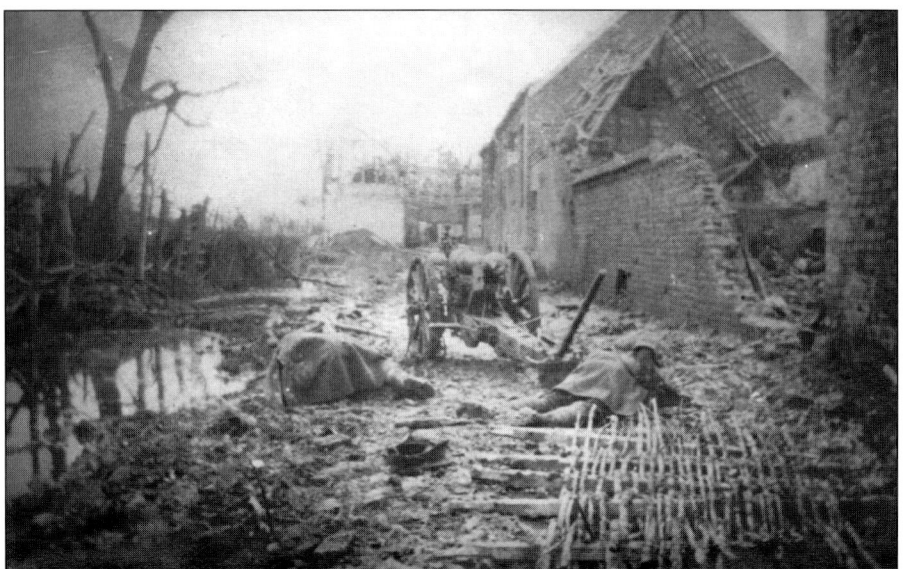

Neuve Chapelle – fighting in the village; photograph taken by an officer of the Worcester Regiment, Lt. M.A. Hamilton-Cox. (Mercian Regiment Museum, Worcester)

10 March 1915: the first day of battle

The battle was timed to start one hour after sunrise. 'Granny' – a 15" howitzer – broke the silence and signalled the start of the battle. At 7:30 a.m., the general fire was opened.[1] One of the British soldiers, who immediately went into action with the 2nd Royal Berkshires – a part of the 4th Corps of the First Army – was 21-year-old Private William S.[2] William had been prone to various physical pains and aches for all his life: before enlisting in the army at the very beginning of the war, he frequently suffered from shakiness and chest pain; nevertheless, he was determined to fight for his country. William was sent to France at the end of December 1914. He still suffered from sudden attacks of excruciating pain, which he tried to ignore, but otherwise he was well until 10 March – his first day of battle. However, his first mission was short-lived: not long into the battle, William's party got into friendly fire, and he was buried by a shell explosion. William had to be dug out and remained unconscious for about an hour. Later, when he had been admitted to hospital, he recounted the experience: he was 'stifled' by fumes and struck on his head by a trench parapet; his left shoulder was dislocated. When he came around, he could hardly stand and his head felt 'giddy

---

1   Bridger, Geoff, *The Battle of Neuve Chapelle* (Barnsley: Leo Cooper, Pen & Sword Books Ltd., 2000), p.26.
2   QSA: Queen Square Records, Dr Turner, 1915, male L-Z: case record Private William S.

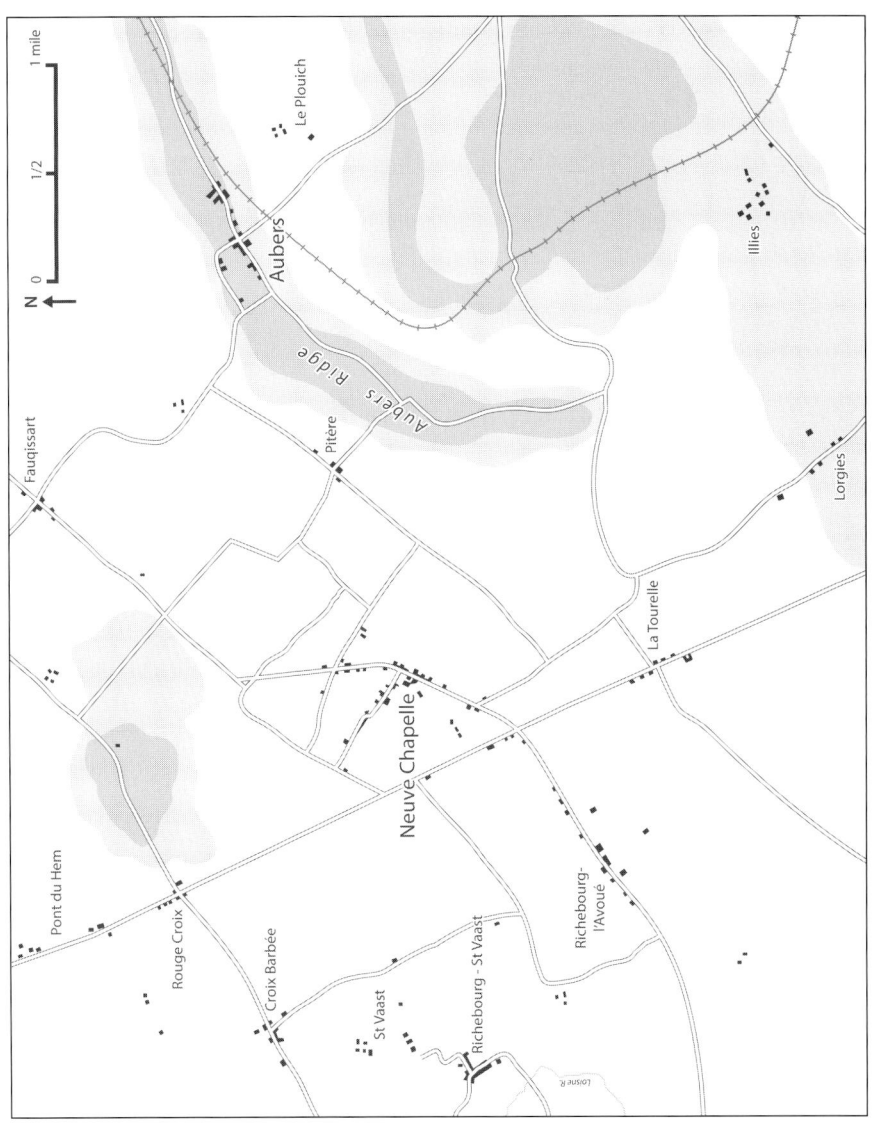

Map 2 Neuve Chapelle. (Map drawn by George Anderson)

and heavy'; he also 'trembled all over'. In this state, he was clearly of no use to his regiment. William was sent behind the front line to the French city of Rouen, where the BEF had established a military hospital – and at Rouen, he continued to suffer from severe heart pains. The attendants also observed strange attacks at night, when his legs and arms trembled for five to 10 minutes – and upon waking up, he was unable to speak and move; he sometimes had several of these attacks in the same night. William was also suffering from severe, constant headaches and complained of a poor vision and 'bug brown patches' that appeared in front of his eyes in strong light. William's mental state did not improve during the month at Rouen – and when he was sent to London to be treated at the National Hospital, it was clear that he was never going to see battle again. Although he recovered from his breakdown, the Queen Square doctors knew that William was not fit for army life; he was one of the first mental casualties of the Battle of Neuve Chapelle.

11 March 1915: the second day of battle

By the end of the first day of battle, the Neuve Chapelle salient – including the village – had been captured and was now in British hands. In order to attempt the recapture of Neuve Chapelle, the Germans sent the 6th Bavarian Reserve Division into the area by train. Although the British Royal Flying Corps had observed the area closely, they failed to spot the German units arriving after dusk. There were now an extra 12,000 enemy soldiers behind the front lines, of which the British were unaware. The new German arrivals were well rested and preparing for action; however, there was very little movement on 11 March. Nevertheless, it was a day of heavy losses on both sides. On that day, Private John W. was awaiting the enemy's attack.[3] John, 23 years older than William, was a strongly-built and experienced soldier, who had already seen action in the Boer War; he had been sent to France with the 2nd Yorkshire Regiment on 14 November 1914. Until the Battle of Neuve Chapelle, he had been both physically and mentally well; however, it took only one shell, which exploded against his trench, to change this. The trench was half-blown in, and all of John's comrades were killed. From then on, John, although physically unscathed, felt shaky, dizzy, frightened and constantly sick; he could not sleep properly and was easily startled; he suffered headaches and bad dreams. When he arrived at Queen Square two months after his breakdown, it was noted that he could not concentrate and that he struggled to remember even basic facts from his life. John's answers to questions were hesitant, as if his mind was preoccupied with something else. He still felt dizzy and frightened; his outstretched hands showed a slight tremor. John was duly diagnosed with 'traumatic neurosis'. Like many of the other traumatised patients at Queen Square, he only needed a few weeks of rest and massages until he made a complete recovery; however, he was still not considered fit for active service and was sent to a convalescent home.

3   QSA: Queen Square Records, Dr Taylor, 1915, male L-Z: case record Private John W.

Stories like John's refute the view of some doctors and military commanders of the time, that shell shock symptoms essentially served the function of getting the soldier out of the dangerous battle zone. If this had been the case, they should have been much more resistant to the relatively gentle therapies that were applied in many cases. They also refute the myth propagated in much of the modern literature that doctors in the hospitals at home saw it as their primary mission to get the soldier back to the front as soon as possible; on the contrary, they were reluctant even to send seemingly recovered patients back to France, because they doubted that they could withstand the renewed stress of battle – and yet, this policy was not widely publicised (certainly not outside specialist medical journals), which makes it unlikely that soldiers malingered shell shock symptoms to ensure permanent release from combat duties.

12 March 1915: the third day of battle

On the morning of 12 March, the German battalions that had remained hidden in the woods and hamlets of the surrounding area moved into position ready for the planned recapture of Neuve Chapelle; a day of fierce fighting with the BEF lay ahead of them. Twenty-two-year-old Private Peter R. from the 1st Battalion of the Seaforth Highlanders was in the midst of battle when a shell burst over his head.[4] Peter was unconscious for about half an hour – and on recovering, found he was deaf and unable to speak. Although 'he could think of the words [he] could not say them'. He felt insecure and did not want to embarrass himself, so he made desperate attempts to speak when no one was listening. It did not take long until it was noticed that something was wrong with him: he was sent back to Britain and arrived at the National Hospital on 20 March 1915. He was still unable to speak, although 'he made a great effort'. Peter felt dazed, frightened and jumpy for some days; he suffered from terrifying dreams at night. Although he was not able to talk about his gruesome experiences at the front line, he was able to write them down in a chronological order, which he did during his rest time on one of the shell shock wards at Queen Square. The neurologist in charge of Peter acknowledged in the notes that Peter had 'a better knowledge of names and places he has been to than the average soldier'.

This is what Peter wrote down:

> I went out to France on the 3.11.14. I was two days at Le Havre. Then we went on to our 1st Batt. When we arrived at our destination the regiment was in the trenches, so we had to go in. It was snowing. I felt it very cold. This was at Givenchy. We were relined the following night and we went back for a rest. The next place we went to was just opposite Neuve Chapelle on the La Bassée road and it was awful. The Trenches were up to the knee in mud and water. The first night was very quiet but the following morning about 9am the Germans

---

4   QSA: Queen Square Records, Dr Batten, 1915, male L-Z: case record Private Peter R.

started shelling and continued all day. The next was the same but about 1 o'clock the Germans were seen to be coming up in masses. They got to within a distance of about 25 yds. Then they turned. They commenced shelling us again and they had another try about 3 o'clock but they did not get far. One of the men on my left had the half of his face blown away and we had about 92 killed and wounded. We got relieved after being in 5 days. Then we went back for 3 days rest. The next place we went to was Rue de l'Efinette and we had an awful time there just before Christmas. We went into the trenches and we were up to our middle in water. In some places it would have taken you over the head. We were in these trenches for 24 hours. There was nothing unusual happening and we got relieved by the Royal North Lancs but we got not far away. We had just got into our billets and were making some tea when we were told that the Germans had broken through the North Lancs. We went into the trenches for another 72 hours. If the Germans had attacked again we could not have fired a shot as we were hardly able to stand for the cold and with the wet kilts on our legs, it was awful. We got nothing to eat except 3 biscuits that some of the men went out and got. When we got out of the trenches at Christmas eve we looked all like old men and a lot of them had to be carried. We went back for a rest to Aumerval about 30 kilometres from the fighting line for a month. When we came back again we went to La Bassée and had a pretty short time there. The next place we were at was at that big fight at Neuve Chapelle when 472 guns bombarded the German trench for 35 minutes at about 7am. The word was passed along that we were to charge the German trench in front supported by the city of Lorduterre. We got the trench all right and I got orders about 4pm to go back to our own trench and bring along the belt-fitting… belonging to the machine gun. There was not a proper ammunition trench. … I was just stepping out of the trench when a shell burst just over my head and I went down. When I came to my senses, I was lying in our support trench where I had been carried by two of the men of the Black watch one of them said something but I could not hear him and I tried to tell him so then I discovered that I could not speak.

Peter had endured all hardship and brutalities at the front line for months before he lost his speech and hearing. His written report demonstrates that he was not confused and quite able to remember what had happened during his active service; he even clearly recalled his actions up to the fateful moment when he stepped out of the trench.

Frederick Walker Mott was particularly interested in soldiers like Peter, who suddenly lost their speech, and he tried to understand why 'these mutes, whose silent thoughts are perfect, [should] be unable to speak? They comprehend all that is said to them unless they are deaf; but it is quite clear that in these cases their internal language is unaffected, for they are able to express their thoughts and judgements perfectly well by writing, even if they are deaf. […] Many who are unable to speak voluntarily yet call out in their dreams expressions they have used in trench warfare and battle.'⁵ Mott emphasised the symbolic meaning of these symptoms, which could not be explained by a direct trauma to the brain. The patient was merely unable to talk about his terrifying experiences; Mott reckoned that there were simply no words for the horrors he had gone through – soldiers were 'dumb with fear'.[6]

The doctors isolated Peter from the other patients at Queen Square, and his speech suddenly returned on the third day in hospital. Like Peter, other soldiers who had gone through unimaginable horrors found it difficult to talk about what they had experienced, and preferred to hand in written accounts. These handwritten reports were often very factual – lacking emotional expression and revealing gruesome facts in a detached, emotionally distant way. Other soldiers had difficulties concentrating, and used handwritten statements to bring order into their thoughts. One of them was 37-year-old regular soldier George D. who, like Peter R., broke down during the third day of the Battle of Neuve Chapelle.[7] When George was in the trenches, a shell exploded near him and he was buried in a mass of brickwork. He was pulled out by the men of his platoon, and when he came to himself after 30 minutes, he carried on with his duties. During the night, his company advanced towards the German trenches and was exposed to heavy shelling. Although George 'was knocked silly and fell', remaining unconscious for a little while, his commanding officer told him to take the men forward. He carried out this order, heard another explosion and was blown back into the trench. George found himself in the trench with a number of wounded comrades, and a man who had lost his sight was on top of him. Even after this attack, he still carried on with his platoon. After the explosion of another shell, he collapsed again and was finally taken to hospital near Armentières – complaining of severe pain in both legs 'like tooth ache from the toes to the knees'. He was taken to a base hospital in Boulogne, where he complained of an intense pain and inability to move his right foot. The military doctors were out of their depth, and George was shipped to England; this was the beginning of a long odyssey through a dozen military hospitals.

George described his painful journey through the British medical system in a handwritten statement, which was attached to the Queen Square Records:

> Sir, I write this statement because I do not seem to be able to concentrate my mind on questions very quick when they are asked. I was discharged [from] the army December 1916 with 15 years' service. The cause of discharge [was] shell shock and deformed right foot. In July 1917 I was sent for to be examined by a Board of Medical Officers. I was ordered further treatment and sent to Military Hospital Richmond. The Doctors there had my foot X-rayed and decided that I should be treated at the Orthopaedic Shepherd's Bush. I was transferred and

---

5   Mott, *War Neuroses and Shell Shock*, p.99.
6   Mott, *War Neuroses and Shell Shock*, p.121.
7   QSA: Queen Square Records, Dr Buzzard, 1917, male and female A-K: Case record George D.

after being examined by 3 surgeons it was decided that my foot was caused by Spasmodic Inversion. Colonel Aeland? (Aitken) came and examined me and he decided to get me a bed here. While under examination I get excited, very often making me tremble. Street noises such as, back fires of cycles, motors, make me jump and send a queer sensation to the head, this brings on pains in the head. My sleep at night is continually broken by sensational dreams.

This makes 10 hospitals in England. At King's College I received Radiant Heat and Massage. At all other Hospitals, Massage. The Hospital from where I was discharged, Fort Pitt Chatham gave me 6 weeks Baines Diselectric Oil Treatment.

George's examination on admission to Queen Square in November 1917 showed that his right foot was still paralysed. George walked on the outside of the right foot – the inside of the foot being turned up. When doctors tried to move his right foot, George turned his head in the opposite direction and wrinkled his face as if suffering great pain. When George himself attempted to move his foot, violent spasms developed: first of the foot, then of the leg, then of the whole body. The hospital notes do not specify the kind of treatment George received at the National Hospital; because George was treated by Lewis Ralph Yealland, the most likely treatment would have been electrotherapy – the application of electric currents to the paralysed foot (see Chapter 12). At the end of this intervention, George was reportedly cured. His journey through the British medical system had lasted two and three-quarter years, from his breakdown in Neuve Chapelle on 12 March 1915 until his discharge from Queen Square on 1 December 1917.

13 March 1915: the fourth day of battle

Many men had lost their lives; others were physical or nervous wrecks after three days of fierce fighting. The 13th of March 1915, the fourth and final day of the Battle of Neuve Chapelle, would mean the end of fighting for many more men who could not stand the pressures of warfare.

One of them was Private Herbert M. of the 4th Battalion of the Suffolk Regiment – a slim man with a long, small face, blue eyes and a light brown moustache.[8] At 34, he had already lost all his teeth. Born and bred in Nottingham, Herbert had left school at the age of 13 – and he soon went to work in the Brough motorcycle factory. Founded in 1899 by William Brough, the factory became well known for its pioneering engine technology – and William's son, George Brough, went on to design a range of high-performance motorbikes that were popular with the great and good (amongst them Thomas Edward Lawrence 'of Arabia', who died riding one of them in 1935).

---

8   QSA: Queen Square Records, Dr Collier, 1916, male and female L-Z: case record Private Herbert M.

Herbert had joined the Territorial Army and was duly mobilised when war was declared. He had to leave his wife and three children – aged 10, eight and seven – behind when he was sent to the Western Front.

At Neuve Chapelle, on 13 March 1915, he was

> … in a bayonet charge, 500 yards from the German trenches, when he was struck by a bullet. He swung round and fell on his back, he felt for the injured arm but could not find it, it was twisted round his back, the feeling had gone. In the course of a few minutes he had a "funny feeling" shooting up the arm "as if the funny bone has been hit." He was pulled back into the trenches, sent to the Dressing Station and then sent to Boulogne, after which he was sent to England… .

Herbert was treated at the First Southern General Hospital in Birmingham for four months. Because he did not regain the power of his left arm, he was eventually discharged from active service and offered a position in a lavatory at Dunstable in Bedfordshire. In May 1916, he had to attend a Medical Board for re-examination and assessment of his military fitness; at this time, Herbert still had no use of his left arm – and he even wanted it to be amputated because he was so upset about this useless limb. The Medical Board did not respond to his request and sent him for further treatment to Hampstead and King's College Hospitals. Treatment failed again, and a referral to the National Hospital seemed the last resort. The Queen Square neurologists did not find any plausible physical explanation for Herbert's paralysis: he had normal reflexes and normal electrical reactions of his nerves and muscles. This clearly pointed towards a functional disorder – shell shock. 'After a little suggestive treatment and electricity', Herbert regained the use of his arm and shoulder.

William, John, Peter, George and Herbert were among thousands of British soldiers who broke down during the Battle of Neuve Chapelle – and their outlook may have been less triumphant than that of the British press, which celebrated the outcome of the battle.

On 19 April 1915, *The Times* reported:

> For the first time the British Army has broken the German line and struck the Germans a blow which they will remember to the end of their lives. The importance of our success does not lie so much in the capture of the German trenches along a front of two miles, a killing of some 6,000 Germans and the taking of 2,000 prisoners. It is the revelation of the fact that the much-vaunted German army-machine on which the whole attention of a mighty nation has been lavished for four decades is not invincible.[9]

---

9   *The Times*, 19 April 1915.

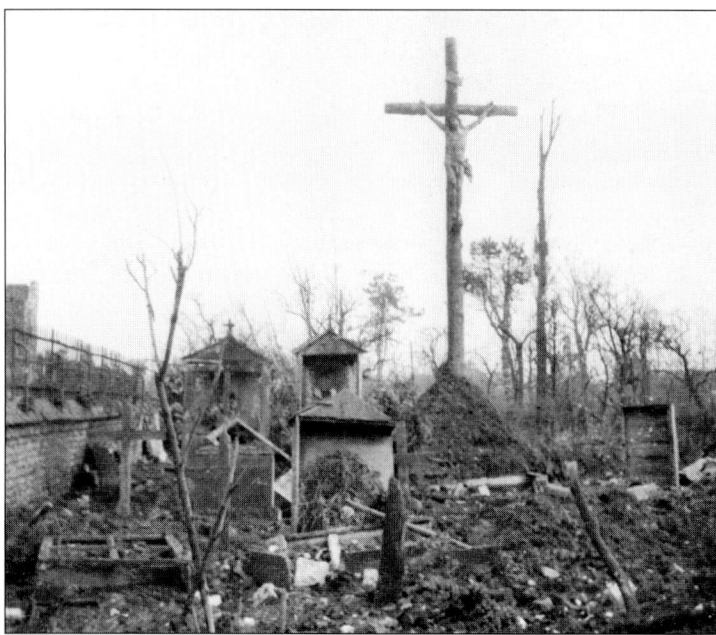

The churchyard, Neuve Chapelle; photograph taken during the battle, 10 March 1915. Note the crucifix standing after the heavy bombardment; Q 56178. (Imperial War Museum, London)

The *Evening Express* struck a slightly more sombre tone in its reporting on the British successes in and around Neuve Chapelle: 'The ground west of this now shattered town, from which the British drove the Germans in the middle of March with such terrible loss of life on both sides, is literally cobbled with German skulls. [...] The scene can best be likened to the site of a western American town razed by a cyclone'.[10] The churchyard, in the heart of the previously idyllic village, bore testimony to the havoc wrought by the endless shell fire: 'Here, the very dead have been uprooted only to be buried again under masonry which has fallen from the church, and crosses from the heads of the tombs be scattered in all directions. The sole thing in the cemetery that has escaped damage is a wooden crucifix still erect amid the medley of overturned graves'.[11]

In four days of fighting, about 12,000 British men were killed, wounded or went missing; German casualties were estimated at a similar figure of 12,000, which included 1,687 prisoners.[12] The British gain of territory – largely, burnt soil – was approximately one square mile.

10 'In and around Neuve Chapelle, Death and Destruction: Ground littered with German skulls' – *Evening Express*, 19 April 1915.
11 'Havoc by Shell Fire Stricken village of Neuve Chapelle, Solitary Crucifix' – *Aberdeen Journal*, 29 March 1915.
12 <http://www.1914-1918.net/bat9.htm> accessed 15 February 2014.

Neuve Chapelle and Hill 60 93

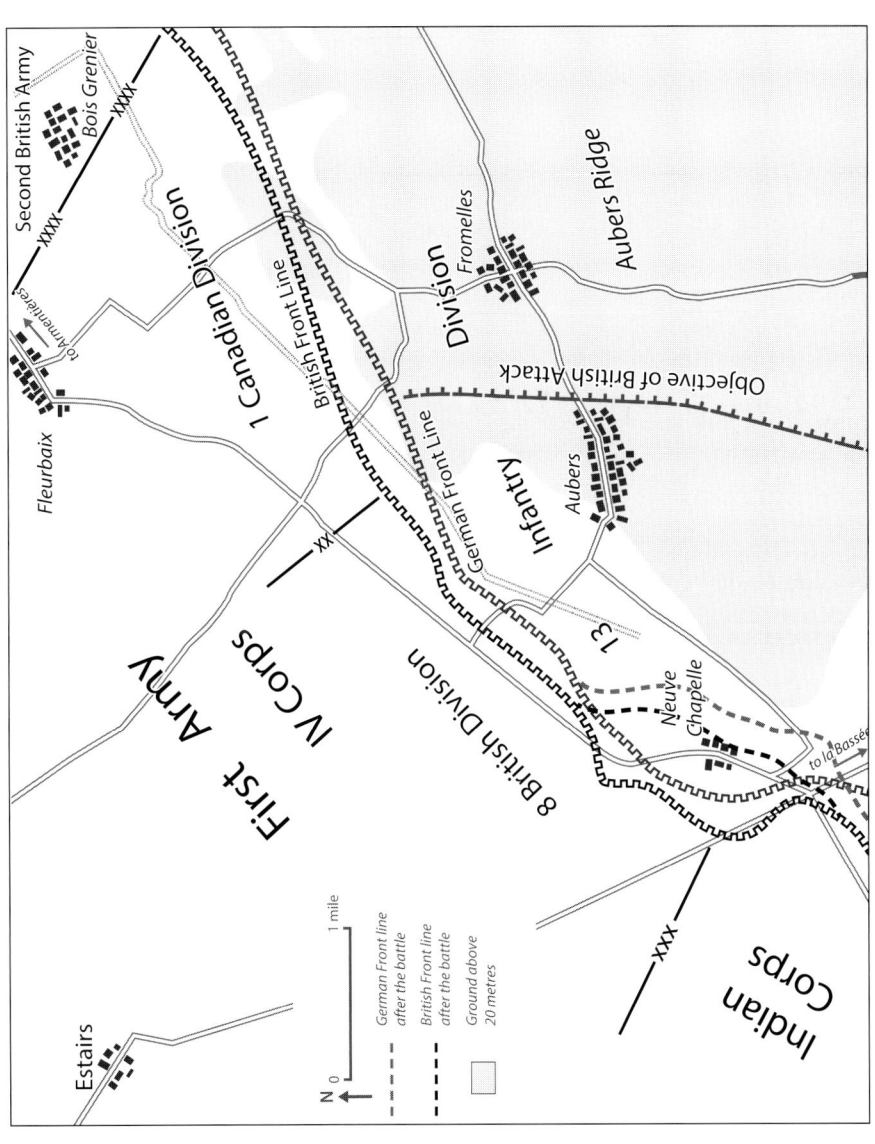

Map 3 'The Battle of Neuve Chapelle, March 10–12, 1915, trench line before and after the battle' (Map drawn by George Anderson)

Officers and common soldiers

'In the midst of death and destruction, in one of the dug-outs, a group of British soldiers carried on as usual. "Excellent tea was passed round, for the British soldier, and especially the officer, wants tea in the firing line just as much as at home."'[13] This was the atmosphere after the Battle of Neuve Chapelle captured by the British press.

William, John, Peter, George and Herbert were far from carrying on as usual: we have heard their voices, or read their personal accounts; followed their movements throughout the battle, and have seen how the trauma of war took over their minds and disabled their bodies. With their paralysed arms and legs, trembling, loss of speech and hearing, nightmares, pains and anxiety attacks, they had to be removed from the theatre of war; however, William and the others were soldiers of lower ranks. Was it true that their superiors, who were generally members of the officer caste, with a middle- or upper-class background, were less affected by the pressure of warfare? Were they less prone to break down, and did mental breakdown manifest in different ways compared to the lower ranks?

Surprisingly, this issue was never discussed in very much detail in the contemporary and post-war medical press. Psychiatrists and neurologists of the time simply declared that hysterical symptoms such as functional paralyses, trembling and shaking, functional seizures and gait disorders were almost entirely confined to privates and non-commissioned officers.[14] The unconscious conversion of ideas into physical symptoms was said to be the common way for lower ranks to react to the unbearable pressures of war; conversely, officers were described as suffering from more subtle symptoms, such as anxiety, exhaustion, pain, palpitations and digestive problems. These symptoms were commonly subsumed under the heading of 'neurasthenia', or 'anxiety-neurosis'. Neurasthenia was presumed to be caused by extraordinary hardship – leading to physical and mental exhaustion. Contemporary doctors agreed that constitutional factors (inborn weaknesses) did not play a major role in the development of neurasthenia – and this way of thinking fitted into contemporary stereotypes of constitutionally strong upper classes and weaker lower classes. Soldiers of lower ranks and lower status in society were to blame for their mental breakdown; the same rules did not apply to well-bred patients. Myers remarked that although 'the forces of education, tradition and example make for greater self-control in the case of the Officer, the overwhelming burden of responsibility inevitably [leads] into his breakdown'.[15] Indeed, historian Peter

---

13 'Havoc by Shell Fire' – *Aberdeen Journal*, 29 March 1915.
14 For example: MacCurdy, *War Neuroses*, p.87: 'These cases [of conversion hysteria] are confined almost entirely to privates and non-commissioned officers. ....'; also Mott, *War Neuroses and Shell Shock*, p.139: 'In non-commissioned officers and men hysteria is common' [as opposed to anxiety neuroses in officers]; Myers, *Shell Shock in France*, p.40: 'The symptoms exhibited by Officers are predominantly of the neurasthenic type, whereas those exhibited by the men are predominantly of the hysteric type'.
15 Myers, *Shell Shock in France*, p.40.

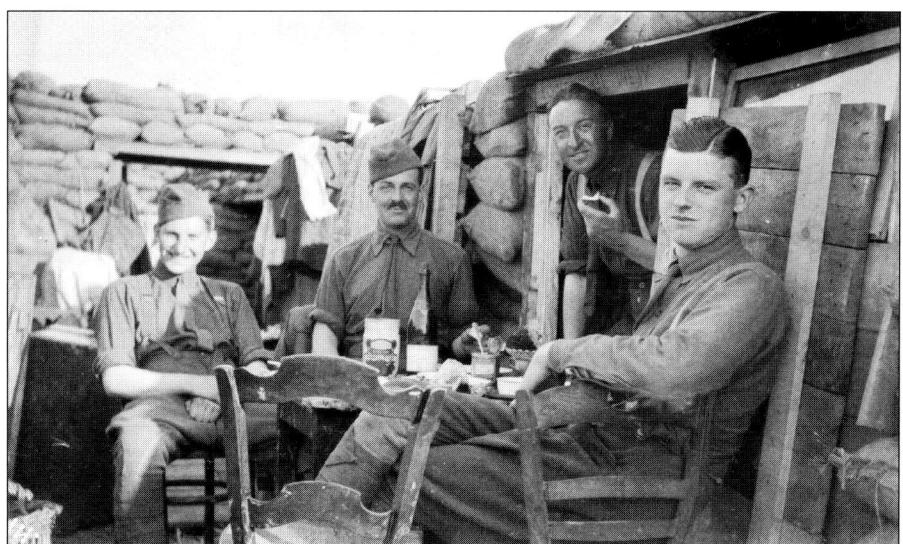

Officers of 'C' Company, 1st Battalion, Cameronians (Scottish Rifles) taking a tea break in the trenches at Grande Flamengrie Farm – on the Bois Grenier sector of the line – in May 1915; Q_51632. (Imperial War Museum, London)

Leese found evidence in officers' medical records – of which not many have survived until today – that little emphasis was placed on hereditary explanations; conversely, 'the use of an hereditary diagnosis for cases in the other ranks was [...] a matter of conventional medical interpretation'.[16] Treatment approaches also reflected this conventional view: officers were 'treated more than disciplined; viewed with sympathy more than suspicion'.[17] Craiglockhart – one of the most important treatment centres for shell-shocked officers during the First World War, and the largest ever established – offered gymnastics, musical and theatrical entertainment, poetry, outdoor activities and memory training to its privileged inmates. Siegfried Sassoon's description of 'Slateford War Hospital' in *Sherston's Progress* – the thinly disguised autobiographical account of his encounters with Rivers at Craiglockhart – provides some insight into the combination of sports, cultural recreation and conversational therapy that was typical of such institutions.[18] 'Where the other ranks did farm work or carpentry, officers at Craiglockhart were allowed therapeutic hobbies, and it is at this point that the officer's hospital experience begins to resemble an extended retreat at a country house';[19] equally,

---

16 Leese, Peter, *Shell Shock: Traumatic Neurosis and the British Soldiers of the First World War* (New York: Palgrave, 2002), pp.108-110.
17 Leese, *Shell Shock*, p.103.
18 Sassoon, Siegfried, *Sherston's Progress* (London: Faber and Faber, 1936).
19 Leese, *Shell Shock*, pp.104-106.

treatment of the lower ranks focused more on discipline, education and reinforcement, as we will learn in Chapter 12 – thus, there is much evidence to support the view that officers enjoyed a different treatment, as compared to the lower ranks. However, to date, there is no clear evidence that officers' symptoms actually differed from those exhibited by their men.

Although the National Hospital was not a primary treatment centre for officers, soldiers of higher ranks were referred to Queen Square whenever a specialist neurological opinion was needed: one of them was 41-year-old Captain Ronald C. of the Suffolk Regiment, who – like the soldiers encountered above – broke down during the Neuve Chapelle offensive in March 1915.[20] What distinguished his case from that of his subordinate, Herbert M., and the other lower-ranking soldiers? Did he present in a different way; did doctors find a different explanation for his symptoms, and was he treated differently? Reading the notes, it becomes evident that in trying to explain the captain's breakdown, doctors indeed put less emphasis on hereditary explanations than in most of their lower-ranking patients. Even Dr Francis Walshe, who was known for this uncompromising stance and harsh treatment of shell-shocked soldiers, emphasised Ronald's strong constitution. Ronald had always been in 'perfect health' – and there was no family history of mental or somatic problems; his parents, seven brothers and one sister were all well and in good spirits. Ronald had 'roughed it in all climes and ha[d] enjoyed unusually good health'. Before the war, he had returned from West Africa; there is, however, a short note about a previous admission to the National Hospital nine years before, 'with sulphonal habit' – an overuse of sleeping remedies.

If Ronald's constitution was not to blame for his breakdown, what had happened to him on the battlefield of Neuve Chapelle? Ronald had been in France since October 1914 as adjutant of a territorial regiment – and being the only regular officer attached to the battalion, 'he had had much work and worry', and for some weeks before his injury, 'had felt that his energy was diminishing, and that he was "getting used up"'. At times he could scarcely pull himself together to carry out his duties'. Like in many of his subordinates, his mental breakdown was triggered by a shell explosion. Although he did not obtain any visible injuries, Ronald was rendered unconscious for about half an hour. When he regained consciousness, he felt 'very dazed', but carried on until the next morning, when he suffered two wounds in the right arm in quick succession. He managed to walk for three miles to the next clearing station, where he received an injection. Of the subsequent events, he did not remember anything until he awoke three days later in hospital at Grosvenor Gardens in London.

In the hospital record, his progress is described as follows:

> His arm was fractured and the surgical aspect of his condition has progressed favourably since, but he complains of constant severe dull headache at the back of

20   QSA: Queen Square Records, Dr Russell, 1915, male A-K: case record Captain Ronald C.

the head, which varies in intensity from time to time, but is always present. When severe this makes him very drowsy and he sleeps for hours without waking. In other respects he feels well, but still used up and not fit to return to the front yet. He has no appetite, and dreams constantly of his recent experiences. Sleeps deeply and cannot be roused to eat or urinate. At other times normal, especially when wife is present. Cannot be found to take any drugs. Has had to be catheterised at times, as bladder has been distended, and has alas been nasally fed. Is losing weight. Surgically is almost well.

When Ronald was admitted to the National Hospital on 10 April, he was a shadow of his former self; the doctors described a pale, thin and 'listless looking man':

He lies in bed on his back with both eyes partly closed. On inspection the lids are seen to be in a constant fine tremor, and are never quite closed. When suddenly touched they tighten and there is slight, but definite resistance to opening them. When this is done the globes at once roll up covering the cornea completely. This always happens. While this is being done pt. makes no sign of being awake or in any way aware of observer's presence. Suddenly he awakes dramatically looks around in a dazed manner, rubs his eyes and fixing observer with his gaze, asks, 'who are you'. He then looks around like one awaking in a strange place.

Dr Walshe, the responsible junior doctor, found Ronald's 'whole performance [...] very theatrical' and suspected simulation. Ronald's strange behaviour, and the need to catheterise his bladder and feed him through a nasal tube, did not seem to fit into the stereotype of nervous exhaustion in officers; the captain may have sensed this antagonistic attitude towards him – and he did not feel the need to stay in hospital for very much longer. Perhaps he did not feel comfortable as a patient, or as an officer among ordinary soldiers; he left hospital at his own request after two days. Dr Walshe concluded that 'once waked he is in every respect a normal individual, talks well and intelligently and shows no amnesia, or other mental defect. In fact beyond a natural 'worn-outness' quite comprehensible in view of his seven months at the front, he is an ordinary individual'.

Officers undoubtedly carried a heavy burden: they were responsible for their men and were expected to be role models. It is well documented that casualty figures were even higher for British officers (17 percent killed) than for ordinary soldiers (12 percent killed) of the First World War.[21] Subalterns – low-ranking (non-commissioned) officers – were even more vulnerable to mental breakdown than commissioned officers, and also than the other ranks, because they acted 'as leaders in the field and were both responsible to higher-ranking officers as well as working closely with men

---

21   <http://www.nationalarchives.gov.uk/education/greatwar/g4/cs1/background.htm> accessed 6 June 2014.

under their own immediate command'.²² This conflict is illustrated by the case of Sergeant Norman H. of the 1st Battalion of the Nottinghamshire and Derbyshire Regiment.²³ He had joined the army in November 1911, aged 18. His regiment left England early in October 1914 – landing in France on 5 November 1914 – and Norman first went into action on 13 November 1914. At Neuve Chapelle, many of his men and every single officer of his battalion were killed. Norman had only obtained a slight scalp wound, for which no intervention was needed – and although he was badly shaken, he carried on for another year. Norman clearly felt responsible for his comrades and was prepared to risk his life for his men: in December 1915 – when at Bois Grenier – he gained the DCM (Distinguished Conduct Medal) for throwing back a trench mortar shell which was about to explode; at Souchez on 24 May 1916, he was buried by a mine explosion, but managed to dig himself out and rescue one of his comrades by carrying him back to safety, for which he later gained a clasp to his DCM. After returning to the trenches, Norman was exposed to another shell explosion. He was only buried for about five minutes when he was dug out by two of his men and taken to a reserve trench. Although he suffered a slight fainting attack, he carried on with his duty; two days later, however, Norman collapsed and had his first fit. At the 2nd Canadian Casualty Clearing Station, he had more fits, which were witnessed by the medical officer, Captain Maywood. Maywood ruled out genuine epilepsy because Norman's fits did not include the typical repetitive (clonic) limb movements of epileptic seizures, and he did not turn blue (cyanosis) during the fit: 'In my opinion a diagnosis of epilepsy is doubtful. He had a more or less typical tonic spasm of epilepsy, but the clonic spasm and cyanosis were not present'.

On 21 June, Norman was transferred to the 1st Canadian Hospital at Étaples, where he only remained for one night. The following day, he was sent to Calais, from where he embarked on a ship to England to be transferred to Queen Square. At the National Hospital, he continued to have fits. Apart from these fits, general exhaustion and nightmares about the war, Norman came across as 'a bright, intelligent youth with a cheerful disposition, not in the least distressed or worried' – and his repeated 'attempts at a fit – obviously functional' were not taken seriously. Norman was also observed 'practising a hemiplegic gait'. The young sergeant must have been relieved when he was finally discharged and recommended for furlough and light duty.

---

22   Leese, *Shell Shock*, pp.43, 109.
23   QSA: Queen Square Records, Dr Russell, 1916, male A-K: case record Sergeant Norman H.

The Battle of Hill 60

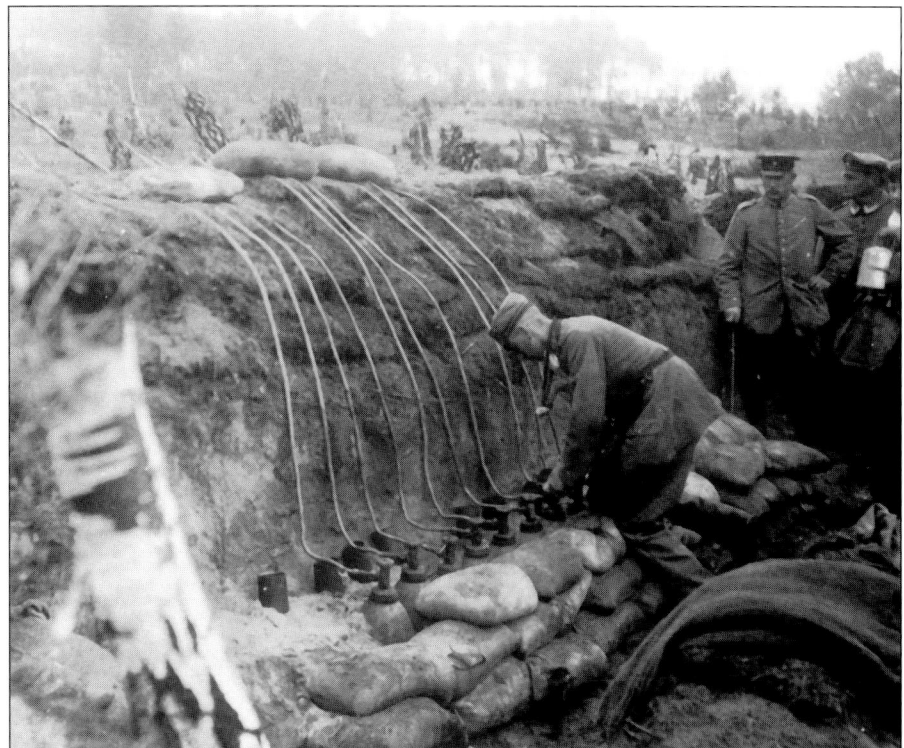

A German battery of chlorine gas cylinders being prepared for an attack, and awaiting the right weather conditions to prevent blowback, similar to the arrangement at Hill 60 in May 1915; open domain. (Private collection)

Gas and glory

> ... If you could hear, at every jolt, the blood
> Come gargling from the froth-corrupted lungs,
> Obscene as cancer, bitter as the cud
> Of vile, incurable sores on innocent tongues,—
> My friend, you would not tell with such high zest
> To children ardent for some desperate glory,
> The old Lie: *Dulce et Decorum est*
> *Pro patria mori.*[24]

---

24 Owen, Wilfred, 'Dulce et Decorum est' – *The Poems of Wilfred Owen* (St Ives: Wordsworth Classics, 1994).

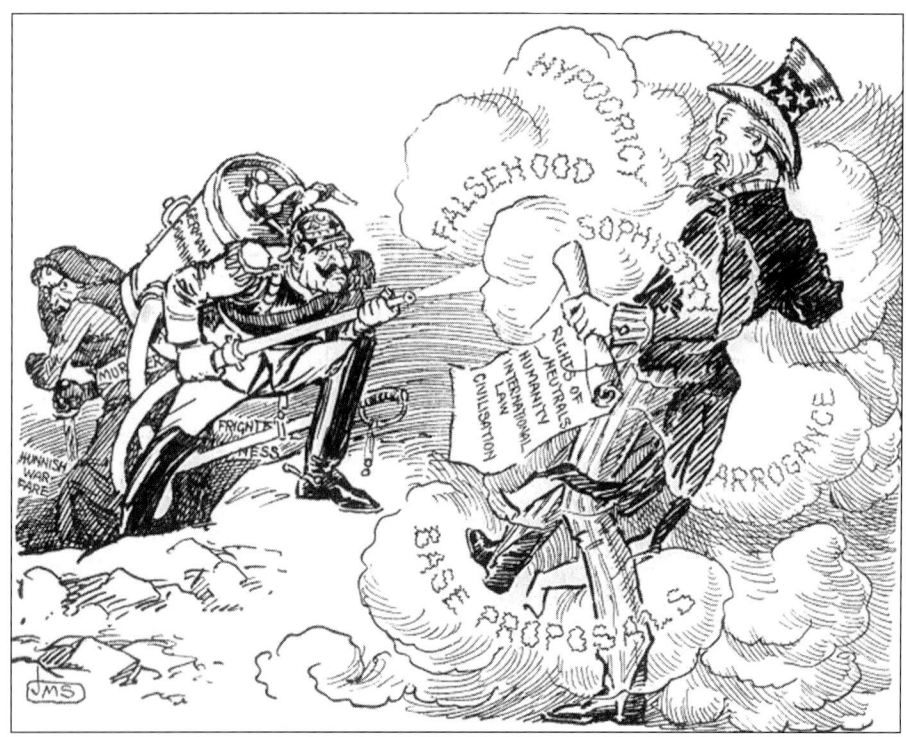

'A Whiff of the Kaiser's Gas' – *Western Mail*, 13 July 1915: '… it was the use of gas by the Germans in the Second Battle of Ypres, which began on 22 April 1915 that caused the greatest condemnation. It went against the 1907 Hague Convention on Land Warfare, which prohibited the use of "poison or poisoned weapons"'; cartoon by Joseph Morewood Staniforth, Cartooning the First World War Project. (Cardiff University)

The use of chemical weapons from April 1915 introduced a new dimension of threat to trench warfare, as stated in an opinion piece in the contemporaneous press: 'We know now that Germany is bound by no principle, no agreement of any sort of kind; that she is actuated by a spirit of savagery, which, if not utterly crushed, will strike at the very root of European civilization; that this is no longer merely a national war, but a struggle of civilisation against barbarism'.[25]

The first gas attacks completely surprised the BEF, and thousands of its soldiers – without any protection – became the helpless victims of the cruel inventiveness of the German chemical industry. It took some time until effective gas masks were available in sufficient quantities – affording some protection against the destruction of the skin, mucous membranes, lungs and digestive system that was described in graphic

25 'Gas on Hill 60' – *Western Gazette*, 14 May 1915.

detail by Wilfred Owen in his 1917 poem; yet, gas also had an enduring psychological effect on soldiers: psychological symptoms often mimicked those of mild exposure to gas, but could also be dominated by anxiety, fears, sleep disturbances, dizziness and tremor.[26] These symptoms could be found in several Queen Square soldiers who had been exposed to gas, and who later described its devastating effects in much detail: one of them was Harry M., a 24-year-old lance corporal with the 2nd Battalion of the Seaforth Highlanders, who was the victim of a German gas attack at Hill 60 (near Ypres) on 5 May 1915.[27] On that day, 'at about 9 am clouds of gas were suddenly issued from the German trenches at Hill 60, evidently ejected under great pressure, for they travelled at once to a considerable distance, though the wind was not strong'.[28]

Harry, not prepared for this attack, described the dramatic physical effects of the chemicals:

> At first the gases caused a severe smarting sensation in the eyes, then irritated the mucous membranes of respiratory tract, causing severe sneezing and coughing. This was followed by severe difficulty in breathing. He made violent efforts to inhale, at the same time there was a feeling of intense and painful irritation in the abdomen, causing sickness, violent retching and severe tenderness so that he felt as though his abdominal organs were being torn from him. Drinking water made the symptoms worse. He got most relief by holding the trunk erect. He noticed that the patients who moved about got most relief.

However, unlike the masses of Allied soldiers who had been caught by complete surprise and immediately died during the earlier German gas attacks, Harry managed to survive. He was taken to a British base in Boulogne on the next day, and sent on to Rouen on 12 May. About a week later, 'he began to feel free from the effects of the gas poisoning'; however, he developed other symptoms that could not easily be attributed to the gas effects – attacks of giddiness, during which all his limbs were shaking. He also felt generally weak and 'had no ambition to do anything; in fact, he could not bring himself to any sustained effort'. His sleep was poor; he was sent back home and arrived at the National Hospital on 6 June 1915.

The doctors in London – consultant neurologist Dr Tooth and house physician Dr Walshe – treated him with 'high frequency back and head daily', which was a standard method of the time involving electrical stimulation of the skin and muscles. His symptoms improved and after a month at the hospital, he was discharged; however, he was not sent back to the front line, but recommended for home service.

26 Jones, Edgar, Everitt, Brian, Ironside, Stephen, Palmer, Ian and Wessely, Simon, 'Psychological Effects of Chemical Weapons: A Follow-up Study of First World War Veterans' – *Psychological Medicine*, 38:10 (2008), pp.1,419-1,426.
27 QSA: Queen Square Records, Dr Tooth, 1915, male L-Z: case record Lance Corporal Harry M.
28 'Gas on Hill 60' – *Western Gazette*, 14 May 1915.

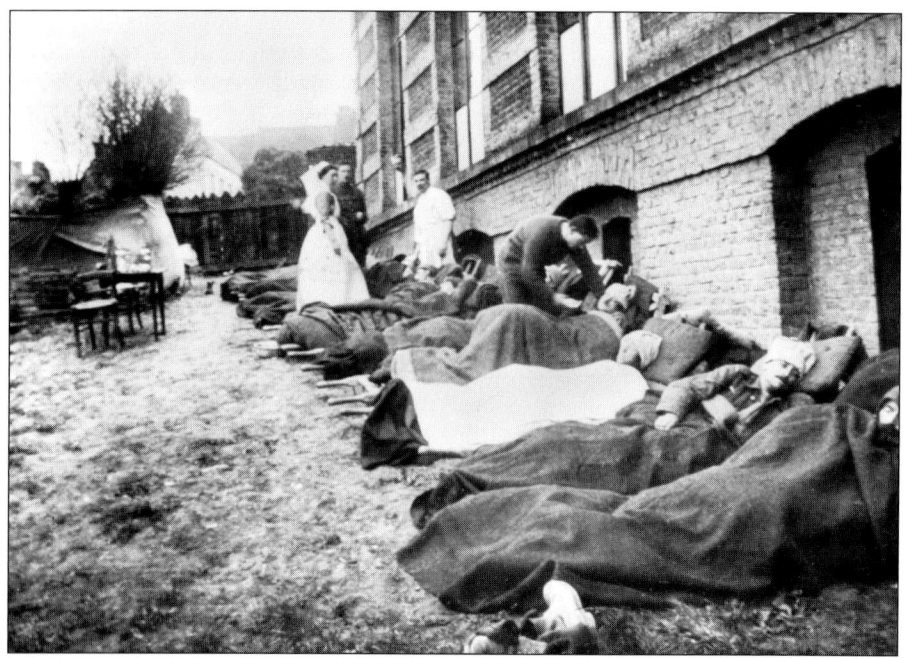

British casualties of the gas attack on Hill 60 receiving treatment at No.8 Casualty Clearing Station, Bailleul; Q 114867. (Imperial War Museum, London)

The doctors had determined that he had suffered nervous breakdowns already before the gas attacks, and therefore probably would not cope with the stress of further military action. They had also taken a detailed personal history and established that Harry had already found it difficult to cope with the mental strain during two years as a commercial representative in Burma – during which he had also suffered dengue fever. His mother, who had died at the age of 45 from a stomach ulcer, had been very 'excitable'. 'Of superior intelligence', he had been an 'unruly' child; his maternal grandfather 'was said to be queer'. During his frontline service, before being gassed, Harry had suffered from episodes of severe shaking, which interfered with rifle firing. This lenient disposal, at a time of extreme strain on British military resources, is all the more remarkable because the doctors clearly suspected Harry M. of malingering.

Like Harry M., Joseph B. was among those men who had been badly shaken by some of the first gas attacks in the First World War.[29] The 28-year-old private from the North Staffordshire Regiment had joined the army at the very beginning of the war, and was sent to France on 4 March 1915; he went into action soon thereafter.

29   QSA: Queen Square Records, Dr Russell, 1916, male A-K: case record Private Joseph B.

The experience of being gassed at Hill 60 deeply upset him and:

> ... he has not felt himself since – he felt depressed and absolutely terrified. He could hardly make himself understood he stuttered so badly, and he shook all over and became very hysterical. He was sent down to H.Q. and given light duty at a Quartermasters office. However, he remained very shaky and was sent down to a base in a few days with others and put in hospital.

When he was admitted to the National Hospital on 15 August 1915, he still had a 'marked stammer accompanied by facial grimacing when he attempted to speak'. All his movements were described as 'feeble and tremulous, and easily fatigued'. Joseph, 'thin, anaemic and delicate–looking [...], in a state of pitiful apprehension', came across as:

> ... a thoroughly frightened and unnerved man. He is very emotional and quite 'strung-up.' The least unexpected sound or cutaneous stimulus gives rise to a grotesque motor and emotional reaction. When tested for sensibility to pinprick he starts violently at each prick, even when he sees it coming. With his increasing emotion his stammer becomes worse and he shakes all over and his eyes fill with tears.

Joseph was so nervous and restless that he was prescribed high doses of sedatives – among them bromides, chloroform and barbiturates. He eventually calmed down, but his stammer and tremor persisted; he was recommended for furlough and home service.

Soldiers who had been confronted with the first gas attacks were deeply traumatised and unsettled – and the mere anticipation of further, similar attacks filled them with horror and crippled them with fear. There was no way of getting used to the gas, as illustrated by the case of Private Frederick R. of the Bedford Regiment:[30] a young man of 19, Frederick was taken by surprise by one of the first attacks involving the use of chemical weapons. He survived several gas attacks unscathed. However, one morning at Hill 60, he was attacking the enemy 'through a cloud of gas'; this time, he lost consciousness and – as he fell – his right leg was pierced by two bullets. It seems that he remained unconscious on the field for four days. When he regained consciousness, he could feel the after-effects of the gas: he was coughing badly; whenever he ate, he tasted the sulphurous fumes of the gas. He also suffered from severe shooting pains in his head, which came on in frequent attacks – lasting a few minutes and occurring about every half hour. Although the wounds took only six weeks to heal completely, he had not been able to straighten the knee to walk properly since the day of the gas attack. When standing, he held the leg rotated out and bent at the knee,

---

30 QSA: Queen Square Records, Dr Tooth, 1915, male L-Z: case record Private Frederick R.

and limped grotesquely, with bent leg and inverted foot. Frederick also suffered from uncontrolled twitching of his eyelids and grimacing when the wounded leg was accidentally touched.

The Queen Square doctors were able to fix Frederick's leg with 'strong moral persuasion' and the application of strong electric currents, exercises and massages – and it did not take long for him to walk 'almost normally' and lose his facial tics. The marks the trauma of war had left on his body had vanished; yet, the terrifying experience of the first gas attacks in the history of modern warfare had forever ended his military career. It was clear that like the traumatised soldiers of Neuve Chapelle, he would never be able to face battle again.

The Battles of Neuve Chapelle and Hill 60 left many soldiers with nightmares and terrifying memories of the extreme danger to their own lives and the gruesome events they had witnessed. Nobody was sheltered from these experiences, and officers were affected by trauma in the same way as their men. The clearing stations and field hospitals were overwhelmed by the challenges posed by the complex neurological symptoms – and for some of the soldiers, Neuve Chapelle and Hill 60 were the start of a protracted journey through numerous military hospitals before they finally received their specialist neurological treatment in the heart of London. The fate of most of them changed dramatically once they had arrived at the National Hospital – and some of the treatment descriptions, in fact, sound like miracle cures: soldiers who had been paralysed for months suddenly regained control of their limbs; soldiers who had entered the hospital on crutches, briskly walked out after just a few days. What exactly happened to them at Queen Square – and whether these cures are credible – will be the focus of Chapter 12.

6

20 May 1917: One Day on the Shell Shock Ward

Sunday, 20 May 1917: the National Hospital at Queen Square operated at full capacity, and beyond; every single bed in the hospital was occupied. The war had enforced many changes in the infrastructure of the world-renowned neurological hospital: four wards accommodated physically and psychologically wounded soldiers, and two adjoining houses at Queen Square had also been made available for the ever-increasing numbers of military admissions. Because so many severely injured and shell-shocked patients lived on the wards for weeks or months, the waiting list for civilian patients grew longer every day – and even seriously ill patients had to be rejected.[1]

The war had affected the hospital in several more ways: the hospital buildings themselves had been targeted by the German war machine.

On Wednesday, 8 September 1915:

> … about 10.45 pm […] a German 'Zeppelin' airship [had] dropped an explosive bomb in Queen Square about 30 yards west of the South West Corner of the National Hospital. The bomb exploded in the gardens of the Square and portions of it and other objects disturbed by the explosion hit the Hospital. […] Many windows were broken by the concussion.

Several inpatients – well-off ladies with hysterical paralyses, who had been bedridden – rushed from their beds and were later found scattered through the hospital.[2] The bombing came just a month after the hospital's Board of Management had resolved to insure the hospital against aircraft risks.

Finally, the war had caused a serious staffing crisis: several consultants had offered their service to the War Office and were absent from the National Hospital. On 10 February 1917, the post of 'Junior House Physician, Salary £150 per annum, with

---

1 Queen Square Archives: minutes from the Board of Management meeting, 9 February 1915.
2 Holmes, *The National Hospital*, p.58.

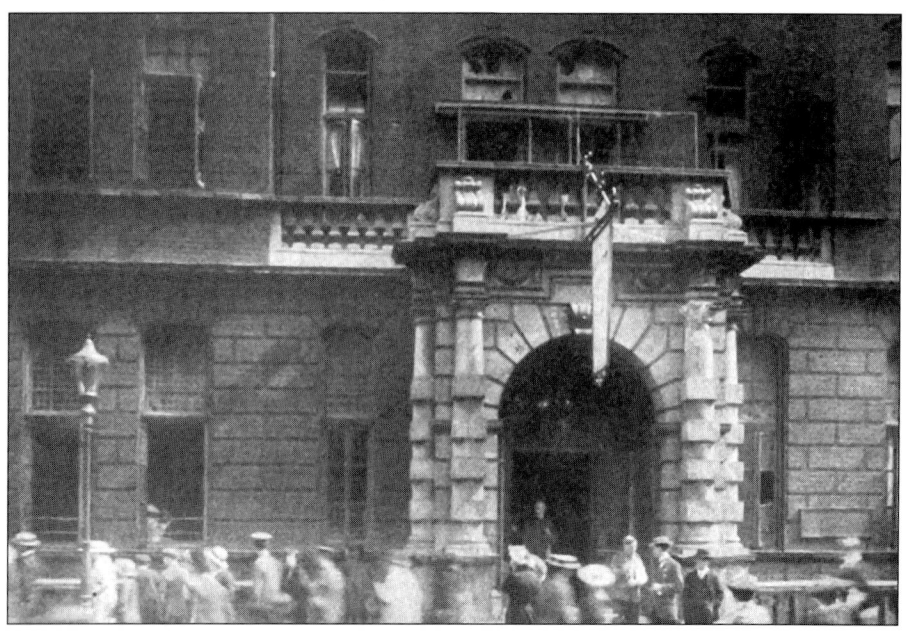

The National Hospital on 8 September 1915 after the Zeppelin raid; photograph, QSA/15429. (Queen Square Archives, London)

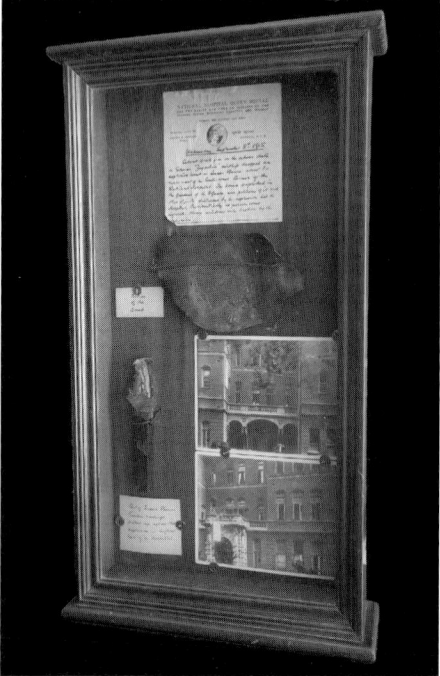

A Zeppelin bomb damage display, with a cabinet containing evidence of bomb damage in Queen Square from a Zeppelin raid in September 1915. It includes a note describing the event, photos, part of a garden railing and a fragment of the bomb; QSA/15424. (Queen Square Archives, London)

board, &c.' was advertised in *The Lancet* – one of the leading medical journals. It was of the highest priority that this post should be filled with one of the most gifted junior doctors – preferably with experience in the field of military medicine. The secretary of the National Hospital did not have to wait for long until he received the application of a promising young doctor.

Thirty-year-old Temporary Captain Clive Farranridge, who in early 1915, had come all the way from Sydney to volunteer for the Royal Army Medical Corps, was offering his services to the National Hospital. He had been with the 8th Battalion of the Gloucestershire Regiment, worked in the 8th General Hospital in Rouen in France, and was eventually posted to the Cambridge Military Hospital at Aldershot in Hampshire – the first base hospital in the UK to receive battle casualties directly from the Western Front. Here, in a unit which had pioneered plastic surgery for soldiers, he had performed demanding surgery on severely wounded, traumatised and disfigured men. His superiors described him as a kind, devoted and 'charming colleague', a 'most conscientious indefatigable worker… [with] good judgement' and also 'a useful pair of hands'.[3] This son of an Australian grazier was the perfect candidate for the advertised job – and soon, Farranridge was introduced as a new member of staff.

Ward rounds

Sunday, 20 May 1917 was of one of Dr Farranridge's first days at Queen Square. At Rouen and Aldershot, he had seen the devastating effects of shells, bombs, bullets and gas on the human body. While he was serving with the Gloucesters, he had witnessed soldiers die from their penetrating wounds, infected flesh and torn bodies, but he had also performed life-saving operations and seen them recover from their combat injuries. He had seen it all, so he thought, and he felt well prepared for the new job.

Equipped with 'excellent practical knowledge of both medicine and surgery', Farranridge took the new challenge. He eagerly cared for the numerous wounded soldiers, young men with debilitating nerve injuries, life-threatening gunshot wounds and head injuries – the victims of the raw violence of modern weaponry. He had seen hundreds of these cases before; however, he was ill-prepared for the patients who were clearly suffering from the effects of the war, but had nothing to show in terms of physical injuries. These patients, termed 'functional' for want of a better word, made up similar numbers to those with documented brain injuries. For many of them, the functional consequences of the war trauma eclipsed what Farranridge had seen in his surgical cases. He was even less familiar with the civilian cases: women, men and children with classical neurological disorders. The more common cases suffered from epilepsy, 'tabes dorsalis' – an advanced stage of syphilis – amyotrophic lateral sclerosis (motor neurone disease), 'spinal caries' – tuberculosis leading to a deformation of

---

3   Farranridge, Clive: Correspondence, March 1917, NHNN/S/2/68, Queen Square Archives.

the spine – and tumours of the brain and spinal cord. 'Disseminated sclerosis', today commonly known as 'multiple sclerosis', was also a frequent diagnosis among both male and female inpatients. Many children with poliomyelitis were scattered over the wards – and then there were the less common disorders, like 'Friedreich's ataxy' (today commonly termed 'Friedreich's ataxia'), which was an inherited disease named after the German physician Nikolaus Friedreich, which caused progressive damage to the nervous system – resulting in symptoms ranging from gait disturbance to speech problems. Diagnoses relied very much on a precise and skilful neurological examination; of course, soldiers were not spared these usually chronic conditions. On 20 May 1917, one soldier was treated for Huntington's chorea – an inherited disease that causes involuntary jerks and leads to increasing disability and early death.

Bentinck ward

When Farranridge entered Bentinck ward on 20 May, he first attended to one of his more unusual civilian cases: this man took up more space than any other patient – occupying two hospital beds and requiring extra food rations. Twenty-five-year-old Frederick Kempster was indeed 'a striking looking individual', measuring 7' 9" (2.36 m) in height, with 'massive' bones, an enormous skull, huge hands and large feet (corresponding to a UK shoe size 14).[4] His voice had a 'peculiar booming quality', his muscles were 'flabby' and his spine was grossly deformed. Frederick had been born in Bayswater in 1889 and begun to grow abnormally when he was 14. As a 'professional giant' and showman, Frederick had been touring in Germany at the outbreak of the war – and because of his physical appearance, he had been placed under house arrest in Berlin by the German authorities. He was released after a month and returned to Britain, where he gave several interviews to the London press. He visited his brother, George, who was recovering in hospital after being wounded in France in 1916. The Queen Square neurologists had no doubt that Frederick was suffering from a medical condition called 'acromegaly' – excessive growth of the extremities. In 1909, the American surgeon Harvey Cushing had established that this condition could be caused by tumours in the pituitary gland.[5] Frederick was suffering from intense frontal headaches. The X-ray of his skull showed a very large *sella turcica*: this saddle-shaped depression in one of the skull bones – named for its similarity with a 'Turkish chair' – houses the pituitary gland, and its widening indicated a tumour of the type described by Cushing. Although the Queen Square surgeons had experience in the operation of such tumours, Kempster was not considered for surgery. Instead, he was treated with

---

4   QSA: Queen Square Records, Dr Steward, 1917, male and female A-K: Case record Frederick K.
5   Mammis, Antonios, Eloy, Jean A. and Liu, James K., 'Early descriptions of acromegaly and gigantism and their historical evolution as clinical entities: Historical vignette' – *Journal of Neurosurgery*, 29:4 (2010), p.E1.

20 May 1917: One Day on the Shell Shock Ward 109

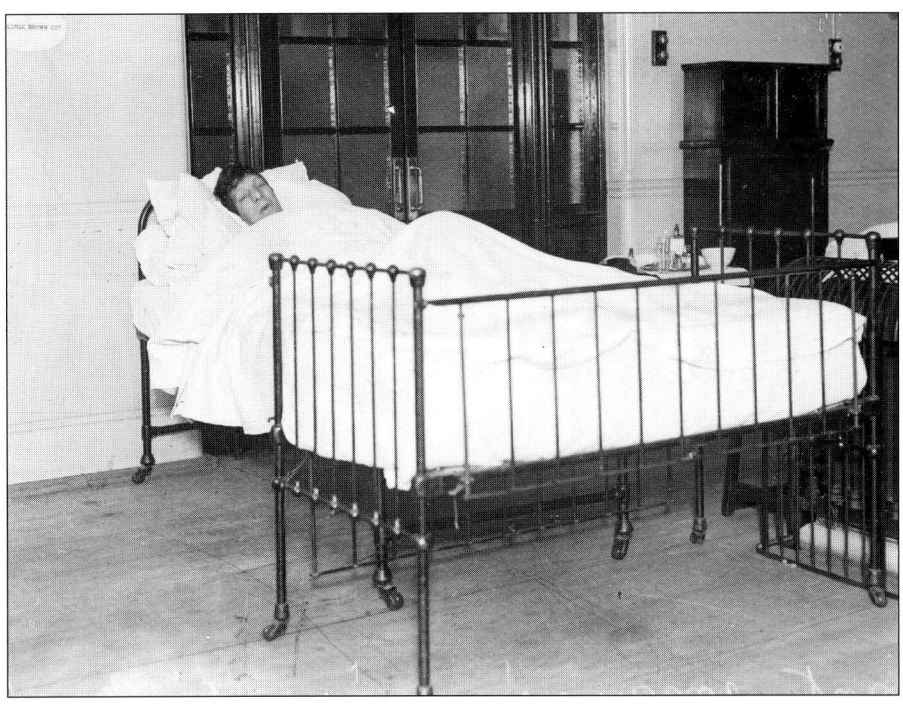

Frederick Kempster – the world's tallest man – occupying two hospital beds; QSA/12389. (Queen Square Archives, London)

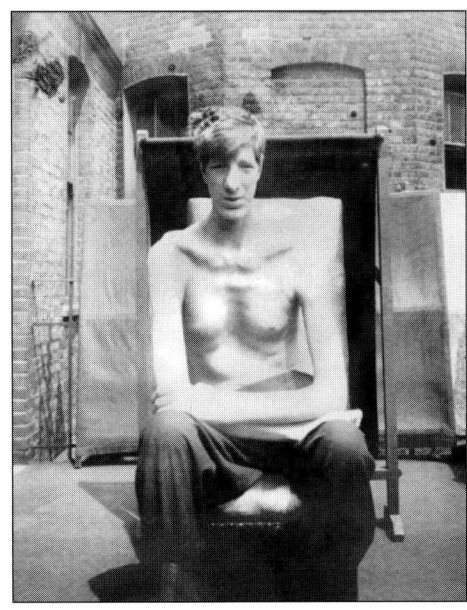

Frederick Kempster – a photograph in the hospital yard at Queen Square. (Queen Square Archives, London)

the medical remedies of the time, such as caffeine and aspirin, and also suprarenal gland extracts. When the press heard about Frederick's admission, they took a picture of him in his hospital bed, which was made up of two beds pushed together.

With his caseload of neurological patients like Kempster, and the many brain-injured and shell-shocked soldiers, Farranridge had very little time for the remaining group of patients – civilians with 'neurasthenia' and 'hysteria'. These patients, without any obvious organic disease or injury – who had not even fought in the war, or been exposed to explosions – presented with paralyses of arms and legs, seizures, dizziness, headaches and involuntary movements (often very similar to the shell-shocked soldiers). Neurasthenic patients had made up a considerable portion of the intake of neurological wards before the war, and they certainly did not disappear with the outbreak of the war. They were usually chronic cases – often demanding and resistant to the wide array of treatments developed for their variable symptoms. Caring for this particular group of patients was not very rewarding, and many neurologists had given up on them. Wartime pressures did not allow Farranridge to spend too much time with this patient population, and it was generally assumed that too much attention and compassion were not beneficial for their cure anyway.

John Back ward

On his ward round on the morning of 20 May 1917, Farranridge enthusiastically entered another ward, John Back, which was named after The Reverend John Back – the previous vicar of St George the Martyr and the National Hospital. The young doctor's attention was instantaneously drawn towards a distant corner of the spacious, yet overcrowded, hall: Private John T., a young exhausted-looking soldier, was trying to get some rest, while his whole body was grasped by violent convulsions.[6] Clearly, there was an opportunity here for the new doctor to learn something about a classical neurological disease, epilepsy; however, ward staff soon informed him that this was anything but classical epilepsy: the 19-year-old from the 5th Seaforth Highlanders

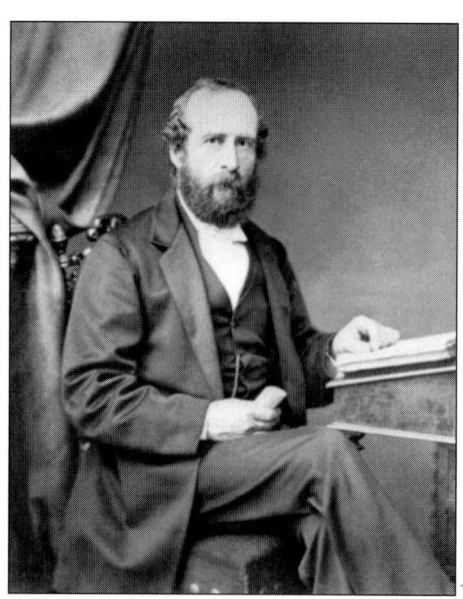

The Reverend John Back, vicar of St George the Martyr and the National Hospital; QSA/1814. (Queen Square Archives, London)

---

6   QSA: Queen Square Records, Dr Russell, 1917, male L-Z: case record Private John T.

suffered these fits of shaking, which usually lasted for two to three hours, since he had been blown up by a mine during the Battle of the Somme on 13 November 1916. During the night, he would wake up the other patients – crying out in his sleep, while living through terrible nightmares; this was a classical case of functional, non-epileptic fits.

On the other side of the ward, another young soldier – 19-year-old Private Edward C. from the 20th London Regiment – was also shaking violently.[7] The convulsions always started in his hands and arms, and then spread to his trunk and head. To Farranridge's surprise, the young electrician had not developed his symptoms during combat, but while on a short leave from the front line: at 7:00 p.m. on 19 January 1917, at home in bed, Edward had been disturbed by a colossal explosion at an ammunitions factory in Silvertown (about half a mile from his home).[8] Although the detonation killed 73 workers and injured a further 400, Edward's house had not been damaged; however, he began shaking all over and 'has continued to shake without intermission ever since'. It was painful to watch these young and physically fit men lose control over their bodies. During his short time at the National Hospital, Farranridge had learned that involuntary movements such as shaking, tremors or tics were the most difficult functional disorders to treat, and sometimes even resisted treatment completely.

On a chair close to the big fireplace sat another military patient: forty-three-year-old Sergeant James E. of the Welsh Pioneers was an experienced soldier, who had joined the army in 1897 and had served in Ireland, Malta and South Africa.[9] He rejoined the army in August 1915; however, without any apparent medical reason, his legs began to feel tired and gave way from time to time. In May 1916, he was sent to base hospital with dysentery and vomiting; the weakness increased so that he was unable to stand on his legs.

James had been confined to a chair for the past six months – and he was not the only soldier to become paralysed: Farranridge came across several patients who were unable to move without assistance, but were classified as 'functional' cases. In addition to their therapies, these bedridden and weakened soldier-patients were encouraged to rest and eat well to regain their strength; however, a petition from the soldiers on John Back ward – asking permission for those who were unable to get up to be allowed to smoke in bed – had been turned down by the hospital's Board of Management, 'in view of the fire risk'.

All of a sudden, another soldier let out a high-pitched shriek. Farranridge and one of his female colleagues, Dr Elizabeth Ashby, rushed to the little man with fair hair and grey eyes, who had turned pale and was breathing rapidly. When he started moving his arms and legs in a most dramatic display, Dr Ashby pressed her thumbs

---

7   QSA: Queen Square Records, Dr Tooth, 1917, male and female A-K: case record Edward C.
8   Silvertown in West Ham, Essex – now part of the London Borough of Newham.
9   QSA: Queen Square Records, Dr Batten, 1917, male A-K: case record Sergeant James E.

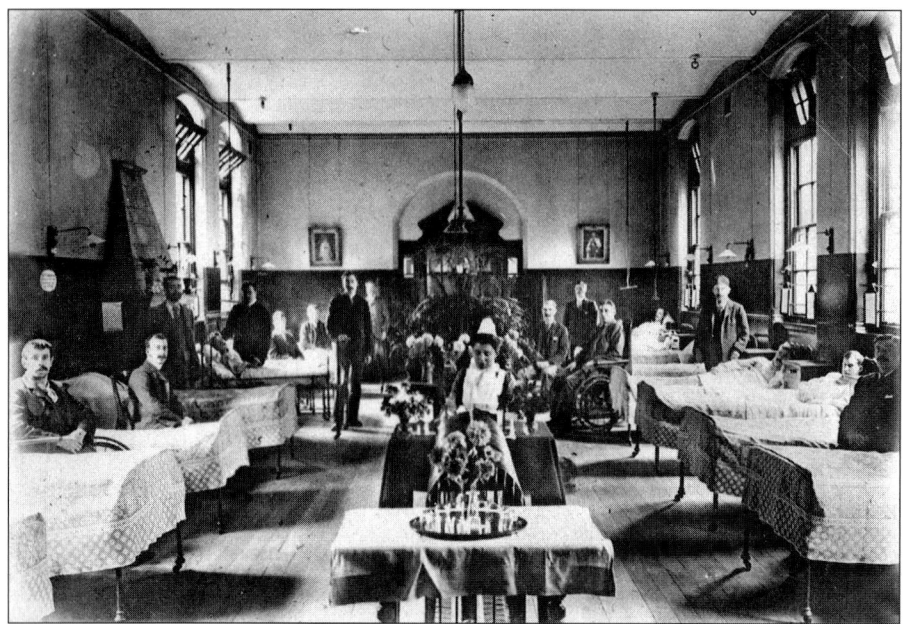

John Back ward, National Hospital; QSA/1328. (Queen Square Archives, London)

hard above the patient's eyeballs. This powerful method of applying 'supraorbital pressure' had been introduced to Queen Square by their senior colleague, Dr Lewis Ralph Yealland – and it worked immediately. The soldier, slightly shocked by the painful intervention, regained his composure. The patient was introduced to Farranridge as 19-year-old George B., a former motor driver who had had his first fit after heavy shelling in the trenches.[10] He was one of the numerous referrals from Étaples, which had become the principal *depôt* and transit camp for the BEF in France.

The patient in the neighbouring bed had also come from Étaples, with a handwritten note by Captain G.G. Steward from the 1st Canadian General Hospital – stating that: 'This is to certify that the accompanying man was seen in an epileptic fit'. The notes also revealed that 29-year-old Private James H. had apparently developed fits long before he was sent to the Western Front, whilst he was still in training in Northumberland.[11] He was, nevertheless, sent to France in March 1917, but soon started having regular fits in the trenches. However, to the Queen Square doctors, these attacks did not look like genuine epileptic seizures: according to the transfer notes, Private James typically developed a headache several hours before a fit. During the attack, he lost consciousness, or seemed dazed for up to an hour. Sometimes, he

10   QSA: Queen Square Records, Dr Turner, 1917, male A-K: case record Private George B.
11   QSA: Queen Square Records, Dr Turner, 1917, male A-K: case record Private James H.

vomited before or after the attack, and he never bit his tongue or passed urine. Since his admission to the National Hospital, James had not suffered any more fits, though. Interestingly, James would later be discharged from the army as 'no longer physically fit for war service'. The pension records reveal that the diagnosis documented by the Medical Board was 'epilepsy not caused or aggravated by service'; the army had obviously overturned the Queen Square doctors' final diagnosis of 'functional fits'. One reason might be that the army doctors were still less receptive to non-organic explanations of the problems of their men than the doctors in civilian hospitals (see Chapter 10); another reason may be that pre-existing conditions did not warrant a war pension, and one of the aims of Medical Boards then, as today, was to limit the number of pension claims.

On another bed, a thin boyish-looking man, with a weary expression, was talking to himself; he did not notice the two young doctors who had approached his bed. He seemed to be in a different world – disconnected from his surroundings. Thirty-three-year-old Corporal William B. from the Sherwood Foresters was having one of his peculiar spells – during which he appeared to be back in the trenches.[12] These episodes could last for several days, and afterwards, he would not be able to remember any of it; it seemed that these episodes of reliving experiences from the front were split off from his conscious mind. During the summer of 1916, at Salonica, William had been blown off his horse and pushed over a cliff by a shell. He had hit the back of his head and been unconscious for four hours. After the accident, William was in a 'total blank'; the trauma had erased all personal memories. He had forgotten his name, that he had fought in the war and that he was happily married with two healthy children; he had even lost his ability to read and write. William's memory recovered gradually on his voyage to England, but when admitted to Queen Square six months after his injury, he was still in the process of recollecting his war experiences and integrating them into his life's story; this seemed to be a difficult and painful process.

Memory problems were common among all soldiers with general physical and mental exhaustion – and they were also common in soldiers who had suffered a major psychological or physical trauma. Many of the soldier-patients who populated the wards on 20 May 1917 were forgetful and suffered from difficulties focusing their mind – and many had even forgotten the events that ultimately led to their breakdown and shipment to England; however, the case of William B. was particularly interesting for two reasons: first, it illustrated that patients could suffer both organic and functional memory problems – and although William's original loss of memory after the injury might well have been a consequence of the physical brain trauma ('retrograde amnesia', which is often observed after brain concussion), his later 'blank attacks' resembled what we would today describe as 'transient global amnesia', which is a dissociative disorder; secondly, William's case was a vivid illustration of the

---

12   QSA: Queen Square Records, Dr Russell, 1917, male A-K: case record Corporal William B.

psychoanalytical model that assumed that unbearable memories were split off from conscious experience. Farranridge was well read and knew about the main psychodynamic theories: according to Janet,[13] feelings and memories associated with traumatic experiences could persist as 'subconscious fixed ideas'. Repressing, or splitting off, the memory of the traumatic event was a desperate attempt to cope with an unbearable trauma; however, although the gruesome memory was temporarily removed from the conscious mind, it persisted in the unconscious and could reappear in form of nightmares or so-called 'dissociative states', as in William's case. Cure could only be achieved if the repressed memory could be recovered and re-integrated into the patient's conscious mind. This was a long and often complicated process, which required a well-trained physician – and at the National Hospital, there was neither enough time, nor manpower, to practice psychoanalytical methods. Although the Queen Square neurologists had embraced psychological interventions, psychoanalysis may also have required an intellectual leap that they were not prepared to make – thus, this method remained confined to even more exclusive institutions, such as the officers' sanatorium at Craiglockhart, where W.H.R. Rivers engaged a number of his patients in this kind of lengthy therapy.

David Wire ward

Farranridge left John Back ward to see his own patients, who had been admitted to David Wire ward. David Wire, Lord Mayor of London, had played a crucial role in raising funds for the establishment of the National Hospital in 1859. Wire, who was partially paralysed after a stroke, had insisted on providing a hospital in which active treatment of disease could be carried out, rather than 'a home for the incurables'.

Like the other wards for male patients, David Wire accommodated a medley of civilian and military patients. Although it had initially been decided that military patients should be separated from the civilian patient population, this regime soon proved problematic: the Hospital Management Board called attention to 'the ill effects which may arise from too close an association of patients suffering from similar ailments';[14] the members of the Board undoubtedly referred to the large group of soldiers with shell shock. The main problem was not that these men, who had sometimes fought side by side on the same battlefield, exchanged their terrifying war experiences, as this could only be cathartic and serve to strengthen their sense of companionship and belonging. The problem, rather, lay in these men's suggestibility; their readiness to take over somebody else's ideas and convictions. Although this could be useful for treatment with suggestive methods, it also meant that shell-shocked

---

13 Janet, Pierre, *L'automatisme psychologique: Essai de psychologie expérimentale sur les formes inférieures de l'activité humaine* (Paris: L'Harmattan, 1889).
14 QSA: minutes from the Board of Management meeting – handwritten note, 9 February 1915.

soldiers mimicked other patients' symptoms and imitated their abnormal behaviours. Farranridge knew from his work at the base hospital in Rouen that one convulsing soldier on the ward could infect a whole group of comrades – thus, a conglomeration of war neurotics was not deemed favourable for the atmosphere and treatment outcomes of the hospital. The Hospital Committee, therefore, gave the medical staff 'discretionary powers as to the distribution of patients' on the different wards.

Like on John Back ward, several soldiers on 'David Wire' were in continuous motion: Private Stanley S. from the Royal Field Artillery – 'a thin youth of 21' – had sudden tic-like movements in his hands and also the left side of his face (involving his eyes and forehead), but sparing his mouth.[15] His hands were also shaking continuously – and all purposeful movements appeared to be jerky and clumsy. He was certainly not fit for military service, nor capable of returning into his pre-war occupation. The former hairdresser had been in this state since being blown up by a shell in the incongruously-named 'Happy Valley' on the Somme in November 1916.

Farranridge moved on to two patients, who were resting on their beds – and he found it difficult to grasp these young men's symptoms: they both complained of dizziness, headaches, forgetfulness and general fatigue. Their sleep was disturbed by nightmares and they seemed to be on the alert all the time – easily startled by the slightest noises. Both men had fought in France and had obtained slight injuries during their active service; however, there was no obvious physical scar left, and both seemed to be in control of their bodies. Sergeant William Henry W., a former heating engineer, who was single and a few years younger than his comrade, had developed symptoms after falling into a 40-foot-deep well on 28 March 1917 while serving with the Royal Field Artillery.[16] Thirty-year-old George H., a married regular soldier with the 2nd Coldstream Guards, had been 'rather badly shaken [on] 15th September 1916 when his battalion made a frontal attack';[17] this was when his complaints started. Farranridge knew that these nervous wrecks were unlikely to be able to fulfil their frontline duties, yet he found their symptoms difficult to comprehend, as Farranridge was not a psychiatrist and he did not possess the vocabulary for a precise description of these vague mental phenomena. All he documented in George's notes was that the young soldier's 'mental state [was] far from normal'. Although both men presented with similar symptoms, William W. was diagnosed with 'neurasthenia', while George H. obtained a diagnosis of 'hysteria'. Farranridge found this slightly confusing: it certainly made sense to him that Sergeant W. – out of respect – should not carry the label of 'hysteria'; Farranridge had noticed that it was general practice to diagnose officers and NCOs with 'neurasthenia'. 'Neurasthenia', as opposed to 'hysteria', was a well-respected diagnosis at the time; conversely, the lower ranks, like Private H., were

---

15   QSA: Queen Square Records, Dr Russell, 1917, male L-Z: case record Private Stanley S.
16   QSA: Queen Square Records, Dr Howell, 1917, male and female L-Z: case record Sergeant William Henry W.
17   QSA: Queen Square Records, Dr Russell, 1917, male A-K: case record Private George H.

labelled with 'hysteria'. The categorical distinction between neurasthenic officers and hysterical men not only mirrored the British class system, but also justified different treatment regimes for officers and lower ranks.[18] Sergeant W. would be referred to a convalescent hospital for officers, while Private H. would be sent back to his command depot. Farranridge quickly prescribed some extra milk for Private H. and arranged for Sergeant W. to see the ENT consultant to remove some wax from his ears; then he continued his rounds.

On the corridor, he bumped into the bookbinder Charles S.[19] With a big scar cutting through the left side of his round face, his abundant hair and enormous brown moustache, he looked wild; it was hard to believe that he was only 31 years of age. Charles had been wounded by a piece of shrapnel in May 1915. From then on, any shell fire had made him shake uncontrollably. He had been discharged from the army in October 1915 to work with the St John's Ambulance Association, but was soon sent home on account of shaking and 'playing the fool'. At home, he was not of much use either: he was 'confused' and could not retain any information given to him – not even names or simple messages. Because he was so absent-minded and inaccessible, his wife was worried that he might harm their four little children. Farranridge put an arm on Charles's shoulder; Charles, who still had not noticed the young doctor's presence, started shaking violently. While Farranridge was supporting him back to Albany ward, Charles was muttering incomprehensibly. On his bedside cabinet, books were piling up – and on top, a textbook of French grammar, which Charles had studied while in the trenches to distract his mind. The book was the only memento of his frontline experience; every other memory had been erased from his mind.

Exercises

Back on the corridor, a group of three soldiers were doing their exercises. One of them, 44-year-old Irish Rifleman Patrick D. from Galway, walked 'with his back bent a little, his arms drawn in front of him, hands somewhat inverted and flexed at the wrist' – reminding Farranridge of the typical gait of Parkinson's disease.[20] Patrick's hands were continuously moving in what could best be described as a 'rhythmic rolling tremor' – and this tremor increased dramatically when he reached out to shake Farranridge's hand. This, after all, did not look like Parkinson's disease, where the tremor typically improved with goal-directed movements – and it did not look like essential tremor either, which was generally more fine-grained; this tremor was most

---

18   Reid, Fiona, *Broken Men: Shell Shock, Treatment and Recovery in Britain 1914-1930* (London: Continuum International Publishing Group, 2010), p.16.
19   QSA: Queen Square Records, Dr Collier, 1917, male and female L-Z: case record Private Charles S.
20   QSA: Queen Square Records, Dr Turner, 1917, male A-K: case record Rifleman Patrick D.

likely in the mind. When Patrick made a step towards the window, all muscles in his legs seemed to be going into spasm. This emaciated man had not even seen active fighting: Patrick had been serving in India in July 1916 when his shaking started. The shaking had not only compromised his military fitness, but also impacted heavily on his everyday life. Feeding himself became increasingly difficult, so that Patrick had lost one and a half stone in weight.

The other two soldiers on the corridor were absorbed in their exercises: the soldier with the dark hair and blue eyes was carefully placing his right foot on the ground and walking 'as though he had no idea of sense of position in the right leg'. The handsome blonde boy – who did not have any obvious physical problems – was cheering him on continuously. This treatment approach had obviously worked. When both young men had been admitted to Queen Square on the same day in early January 1917, their symptoms had been peculiarly similar: their right foot was markedly inverted and contracted, and it could not be passively moved at the ankle joints; they could not move their right hip, knee or foot; when their right leg was moved passively, this induced a 'severe clonus [a series of involuntary muscle contractions], beginning in the right leg and extending to the left and then all over the body'. This caused excruciating pain – sharp and of a stabbing nature. Both men had fought during the Battle of the Somme and had, eventually, been sent to the 4th London General Hospital, where they were treated with massage, electricity and radiant heat. Doctors there had even tried to put their feet into the right position under general anaesthesia, but without success. Twenty-one-year-old Private Frederick C. from the 5th King's Own Yorkshire Light Infantry – the blonde soldier who was urging his comrade on – had been the first to recover after one session of electrical treatment.[21] He was living proof that a miracle cure was possible – and he was, consequently, given the task to practise with his comrade, 25-year-old Private Frederick J. from the 2nd Durham Light Infantry.[22] The two young Fredericks had never met before their admission to Queen Square, but they had already formed a close bond – and it was this case which convinced Farranridge that it could actually be beneficial to treat shell shock patients on the same ward. This role-model effect of the cured patients, the 'propaganda of the cured', as it was called by the Germans, could be a very powerful catalyst for cure.

A clinical lesson

Farranridge had to hurry up, as he wanted to attend a treatment session by one of the most famous shell shock doctors of the time: Dr Lewis Ralph Yealland. Yealland, the Canadian doctor (who was only two years older than him), had been working at

---

21 QSA: Queen Square Records, Dr Collier, 1917, male and female A-K: case record Private Frederick C.
22 QSA: Queen Square Records, Dr Collier, 1917, male and female A-K: Case record Private Frederick J.

the National Hospital for one and a half years. This enthusiastic doctor knew all shell shock patients on the wards, and he was working day and night to perform his miracle cures; patients were scheduled for therapy even on a Sunday.

Two patients were waiting on a bench in front of the treatment room. There was no sign of Dr Yealland yet, and Farranridge took the opportunity to enquire about the patients' symptoms. This was not straightforward, because both men could neither hear nor talk, after being blown up in a shell explosion at the Western Front. Although both of them had become proficient lip-readers, written communication was more efficient and obviated misunderstandings. Farranridge took a piece of paper, turned to the younger, sullen-looking man – a private called James John S. (the 25-year-old machine gunner from the Royal Fusiliers, who was introduced in Chapter 2) – and wrote down an open question: 'What is the matter with you?' (See image on p.36) The handwritten conversation was in full flow, and the young man dutifully scribbled down his answers; however, all of a sudden – and without an explanation – James got up from the bench and rushed out of the room with quick, short jerky steps, with 'one leg following the other in spasms'.[23] Before Farranridge could address the other soldier, who was wearing thick glasses, the door to the treatment room opened and a young clean-shaven doctor, with dark brown hair that was parted deep to one side, appeared: Dr Yealland had expected them. The soldier, a rather poorly-nourished pale man with light brown hair, a brown moustache and blue hazy eyes, got up from the bench and – bent forward and shaking violently – made his way into the cramped room, which was filled with electrical machines and cables. Yealland introduced the soldier as 35-year-old Private John P. of the Queen's Royal West Surreys.[24] About two years before the treatment, he had been blown up by a shell in France – and since then, he had been 'deaf and dumb' and paralysed from his waist down. John, who had worked on a farm before the war, was initially referred to King's College Hospital, but did not respond to any of the treatments he received there and, consequently, became very depressed. Yealland had taken a personal interest in this young man, who seemed to have given up hope. On that day – 20 May 1917 – they had agreed to focus on his hearing and speech; in a previous session, Yealland had tried his standard treatment to cure John's deafness: he had applied electric currents to John's mastoid processes (the bony protrusions behind John's ears). Because this treatment had 'made him extremely tremulous and excited and appeared to do him a great deal more harm than good', Yealland had decided to try a different approach: he wanted his junior colleague to witness a particularly impressive therapy session. The patient was sitting on a reclining chair in the centre of the room. Yealland reassured John – in writing – that this would be the final therapy session and that John would be able to hear and talk by the end of

---

23   QSA: Queen Square Records, Dr Holmes, 1917, male and female L-Z: case record Private James John S.
24   QSA: Queen Square Records, Dr Collier, 1917, male and female L-Z: case record Private John P.

the day; then Yealland applied tuning forks of different frequencies to John's mastoid. At the beginning, he took the largest tuning fork, struck it on the table and placed the handle on the bone behind John's ear. Large tuning forks generate very slow vibrations that can be easily felt; however, the sound they produce is rather low-pitched and difficult to hear. Yealland then applied smaller tuning forks, whose vibrations are faster and thus, more difficult to feel, but whose sound has a higher pitch. John could only feel the vibrations of the tuning forks at first, but when Yealland gradually reduced the size of the instruments, he could eventually hear the sound. John burst out into tears – overwhelmed with the unexpected treatment success. After all, he had not been able to hear a sound for the past two years. However, Yealland had not yet finished his therapy session: he took a stethoscope, put the earpieces into John's ear canals and shouted words into the bell. Although John was able to hear the sounds, he was initially unable to interpret them. Over time, John got used to the sounds and was able to understand their meaning. Yealland then removed the stethoscope and continued shouting words into John's ears; he gradually lowered his voice and went farther away. Whenever John reported that he was able to hear the sounds, Yealland lowered his voice further until John was able to hear a whisper. John was sweating profusely, but looked relieved. He had obviously had enough and was keen to return to his ward; however, John – who had clearly given in to Yealland's treatment methods and was in a highly suggestible state – would not be allowed to leave the room until he was completely cured. Yealland took a big spatula and asked John to open his mouth. By depressing the tongue with the spatula, 'pushing it well backwards to the posterior wall of the pharynx', he made John give a 'groan'; this was the first sound he had made in two years. It was followed by a long session of what Yealland called 're-education': this involved teaching the patient to make sounds, then phonate simple words and, ultimately, talk in a normal voice. This was a tedious process – strenuous for the patient, but also exhausting for the spectator. After two hours of therapy, Yealland seemed to be happy with the result. Later, Yealland would sit at his desk in his cold bedsit at the hospital and write up John's case for his book on *Hysterical Disorders of Warfare*,[25] which was close to completion.

Farranridge had seen enough for the day: he had expected that his new job would be much more straightforward; he had seen it all, so he had thought. He had been wrong – and clearly, there was a great deal for him to learn in this borderland between the mind and the brain.

---

25 Yealland, *Hysterical Disorders of Warfare* – case B2, pp.39-43.

7

The Mental World of Terror

>The dreams of soldiers ... exhibit in a striking manner how an incident of war associated with emotional shock is graven on the mind, for it continually recurs in a vivid and terrifying manner in their dreams, half-waking state, and in some few cases even in the waking state, constituting hallucinations.[1]

Most soldiers who had gone through the horrors of frontline fighting could not let go of their terrifying experiences – and if they managed to suppress some of their trench memories, the gruesome pictures haunted them in their dreams; yet, even in bright daylight, some soldiers drifted into dream-like states, in which they relived – and even re-enacted – combat scenes. About five percent of soldiers treated at the National Hospital at Queen Square slipped in and out of these peculiar states: William Aldren Turner, Queen Square consultant and shell shock specialist, noted that unresponsiveness to the surroundings – accompanied by flashbacks of combat experiences and the re-enactment of battle scenes – were relatively common, particularly in young soldiers in their early twenties.[2]

The re-experiencing – and sometimes restaging – of traumatic events in twilight or confusion states, in dream-like episodes, and also in the fully conscious individual, had already been described by Charcot's pupil, Janet, at the end of the 19th century.[3] However, it was Karl Kleist, a German neurologist and psychiatrist, who first systematically described these acute and transient psychological reactions in soldiers, which he called 'terror psychoses' ('*Schreckpsychosen*').[4] During the war, Kleist was head of the

---

1   Mott, *War Neuroses and Shell Shock*, p.118.
2   Turner, 'Remarks on Cases of Nervous and Mental Shock', p.833.
3   Janet, Pierre, *The Major Symptoms of Hysteria*, 2nd edn (New York: The Macmillan Company, 1924), pp.30-37; here, Janet described the involuntary reliving and re-enactment of elements of the trauma in 'somnambulistic crises'.
4   Kleist, Karl, 'Schreckpsychosen' – *Allgemeine Zeitschrift für Psychiatrie und psychisch-gerichtliche Medizin*, 74 (1918), pp.432-510.

The Mental World of Terror

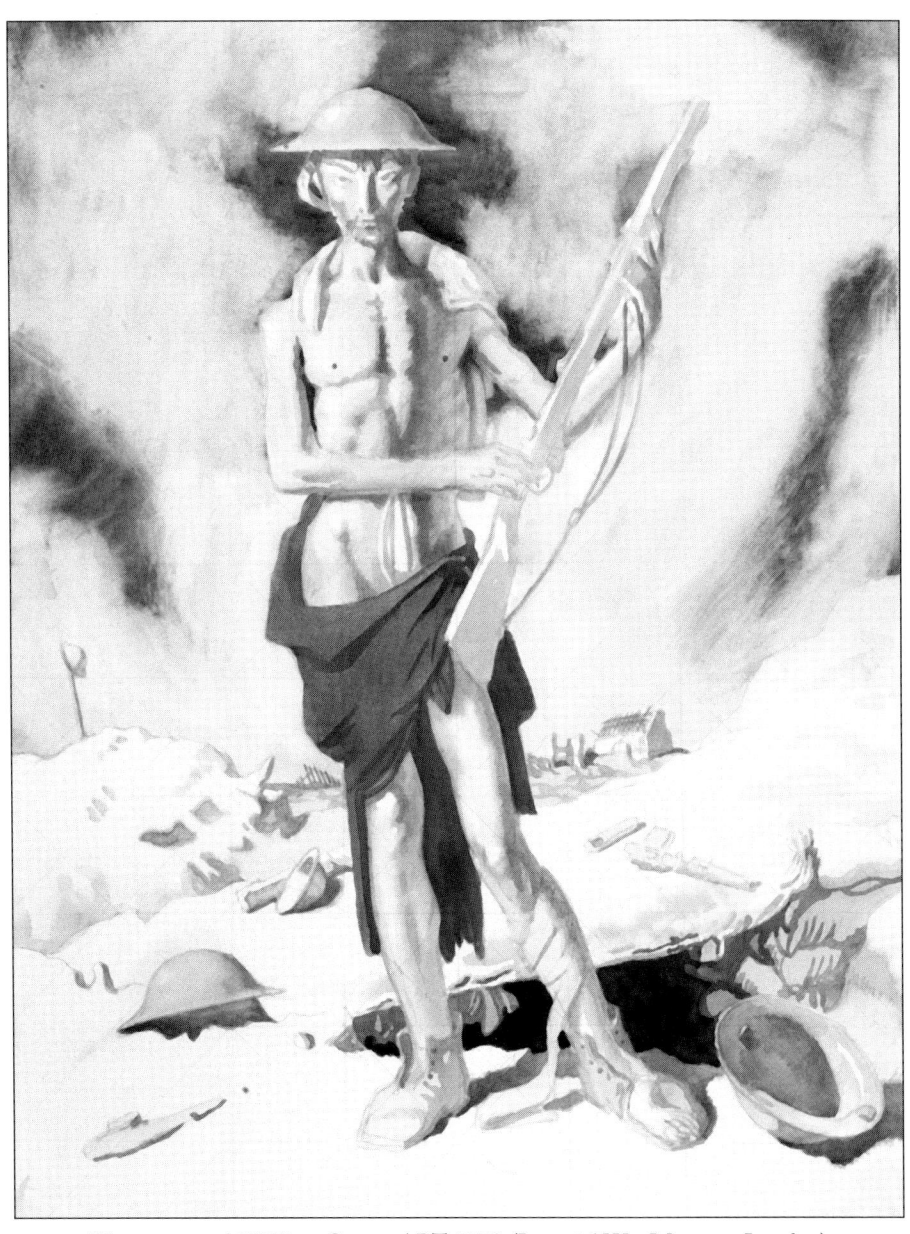

Blown up, mad. William Orpen; ART 2376. (Imperial War Museum, London)

122 They Called It Shell Shock

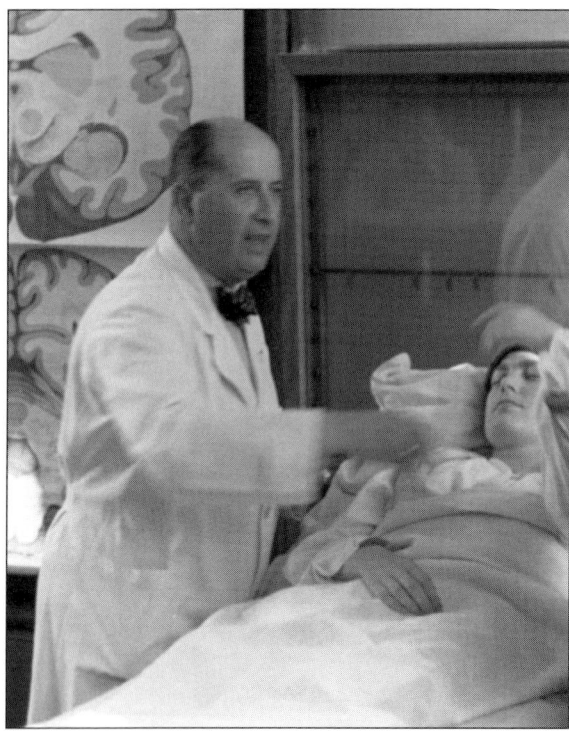

Karl Kleist, during a lecture at Frankfurt University, demonstrating a catatonic state; photograph taken by one of his students circa 1939. (Author's own archive)

neurology section of the German field hospital in Lille, and later in charge of a military hospital in Rostock, where he was chair of psychiatry from 1916-1920.[5]

Kleist encountered frequent scenes of soldiers re-enacting battles on his wards: he described soldiers hiding in imaginary dugouts, during ward rounds, because they were convinced that the hospital staff were a party of Allied soldiers. Some soldiers also fired imaginary guns or, if they could get hold of them, even real ones. Soldiers often showed intense reactions to cues that reminded them of the traumatic event: one of the soldier-patients described by Kleist suffered a recurrence of symptoms during a thunderstorm; another soldier relapsed while witnessing a battle scene during a theatre performance.[6] Others would hide under their beds whenever they heard a loud noise, because they mistook the sound for that of a shell explosion. These symptoms, which resemble the increased arousal of today's post-traumatic stress disorder patients, were common among soldiers who had

5 Bartsch, Andreas J., Neumärker, Klaus-J., Franzek, Ernst and Beckmann, Helmut, 'Karl Kleist (1879-1960)' – *American Journal of Psychiatry*, 157:5 (2000), p.703.
6 Kleist, 'Schreckpsychosen', p.505.

been through traumatic experiences.[7] Although these 'subjective' disturbances could be easily overlooked in a cursory examination, they could cause considerable suffering and 'make life for some of their victims a veritable hell'.[8] Although Kleist was also an eminent neuroanatomist – and always inclined to search for organic causes of neurological deficits – he considered terror psychosis to be the result of a subconscious persistence of the traumatic experience. His almost psychoanalytical explanation centred on the unprocessed trauma, which could be re-experienced in dreams, in states of reduced responsiveness ('twilight states'), or even in the fully awake, conscious individual.

Twilight states

The majority of soldiers with terror psychosis were in a delirious state, which made it difficult to tell them apart from those with actual physical injuries or infectious disease; yet, they did not have a high temperature and were physically unscathed. Soldiers with terror psychosis drifted in a timeless space: cut off from the real world, they were caught in their horrid memories. They had to relive gruelling combat scenes again and again, were haunted by pictures of death and destruction in their dreams, or during bright daylight. Because these soldiers felt threatened and unsafe, they were anxious and sometimes aggressive. A classical example of this form of terror psychosis was 18-year-old infantryman Ernst R., a joiner in civilian life, who was admitted to the Jena Military Hospital on 23 December 1915.[9] Ernst had fought in Belgium, Russia and France. On 1 November 1915, he was in the trenches when a shell exploded close to him. He felt a stabbing pain in his right ear and realised that he could not hear on this side; he also expe-

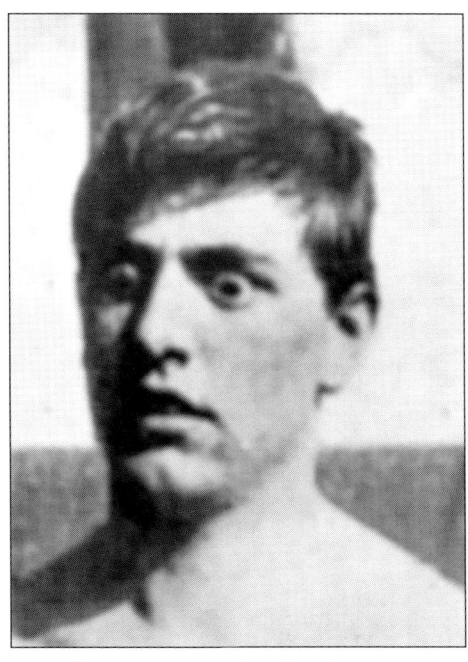

Shell-shocked soldier; Pte E., severe hyperadrenalism and hyperthyroidism with exophthalmos, resulting from prolonged terror; Fig. II, 1; Hurst, Arthur, *Medical Diseases of the War*. (London: Edward Arnold, 1918)

---

7 Hurst, *Medical Diseases of the War*, pp.41-43.
8 Smith and Pear, *Shell Shock and its Lessons*, pp.12-13.
9 Universitätsarchiv Jena, Bestand S/III Abt. IX, Kriegsarchiv, Nr. 316.

rienced buzzing noises in his head. Because the pain became intolerable, Ernst was referred to a field hospital. Soon after his admission, he received an urgent telegram from home – informing him that his mother was dying. Ernst was granted leave and hurried back to Germany; however, his mental state deteriorated and he had to be admitted to a military hospital in Karlsruhe, which was close to his home town. Because Ernst was suffering from fits, he was soon sent to the Jena Military Hospital, which was a specialised seizure centre. In Jena, Ernst regularly left his bed in the middle of the night in a state of trance; he bundled up his bedding and talked to himself. He then behaved as if he was still in the trenches – ducking and hiding under his bed, and imitating the firing of a machine gun. The next morning, he could not remember anything; he only knew that he had dreamt of the war. During the day, he felt utterly exhausted and complained about headaches.

Forty-four-year-old British Gunner Frederick J.W. from the Royal Field Artillery, who was admitted to Queen Square on 8 December 1915, suffered similar episodes:[10] on admission, Frederick looked exhausted; he had not slept for a week and heard shouting and other noises in his head.

On 9 December 1915, after a good night's sleep, Frederick provided some information about what had happened to him:

> Says he does not remember the incident prior to his coming down but he saw last week – one of our own snipers shot through the head. The sight upset him very much and he went to get the enemy who had fired the shot and remembers nothing until he found himself in hospital. ... Accompanying the certificate from headquarters there is a story of his delusions. He was in the 134th Battery Gun Position Camp – left it with two dogs and took a rifle with him. He discharged rifle without apparent cause. He was told to stop by a sergeant but did not seem to understand and was made to do so by the Sergeant who disarmed him after a struggle. After this he was violent for some time. He soon quieted down and regretted what he had done and made rash promises. It was thought that he was drunk. He has been a game keeper, passionately attached to his dogs, fears people will rob him of them.

Frederick was confused for a few days. His speech was incoherent and he had bouts of aggression and shouting; after a few days, he calmed down. At Queen Square, he was assessed as 'a perfectly normal individual, memory perfect – physically powerful'. Apart from sleeping medication, he did not require any treatment – and he was discharged from hospital after three weeks.

Why was Frederick spared the gruelling electrotherapy regime that Lewis Yealland and his colleagues meted out to almost all of their other patients? First of all, there

---

10 QSA: Queen Square Records, Dr Tooth, 1916, male L-Z: case record Gunner Frederick J.W.

was no focal point for electrical stimulation to attack. His trauma did not manifest through localised neurological symptoms, but through confusion and delusions; secondly, the Queen Square doctors soon realised that minimal intervention and rest worked best in these cases, which had a strong tendency to fast and spontaneous improvement.

In some twilight states, the mood fluctuated between elation, anxiety, aggression and irritability. Some soldiers with terror psychosis seemed to be playing a comical character: their gestures were grossly exaggerated and their behaviour was childish or theatrical.[11] These patients were often suspected of malingering, or at least exaggerating their symptoms, as in the case of 19-year-old German Musketeer Walter S., a waiter in civilian life, who had fought at the Eastern and Western Fronts.[12] After an injury to his left foot, he was admitted to several military hospitals. Walter experienced classical twilight states – during which he behaved inappropriately and, on one occasion, even tried to jump out of the window. Classically, he did not remember anything afterwards. At the Jena Military Hospital, where his condition was attributed to 'moral inferiority', he was wandering around in a daze; his behaviour was strange and unpredictable: Walter often started to bark, crow and meow; he disturbed a theatre performance by barking. One time, he was jumping on his bed and dancing in front of the mirror; at a moment's notice, his mood could swing from one extreme to the other. On the ward, Walter laughed uncontrollably, then lashed out and started crying. His strange performances could be infectious: one night, Walter had fits of laughter and crying; in the same night, several soldiers in the same dormitory started having hysterical seizures. This was a well-known phenomenon: a conglomeration of traumatised patients was never favourable for treatment outcomes of a hospital, and the limited space and overcrowding on most hospital wards provided a perfect breeding ground for hysteria. In Jena, where accommodation for traumatised soldiers was more generous than in most hospitals, isolation treatment was successfully used to prevent symptoms from spreading.

Other twilight states were characterised by grandiose ideas ('expansive twilight states' in Kleist's terminology):[13] when 38-year-old militia man Nikolaus K., painter and father of four healthy children, was admitted to the Jena Military Hospital on 23 October 1915, he was extremely agitated – lashing about with his hands and feet, and letting out piercing unarticulated shrieks.[14] Confused and blind with rage, Nikolaus hit everybody who came near his bed. When several attendants tried to lock him into the observation room, he screamed: "I am the Pope, I want to tell the world… A miracle has happened." At the same time, Nikolaus did not know his name and was disoriented to time and place. Because he did not calm down and repeatedly

---

11   Kleist, 'Schreckpsychosen', p.461.
12   Universitätsarchiv Jena, Bestand S/III Abt. IX, Kriegsarchiv, Nr. 1758.
13   Kleist, 'Schreckpsychosen', p.465.
14   Universitätsarchiv Jena, Bestand S/III Abt. IX, Kriegsarchiv, Nr. 194.

attacked hospital staff, he had to be tied to his bed – and the singing, shouting and proclaiming of religious ideas continued for a few days. What brought Nikolaus back into the real world was not one of the various therapies on offer, not a drug or a behavioural intervention, but a visit of his wife to the hospital. Nikolaus gradually regained consciousness and started talking sense again; he complained about a 'misty' feeling in his head. Strikingly, he could not remember anything of the previous three weeks. The last thing he could remember was an argument with his sergeant – and then, all of a sudden, the world around him had changed: people appeared to have abnormally big heads and mask-like faces. He had felt very anxious, but now he could see clearly again. Nikolaus had a brief relapse of symptoms a few days later, but finally recovered from his 'hysterical psychosis' (the term the Jena doctors used for terror psychosis).

The Ganser syndrome – 'strange hysterical twilight states', or the patients who (almost) lied

Twilight states were not confined to war psychiatry: civilian alienists had reported occasional encounters with patients who inhabited a borderland between dream and reality – not quite psychotic, but not quite sane either. One of these ambiguous states had been described by German psychiatrist Sigbert Ganser in 1898:[15] Ganser's patients gave approximate answers to familiar and simple questions; for example, Ganser asked one patient how many fingers he had. The patient answered: "Eleven." And to the question: "How many legs has a horse?" the patient replied: "Three." Then, asked about the number of legs of an elephant, he said: "Five." Because these answers were not random, but close to the correct reply – a phenomenon Ganser called 'paralogia' – the interviewer got the impression that the person had actually understood the question.[16] In addition to this striking symptom, all cases showed clouding of consciousness and sensory deficits, such as loss or disturbance of touch, or pain sensation; hallucinations were also common. Ganser was stunned by these 'strange hysterical twilight states', which resolved within a few days and left patients with a memory gap for the whole episode.

Before the war, Ganser's syndrome had been reported very rarely – and most psychiatrists had never seen a single case. The war changed this, as with so many previously rare conditions: several of the London, Berlin and Jena patients presented with Ganser syndrome.

---

15 Ganser, Sigbert J.M., 'Über einen eigenartigen hysterischen Dämmerzustand, Vortrag, gehalten am 23. October 1897 in der Versammlung der mitteldeutschen Psychiater und Neurologen zu Halle' – *Archiv für Psychiatrie und Nervenkrankheiten*, 30:2 (1898), pp.633-640.

16 Ganser, Sigbert J.M., 'Zur Lehre vom hysterischen Dämmerzustande: Vortrag, gehalten in der VIII. Versammlung mitteldeutscher Psychiater und Neurologen zu Dresden am 25. October 1902' – *Archiv für Psychiatrie und Nervenkrankheiten*, 38:1 (1903), pp.34-46.

Forty-year-old Grenadier Hermann G. was admitted to the Charité after a shell injury that had resulted in rather unusual mental symptoms:

> On admission the patient demonstrates an emotionally cold behaviour, does not look at doctor. Answers questions slowly, hesitantly, often only after repetition: "I don't know". Makes tic-like movements with his brow muscles, wrinkles his forehead, opening his eyes widely, makes shaking movements with his head. On physical examination staring into space, asks: "Shall I now do the same thing with you, you lie down on the sofa, I can also tap you with the hammer", at the same time trying to take the doctor's reflex hammer out of his pocket. [...] Asked for the number of his siblings, he says: "4 sisters and 9 brothers, all together 6". Cannot do the simplest calculations (e.g. 7+5, says 14; 3×3, says 11). [...] How many legs has a horse? – calculates with his fingers, then says: "2 in front and 2 at the back, together this is 6 legs"; What colour is the grass? – "Yellow as a tree"; What colour is blood? – "Pink". Does not know when Christmas and New Year is. Says it is March 1819. [...] The next day the patient cannot recall any of this.[17]

Another soldier, 36-year-old militia man Jakob B. – an inpatient at the Charité in early 1918, who had left his sentry without permission:

> ... gave wrong answers to the simplest questions. He stated that he was 46 years old (correct is 36), that he was born in 1975 (correct is 1872); he did not know the present year and said that he had to consult his wife. He did not know the emperor's name either and claimed that there was no emperor. [...] How many marks has a thaler [ancient German currency unit]? – "I don't have a thaler". – After two days he was completely back to normal, answering all questions correctly.[18]

In fact, many German psychiatrists described Ganser-like syndromes in traumatised First World War soldiers.[19] Jena psychiatrist Hans Berger noted that 'one always gains the impression of the mannered and contrived when the patient behaves like that without an obvious clouding of consciousness'.[20] The genuineness of these

---

17   Historisches Psychiatriearchiv Charité M9424/1918: Krankenakten.
18   Historisches Psychiatriearchiv Charité M8993/1918: Krankenakten.
19   For example, Berger, Hans, *Trauma und Psychose: mit besonderer Berücksichtigung der Unfallbegutachtung* (Berlin: Springer, 1915); Wetzel, A., 'Über Schockpsychosen. Ergebnisse von Untersuchungen an ganz frischen Fällen' – *Zeitschrift für die gesamte Neurologie und Psychiatrie*, 65:1 (1921), pp.288-330; Schioldann, Johan, 'Classic Text No. 87: "Psychogenic Psychoses" by August Wimmer (1936): Part I' – *History of Psychiatry*, 22:3 (2011), pp.347-367; Jaspers, Karl, *Allgemeine Psychopathologie*, 9th edn (Berlin: Springer, 1973), pp.325-326 (1st edn, 1913).
20   Berger, *Trauma und Psychose*, p.143.

presentations was indeed often doubted by the medical profession – leading to harsh disciplinary measures such as confinement to the locked psychiatric ward, or strict isolation in the Berlin and Jena patients.

British doctors, too, were aware of Ganser syndrome, which is not surprising, considering their pre-war admiration for German psychiatry and psychiatric literature.

One of their Ganser cases was 26-year-old Private Harry D., a married miner from Newcastle, who was admitted to the National Hospital at Queen Square with 'shell shock' on 1 July 1916:[21]

> On admission to the National Hospital it was impossible to obtain any history as to his illness or his past life on account of great mental confusion. When asked a question he looks blank and usually repeats the last word of the sentence, for instance when asked when he went to France he looked vacant, handled his identification disc and repeated the word "France". When asked where he lived he was able to say Newcastle but went on repeating it in an aimless way. Cerebration is very slow, when asked if he had any children, he repeated children and after a few seconds said "Yes". When asked if he had a headache, he put his hand across his forehead but said nothing. He called a watch a clock; a canary a mouse, and a pen a pick. When left alone he is quiet quiet but has a rather strained expression. He looks between 35 and 40 years of age and is going bald. On the day after admission he was depressed, not emotional but asked the sister of the Ward to be kind to him.

Two weeks later the patient was:

> … much improved. Knows his regiment – remembers he was in France in the Albert district. Says when he became ill, there was "a lot of shells" and many killed – almost 12 – lot of them ran away further back. Then went into trench higher up line – thinks it was March – and his pal was killed "Isaac" by a sniper – This was "a long time" before he came away. After this he was always frightened. Could not get used to it. Later "a big thing" came over. Killed a lot of his men. One man cut right in two. Had to pick the bits up and bury them. Remembers "a chap" telling him he was "daft" and should not "speak tongues". Told him he was "frightened" – he remembers no more – he found this morning he was getting his memory back. Is afraid of his "head". Never wants to go back to France again. Has always worked hard. "Everyone liked me the Captain and all. Was in charge of the sanitary arrangements". Now remembers coming home on leave in May. His wife told him he was "funny" and would not speak to people – remembers going back and hearing the guns and feeling frightened. He keeps on repeating "I was frightened".

21   QSA: Queen Square Records, Dr Russell, 1917, male A-K: case record Private Harry D.

Harry's approximate answers – paralogia – marked him out as suffering from Ganser syndrome; however, Harry was also suffering from a more deeply entrenched condition: catatonia. He kept repeating the last word of any question addressed to him – a phenomenon called 'echolalia'. His movements seemed to be frozen and his facial expression was 'blank' and 'vacant'. The cessation of all movement and the automatic repetition of another person's words were typical of the syndrome of catatonia, which had first been described by the German psychiatrist Karl Ludwig Kahlbaum in 1874, and could be part of various psychiatric disorders.[22]

The vacant stare

States of stupor, in which patients did not move or talk, and showed no emotional expression, were yet another variant of terror psychosis. The recovery from these conditions was often gradual, with a 'residual' state of general slowing of movement and thinking, which lasted for some time, but was not permanent.

Twenty-one-year-old John N., a private from the 2nd Irish Guards, was admitted to Queen Square on 23 December 1916.[23]

He had lost consciousness after a shell explosion and remembered nothing from that explosion until the time of his admission to the 12th General Hospital in Rouen:

> On admission he was in state of complete stupor and did not answer or pay attention to anything said to him. His expression was very startled and vacant. After a few hours he was again examined. He looked less frightened but only said "I don't know" occasionally. A letter in his kit was read to him and the name Belfast (his city) was repeated until he showed signs of recognising it. Next morning (16th) he showed more intelligence and began to speak a little. On the 17th he has brightened up almost completely and can give a clear account of himself, save the circumstances under which his present state arose. He remembers part of the shelling in the trenches and then nothing more till being here. He states that he was a patient in this hospital in October 1915 for the same condition and that he suffered from the effects for about 6 months and when he went back to the front he felt that if he was subject to the effects of close bursting shells it was very likely he would have concussion again, though he intended to stick it so long as he possibly could. He presumes he was again blown up.

---

22 Kahlbaum, Karl L., *Klinische Abhandlungen über Psychische Krankheiten, I. Heft: Die Katatonie* (Berlin: August Hirschwald, 1874).
23 QSA: Queen Square Records, Dr Turner, 1917, male L-Z: case record Private John N.

Combat, exhaustion and paranoia

Most soldiers struggled to shake off the horrors of trench warfare; they were tormented by unimaginable pictures of destruction, mutilation and dying. Even in a place of safety, far away from the battlefield, they were drawn back into the world of violence and barbarity. The trauma of combat could also affect the soldier's judgement, and distort his thinking and perception of the world without an actual impairment of consciousness and orientation. These men – for whom the entire world had become an unsafe and threatening place – developed strong paranoid fears after long-lasting deprivation and hardship; Kleist called this phenomenon 'exhaustion psychosis'. They lived in a world of phantasised conspiracy and intrigue, in which nobody could be trusted, not even their comrades. One of the soldiers suffering from exhaustion psychosis was 30-year-old Irish-born Sergeant Samuel D. of the 20th Durham Light Infantry.[24]

On 20 July 1916, Samuel was carrying rations to the trenches at Armentières, when:

> … there was great shelling of the British positions. Day after day he was passing where bombs were bursting and by towns that were being continually shelled. This 'got on his nerves'. When he returned at night he was unable to sleep for the noise of gun-fire and on account of his condition. At one time he completely lost his memory.

The sergeant could no longer bear life in the trenches: he became distant and detached from the world, and no longer participated in everyday tasks. At St George's Hospital in Tooting, he tried to strangle himself – and on admission to the National Hospital:

> … he was absolutely inaccessible, sitting up in bed staring round from one place to the other, and it was obvious that he was troubled with delusions and hallucinations. At this time his beard had grown quite long and he had a wild look in his eye. He persisted in keeping his attention on a window directly opposite his bed, and would look around, twitch his head, put his hand to his ear as though he were hearing voices. However he did not utter a sound. There was a tendency present for him to get out of bed, and it was difficult to manage him for a time.

It was hard to know what was going on in the young sergeant's mind. Because he appeared to be frozen with fear, not able to talk or communicate in any other way, it was not possible to get access to his psychotic ideas and experiences. From his behaviour, however, it was quite clear that his judgement was impaired and that he was hearing and seeing things that were not actually there.

---

24 QSA: Queen Square Records, Dr Collier, 1917, male and female A-K: case record Sergeant Samuel D.

Not only Samuel's thoughts and feelings had been affected by his frontline trauma, but also his motor functions: when he tried to stand up, his legs bent under his weight, he started trembling and fell backwards. Samuel was brought back into reality when a little girl of about 10 came into the ward to see her father. When Samuel saw the little girl, he spoke for the first time since his admission and 'gave vent to his emotional depression and cried' for the first time since enlisting. About three days after his admission, he was considerably improved. He replied to questions in a collected way and continued to recover until he was discharged from the National Hospital 'completely cured' four months later. He nevertheless was considered unfit for military service – presumably owing to his high risk of relapse.

German medical records likewise abound with cases of soldiers who developed symptoms of exhaustion psychosis while serving at the front line: like Samuel D., Reservist Edward E. could not bear the continuous shelling at the Western Front.[25] He was upset by every noise, and he started trembling uncontrollably whenever he heard an explosion. He had been sent to France in November 1914 and fought at Arras and in the Champagne region. In May 1915, he was sent nearly 2,000 kilometres to the East, to the region around Brest-Litovsk in Russia (now in Belarus), where he worked as a stretcher bearer. After only three months on the Eastern Front, he was moved to the Western Front again. He barely coped with the stresses of trench warfare: every shell explosion put him in a state of panic and agitation – and his head felt as if it was going to burst; then Edward started seeing enemy soldiers everywhere. On several occasions, he fired his rifle in the trenches, because he was convinced that he had seen a French soldier; however, when he approached the imaginary enemy, he realised that nobody was there. Edward's comrades noticed that he was absent-minded and distracted, and refused to stand sentry with him; his superiors became concerned as well. In November 1915, Edward was sent to the base hospital in St Quentin, from where he was transferred to a military hopital in Frankfurt. He continued to be confused and extremely anxious – wandering around the wards at night and imagining that he was still in the trenches; he also complained about ghosts knocking at the ceiling of the hospital ward. He did not talk much, but repeated 'for the sake of justice' all day long. When Edward was eventually admitted to the psychiatric unit of the Charité, he complained about anxiety and headaches. He made strange grimaces – wrinkling his forehead and averting his eyes – and it took him a long time to answer any question; yet, he was oriented and did not seem to experience hallucinations anymore. The Berlin doctors found strong evidence of Edward's psychopathic constitution: he had already been anxious and timid as a child, talked in his sleep and wet his bed until the age of 12. His cognitive development had not been normal either: he had to repeat the same school year three times. Most importantly, he did not tolerate woollen socks – a peculiar criterion often used by Bonhoeffer's team to determine the degeneracy of their patients. It also came to light that Edward had

25 Historisches Psychiatriearchiv Charité, M4956/1916.

frequently changed jobs. Originally trained in the diamond-cutting industry, he later worked as an orderly and as an unskilled worker in various factories. At the age of 15, Edward had developed a transient paralysis of his legs after an argument with a friend and required six months of hospital treatment.

Edward had not been drafted for regular military service; during his war service, he had not received any promotions or honours. Other evidence that was adduced – and shows the medical and cultural biases of the time – was that Edward's mother had suffered from seizures and that Edward himself was married to a Jew. Karl Bonhoeffer, head of the psychiatric department, concluded that the war had aggravated Edward's pre-existing constitutional traits and had only triggered, but not caused, his hysterical symptoms. Edward was not fit for military service and could only be useful in his civilian occupation. Although his criteria were outlandish, Bonhoeffer may not have been completely wrong about the role of a pre-existing vulnerability to exhaustion psychosis in Edward's case.

Another German soldier who developed paranoia on the battlefield had actually been rejected for military service because of his nervous predisposition: Private Wilhelm H. from Osnabrück, who had just qualified for university when the war broke out, was nevertheless determined to find a way to serve his country.[26] He volunteered for the Red Cross, was sent to France and was, eventually, accepted for military service. Not long into his active service, Wilhelm's older brother was killed in action. It does not become clear from the hospital notes if his brother's death triggered Wilhelm's mental breakdown, but what does become clear is that Wilhelm was soon physically worn out by 'long marches, shortage of food, lack of sleep and cold and wet conditions'. His problems started with a bout of diarrhoea; to ease his symptoms, his comrades advised him to drink three glasses of tea with rum. Later that evening, Wilhelm heard his comrades talking and complaining about him. During the night, he sensed that they were standing below his window – planning to throw stones at him. The next day, Wilhelm was still convinced that his comrades were plotting against him, and had now made plans to kill him. At night, he saw an ape being pulled up to his window – trying to throw stones at him. He noticed other strange things going on: some of his clothes were missing, and somebody had smeared faeces into his trousers. People were playing tricks on him; they wanted to declare him insane to blemish his reputation and put shame on his family. Wilhelm's superiors tried to calm down the young man and reassured him that he was safe; however, Wilhelm became unmanageable in the army base and was referred to the Jena Military Hospital. Very soon after his admission, he started questioning his paranoid ideas. Following a visit of his mother and sister, Wilhelm improved considerably: he became cheerful and open to conversations with the medical staff – and he also enjoyed his food, which he had previously refused, because he had been convinced that people were trying to poison him. After four days of inpatient treatment, he had completely recovered from his paranoid state.

26 Universitätsarchiv Jena, Bestand S/III Abt. IX, Kriegsarchiv, Nr. 405.

Most twilight states and paranoid reactions started suddenly and dramatically – following an event or circumstance that had been profoundly upsetting. The acute phase seldom lasted longer than a few days or weeks, and usually receded as suddenly as it began – leaving practically no residue. Although the outlook was generally favourable, relapse was possible – in particular, when situations similar to the triggering event had to be faced.[27] The Berlin and London doctors were wise not to send these men back into battle.

Terror and psychosis – then and today

Psychological reactions to stressful life events and traumatic experiences have fascinated psychiatrists long before the outbreak of the First World War: the theoretical framework to this concept was provided by philosopher and psychiatrist Karl Jaspers in his famous book on general psychopathology which was published in 1913. According to Jaspers, 'genuine reactions' were closely linked to a specific triggering experience; they would not have developed without this experience, and their presentation and course were closely related to it.[28] Furthermore, Jaspers assumed that the reaction had a purpose – mainly in form of a wish fulfilment. 'Instead of suffering, working through and adapting to an experience, it [was] replaced by physical illness, or by a wishfulfilling psychosis', although this latter idea was not universally accepted. According to Jaspers, the course of reactive disorders was favourable with remission of symptoms after removal from the traumatic situation.

Kleist was not the only psychiatrist who described acute reactions to traumatic experiences that were characterised by clouding of consciousness, confusion, stupor and re-experiencing of the triggering event: many of his German and British colleagues reported on similar reactions to combat trauma.[29]

Twilight states which are at the core of Kleist's concept would today be subsumed under the heading of 'dissociative disorders'. In dissociative disorders, the individual is temporarily detached from his surroundings; when re-connected with the real world, the dissociative experiences are usually forgotten or suppressed. In their dissociative worlds, First World War soldiers relived traumatic experiences; they re-experienced and sometimes even re-staged scenes of violence and destruction. Dissociation, as discussed in the previous chapter, was a desperate attempt to cope with an unbearable trauma; however, although the gruesome memory was temporarily removed from

27 Hollender, Marc H. and Hirsch, Steven J., 'Hysterical Psychosis' – *American Journal of Psychiatry*, 120:11 (1964), pp.1,066-1,074.
28 Jaspers, *Allgemeine Psychopathologie*, pp.320-321.
29 Fauser, 'Kriegspsychiatrische und -neurologische Erfahrungen und Betrachtungen', pp.271-272; Hübner, A.H., 'Über Kriegs- und Unfallpsychosen' – *Archiv für Psychiatrie und Nervenkrankheiten*, 58:1 (1917), pp.324-400; Hurst, *Medical Diseases of the War*, p.13; Mott, *War Neuroses and Shell* Shock, p.119.

the conscious mind, it persisted in the unconscious and could reappear in the form of nightmares, flashbacks or dissociative states.

Kleist's dissociative states bear some resemblance with modern conceptions of post-traumatic disorders, such as post-traumatic stress disorder (PTSD) and acute stress reaction. The resemblance to modern concepts of post-traumatic reactions – in particular PTSD, where flashbacks take centre stage – is striking. The question if PTSD existed before it was officially recognised as a psychiatric disorder after the Vietnam War, has not yet been answered satisfactorily (we will address it in Chapter 15). Kleist's concept might be an important clue towards an answer to this question.

Kleist's terror psychosis not only incorporates dissociative phenomena, but also psychotic reactions to traumatic experiences. This is all the more remarkable, as psychotic and dissociative phenomena have been artificially separated for a long time. We must not forget that the disease model in 19th and early 20th century German psychiatry was overwhelmingly biological: Kleist's teacher, Carl Wernicke, had been one of the founding fathers of this biological model – and Kleist himself was, at least, as much a neuropathologist as a psychiatrist (not unlike Mott). The observation that psychotic episodes could be caused, or at least triggered, by traumatic life events posed a challenge to this biological disease model (and equally to the genetic disease model prevalent in today's psychiatry). It is, therefore, a credit to the scientific spirit of Kleist and Mott that they paid detailed attention to the psychological mechanisms that could contribute to psychosis.

The idea that traumatic experiences could trigger psychosis was very much at odds with traditional psychiatric thinking: psychosis was believed to be a chronic disorder – inevitably leading to intellectual decline and requiring lifelong confinement to a mental institution; yet, many soldiers who developed psychotic ideas recovered within a short period of time. This observation was partly responsible for the introduction of the Mental Treatment Bill on 20 April 1915, as discussed in Chapter 3;[30] however, some soldiers with these post-traumatic reactions – with confusion, stupor and psychosis – were still transferred to asylums, which usually accommodated patients with treatment-resistant chronic mental disorders. There were still nerve specialists who had not realised that these symptoms were likely to be self-limiting – and therefore, did not require long-term asylum care.[31] In fact, most people's concept of psychosis has remained rather monolithic until the present time: there is mental normality on one side and insanity, considered to be a chronic problem, on the other. The cases of shell shock psychosis, and their often impressive recoveries, tell another story: life events can trigger psychosis – and although the psychotic illness can, subsequently, take a chronic course, it can also be limited to a single, brief episode. Patients with a clearly

---

30 'Nerves and War', pp.919-920.
31 Barham, Peter, *Forgotten Lunatics of the Great War* (New Haven, London: Yale University Press, 2004), pp.239-241.

identifiable trigger (such as combat stress) and a good initial treatment response have a tendency to recover well and only suffer a small relapse risk.

Psychotic and dissociative reactions to the trauma of war could prolong and aggravate the suffering; yet, dissociation and psychosis can also be regarded as coping or defence mechanisms; they could create alternative realities and provide an escape from unbearable circumstances. The next chapter will introduce the reader to these dream worlds of the Tommy and the Boche.

8

Dream Worlds

The Angels of Mons

> [I]n mid-air [appeared] a strange light which seemed to be quite distinctly outlined, and was not a reflection of the moon, nor were there any clouds in the neighbourhood. The light became brighter, and I could see quite distinctly three shapes, one in the centre having what looked like outspread wings. The other two were not so large, but were quite plainly distinct from the centre one. They appeared to have a long loose, hanging garment of a golden tint, and they were about the German line facing us. We stood watching them for about three quarters of an hour. All the men with me saw them, and other men came up from other groups, who also told us that they had seen the same thing. I am not a believer in such things, but I have not the slightest doubt that we really did see what I now tell you. I remember the day because it was a day of terrible anxiety for us... we later drove the Uhlans back with heavy loss. It was after this engagement, when we were dog-tired, that the vision appeared to us. I shall never forget it as long as I live. I lie awake in bed and picture it all as I saw it that night.[1]

The lance corporal, who recalled this memorable day in August 1914, was one of many British soldiers dazzled by a cloud of angelic warriors who floated across the ruins of the once bustling town of Mons and halted the German advance against a vastly outnumbered British force. It was, indeed, a miracle that the BEF held their lines in this first engagement for several days before being eventually forced to retreat – causing a crucial delay in the advance of the German First Army. The news about a supernatural force fighting alongside the men of the BEF spread like wildfire among

---

1 The *Liverpool ECHO* – 'The Angels of Mons: Strange confirmation by wounded soldiers, NOT A LEGEND. RESPONSIBLE MAN VOUCHES FOR THE STORY'; eyewitness statement, 12 August 1915.

Dream Worlds 137

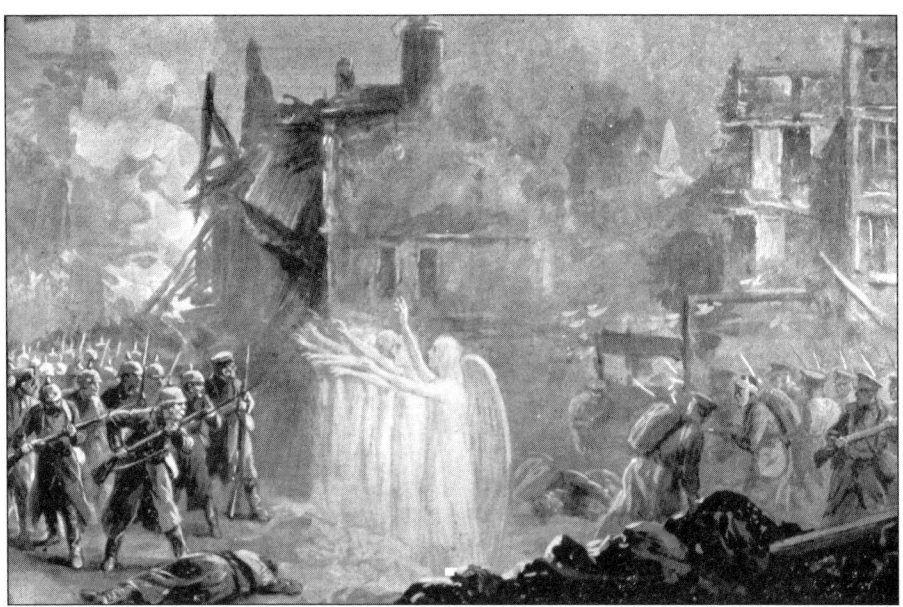

'Shining Angels throw a protective curtain around men from the Lincolnshire Regiment at Mons'; Alfred Pearse, published in *The Chariots of God* by a churchwoman in 1915. (London: AH Stockwell, 1916)

the troops, and became a popular anecdote at the Home Front. It did not matter that some soldiers had seen gigantic angels and others had sighted the longbow men of Agincourt: God had sent superhuman reinforcement to thwart the barbarous Huns.

Twenty-four years later, just before the start of the Second World War, British neurologists revisited the occurrences at Mons. Macdonald Critchley, an eminent Queen Square consultant, spoke about this topic at the British Medical Association conference in Aberdeen on 27 July 1939. He expressed the view that the Angels of Mons were a 'mass or collective hallucination'. According to Critchley, this was a phenomenon well known to the neurologist and psychiatrist: he thought that such hallucinations and distortions of reality could be largely explained by the physiological changes that occur when the body is exposed to extreme conditions – exhaustion, dehydration or agony. Such physiological changes in the many completely unprepared volunteer soldiers of the BEF could have been an explanation for the sighting of heavenly creatures at Mons. The angels might have originated in an odd cloud formation seen by weary troops – a mirage of the Belgian plains; alternatively, the Red Cross nurses – in their white robes (taking care of the wounded and exhausted) – could have been mistaken for angels. All these theories were discussed in the contemporary and post-war press. Critchley also emphasised that certain drugs (for example, those extracted from plants in Brazil and consumed in religious orgies) could produce states

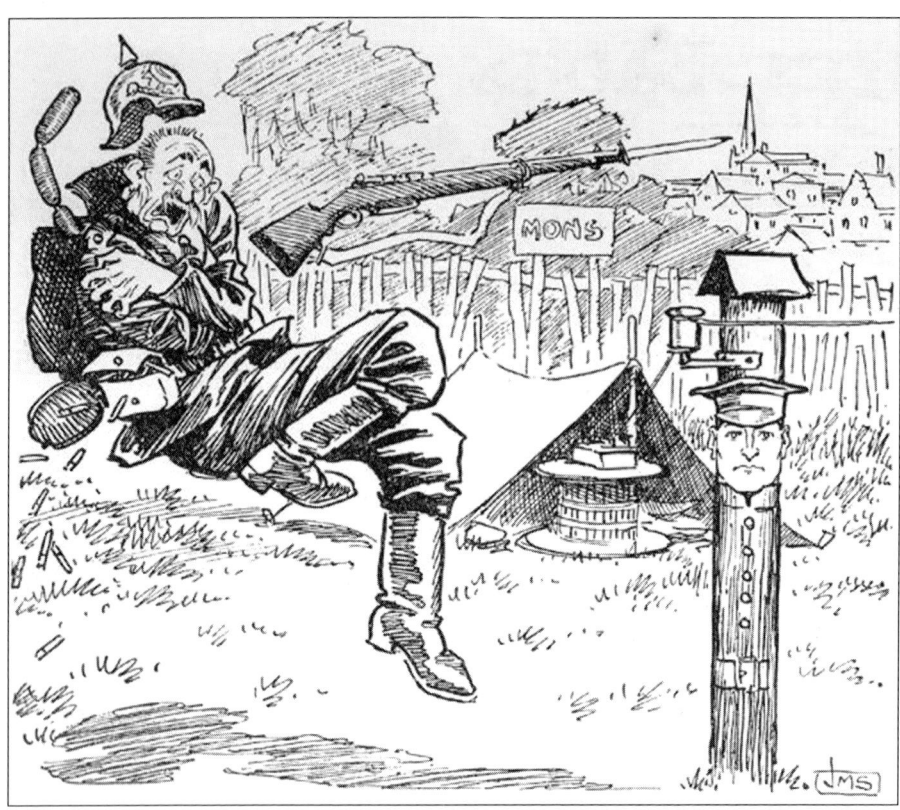

'Gott in Himmel! I am shocked!' – *Western Mail*, 1 September 1914: 'In this cartoon, a German soldier recoils with shock and surprise, as he touches the "live wire" of British resistance at the Battle of Mons. The battle itself has gained a mythic status as victory against overwhelming odds, and this is perpetuated by the reported sighting by soldiers of the Angels of Mons. In this cartoon, an elderly German soldier is clearly dismayed, as he confronts the steady gaze of a youthful British Tommy. The shock has caused him to fall backwards – losing his rifle, helmet, ammunition and a string of sausages.' Cartoon by Joseph Morewood Staniforth, Cartooning the First World War Project. (Cardiff University)

of excitement and vivid visual hallucinations, although he did not imply that these substances would have been used in any major way by the BEF servicemen.[2]

This was the medical explanation, but there was, of course, a religious explanation too: some churchmen referred to the Angels of Mons as a miracle and proof that God was 'on the British side'; however, the Anglican Church was deeply divided regarding these supernatural experiences. The dean of Durham, Dr Hensley Henson, preached

---

2   Reported in two articles published on 28 July 1939: *Press and Journal* and *The Courier and Advertiser*.

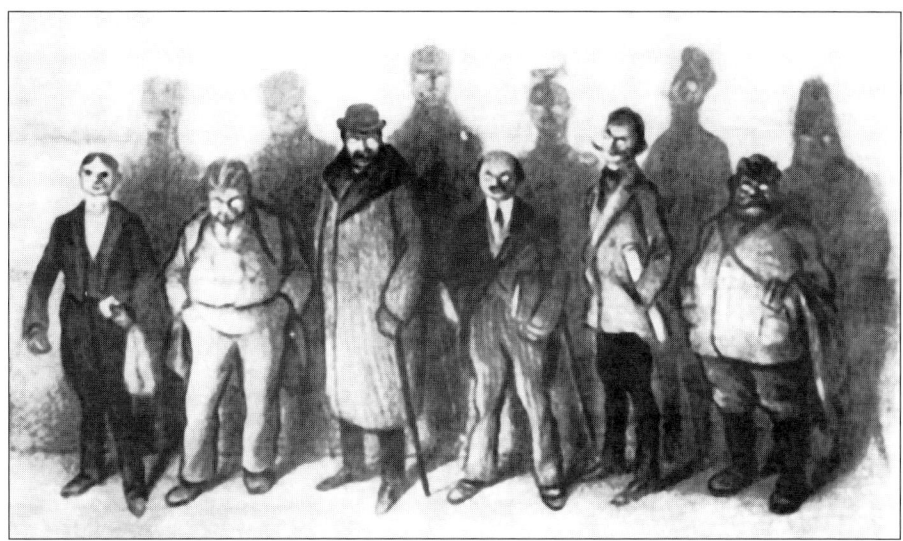

A collection of German spies, cartoon; from Hirschfeld, M. and Gaspar, A., *Sittengeschichte des ersten Weltkrieges* (Hanau: Müller & Kiepenheuer, 1929; re-print of the 2nd revised edition, 1980), p.399.

on these appearances in a service at Westminster Abbey on Sunday, 25 July 1915 and called the reports about the miracle of Mons 'grovelling superstition'.[3] The divided opinion within the Anglican Church reflects the difficulties religious people faced when trying to understand the war.

The 'Angels of Mons' were not the only vision reported by large groups of servicemen during the war: Arthur Machen, a former writer of popular gothic horror stories, published a short story called 'The Bowmen' on 29 September 1914 in the *Evening News*. In this story, 'St George and a host of English bowmen come to the succour of the hard-pressed British Army and rout the German hordes'.[4] Although Machen stressed from the beginning that this story was 'wholly imaginative', the fantasy was widely embraced by members of the public who wanted to believe in a miracle. Soldiers reported that they had actually seen bowmen in the sky – and Machen came to believe that the popularity of his story on ghostly archers at Mons led to the emergence and embellishment of the 'Angels of Mons' legend. In August 1915, he re-published the story in an anthology, and included in the preface a clear statement that 'The Bowmen' story was fictional and not based on true events;[5] yet, such stories had receptive audiences: 'mass hysteria' existed in both Britain and Germany,

---

3 *The Southern Reporter* – Thursday, 29 July 1915.
4 *Evening Telegraph and Post* – Monday, 15 December 1947.
5 Obituary Arthur Machen: *Evening Telegraph and Post* – Monday, 15 December 1947.

and rumours and fictional accounts resonating with the general mood (and playing on the fears, hopes and despair of a whole generation) spread easily. The most prevalent rumours centred on the suspicion that spies were active to undermine the war effort: 'It was a period when many otherwise sensible people in England came to believe that a vast network of German spies existed who used carrier pigeons, radio messages and signalling apparatus to send messages to the enemy'.[6]

The hardships of trench warfare

Many states of extreme mental alteration that we encounter in the soldiers of the Great War were begotten by the extreme stresses of trench warfare. Soldiers had to endure truly unbearable conditions, as 18-year-old Private Steward B. – one of the first military patients referred to the National Hospital at Queen Square (see Chapter 2) – recalled: 'There was considerable rain. They were not able to get water. The diet consisted of "bully beef", jam, cheese and bread. The sand would come into the food and this increased the thirst. They had little chance to sleep; the eye-strain was very severe'.[7] Physical exhaustion – caused by sleep deprivation, starvation and the forces of nature – was only one aspect of trench hardship; the nature of modern industrialised warfare – with its new weapons, bigger armies, increasing casualty figures and anonymity of fighting – had considerably increased the stresses imposed on the individual soldier. Static or trench warfare, as opposed to mobile warfare, often forced the soldier to remain in one position for days – sometimes barely able to move, because any twitch turned him into an easy target for enemy snipers. Boredom and monotony, passivity and a lack of distraction were the result; the individual soldier was left alone with his thoughts and fears. There was also the sight of destruction; of mutilated bodies and of corpses; and then there was the continuous shelling – sometimes going on for hours and hours, day on day. Men exposed to these stresses were under continuous pressure and felt out of control: 'The noises made by shells and the uncertainty of where they would strike caused great uneasiness and strain'. Arthur T., a 28-year-old corporal from the 1st Rifle Brigade, described the 'continual bombardment by trench mortars with aerial torpedoes'.[8] The Germans had used short-range mortars from the very beginning of the war: these mobile devices – short, stumpy tubes – could fire projectiles at a steep angle so that they fell straight down on the enemy. Projectiles could be fired from the relative safety of the trench – avoiding exposure of the mortar crews to enemy snipers. The British only caught up in their mortar production much later in the war – and this continuous threat took its toll on Corporal T.: when admitted to the National Hospital on 29 July 1915, he spoke 'of the feeling of

6   Clarke, David, *The Angel of Mons: Phantom Soldiers and Ghostly Guardians* (Chichester: John Wiley & Sons, 2004), p.69.
7   QSA: Queen Square Records, Dr Batten, 1915, male A-K: case record Private Steward B.
8   QSA: Queen Square Records, Dr Tooth, 1915, male L-Z: case record Corporal Arthur T.

helplessness engendered by the sight of the large lethal objects coming over from the adjacent trench'. The corporal became more and more depressed and had 'frequent and facile attacks of crying'. Even in his sleep, he could not escape the horrors of battle, but found himself in the trenches under bombardment – waking in a state of terror. While 'the life had done him good and he had thoroughly enjoyed it', the trench experience had turned him into 'a gaunt harassed-looking man, […] [lying] in bed without speaking or displaying initiative in any direction, with a look of fixed melancholy, [starting] apprehensively at any unusual sensory stimulus'.

Coping: strategies to bear the unbearable

How could soldiers bear these circumstances in the trenches? Did they develop strategies to cope with the unbearable? Kurt Schneider, a German military psychiatrist who later rose to fame for his systematic account of the symptoms of schizophrenia, argued that soldiers used psychological strategies to avoid mental breakdown: because soldiers could not get away physically they often escaped into a different mental space.[9] Some of them indeed saw angelic saviours and drew comfort from strong religious attachments; others brought themselves into a state between sleep and wakefulness – a twilight state that enabled them to keep a certain distance from the outward world. This temporary withdrawal from the horrors of warfare and retreat into one's inner self served to protect the individual from the intense emotional states of fear and helplessness.

Steward B., the 18-year-old private from the London Scottish Regiment (see Chapter 3), was in just such a state before being sent home from the trenches:

> … he was 5 days and 6 nights in the trenches at a stretch under [terrifying conditions]. The noises made by shells and the uncertainty of where they would strike caused great uneasiness and strain. Patient's comrades remarked that he did not answer when they spoke to him and appeared not to realize that they were speaking to him. Of this he knew nothing until told later on.[10]

When Steward was relieved from his frontline service, he appeared absent-minded and detached from what was going on around him. At the National Hospital, he was initially diagnosed with 'exhaustion psychosis', but made a rapid and complete recovery.

Kurt Schneider was not the only contemporary psychiatrist who described the tendency of an individual exposed to long-lasting adversity to drift into an altered mental state: doctors often described these stress reactions as 'dissociative states'

---

9 Schneider, Kurt, 'Schizophrene Kriegspsychosen' – *Zeitschrift für die gesamte Neurologie und Psychiatrie*, 43:1 (1918), pp.420-429.
10 Steward B., Queen Square Records, Dr Batten, 1915, Queen Square Archive.

because patients were detached from their surroundings – and sometimes, even felt detached from their own bodies. Through dissociation, they were able – at least temporarily – to protect themselves against unbearable or traumatising thoughts and feelings. The eminent Cambridge psychologist Charles Myers, who had coined the term 'shell shock' – and later founded the British Psychological Society – tried to integrate the physiological and psychological explanation of these dissociative states: 'Nature's purpose in repressing the patient's painful experiences is obvious. They demand temporary relief like any painful region or overworked organ of the body'.[11] Some soldiers drifted in and out of a semi-conscious state and plunged into a dream world – often clinging to memories of their pre-war life. This gave them a sense of control – escaping the feeling of helplessness and lack of power, and entering a more agreeable world. These men, who were not in control of the present and were facing an unforeseeable future (if any at all), took comfort in past memories and the prospect of regaining their previous life.

Siegfried Sassoon, the officer-poet who was treated for shell shock at Craiglockhart in Scotland, might have had these dream-like dissociative states in mind when he wrote one of his most famous war poems:

'Dreamers'

Soldiers are citizens of death's grey land,
Drawing no dividend from time's to-morrows.
In the great hour of destiny they stand,
Each with his feuds, and jealousies, and sorrows.
Soldiers are sworn to action; they must win
Some flaming, fatal climax with their lives.
Soldiers are dreamers; when the guns begin
They think of firelit homes, clean beds and wives.

I see them in foul dug-outs, gnawed by rats,
And in the ruined trenches, lashed with rain,
Dreaming of things they did with balls and bats,
And mocked by hopeless longing to regain
Bank-holidays, and picture shows, and spats,
And going to the office in the train.[12]

---

11   Myers, *Shell Shock in France*, p.70.
12   Craiglockhart, 1917.

Dream psychosis as alternative reality

While some soldiers slipped in and out of dream-like states, others gradually lost all contact with the real world: they developed strange ideas, behaved in odd ways and had experiences nobody else shared. These psychotic symptoms were not an active, conscious survival or coping strategy: rather, they overwhelmed the individual and replaced reality with an alternative world. Sigmund Freud, the father of psychoanalysis, regarded psychotic symptoms as a defence against unbearable images, ideas and feelings – enabling the 'flight' from a disturbing life situation. Other psychoanalysts described psychotic reactions as a form of 'waking dream', which could have a temporary problem-solving and wish-fulfilling function, and serve as an escape from a disturbing life situation.[13] Karl Jaspers, the German psychiatrist and philosopher, provided the classical account of this phenomenon in his *General Psychopathology*: 'Through delusions and hallucinations the individual's fears, needs, hopes and wishes seem to become alive and real. […] Reactive psychosis serves as a defence, a refuge, an escape as well as wish fulfilment. It derives from a conflict with reality which has become intolerable'.[14]

These wish-fulfilling psychoses sometimes took an epidemic course – spreading like wildfire from one soldier to the next. The Angels of Mons were the most famous occurrence, but many other similar legends of supernatural warriors, magic castles and mysterious clouds developed during the Great War; yet, many soldiers also developed their own comforting phantasies and religious delusions: for example, the German Pioneer Alfred P., who was injured in Verdun on 20 April 1916.[15] A shell splinter had travelled through his right thigh and left him with two purulent wounds. Alfred suffered from excruciating pain, which was so intense that he passed out on several occasions. Because he became increasingly restless and agitated, Alfred was transferred from a surgical unit to the Charité psychiatric department on 1 May 1916. Soon after his admission to the psychiatric unit, he developed a high temperature; then he saw God: 'God came through the ward, looked at the patient, called his name and said that his wound would be healed'.

Alfred started singing and told the ward staff that God had chosen him to be the Messiah and that he had suffered pain on behalf of all mankind; God had chosen him because he was a true believer and had borne the suffering for the world; God had told him to deliver the good news that the war was going to end soon. Alfred, strongly believing in his recovery and an imminent end of the war, felt calm and euphoric.

---

13 Bornstein, Maurycy, 'Über einen eigenartigen Typus der psychischen Spaltung ("Schizothymia reactiva")' – *Zeitschrift für die gesamte Neurologie und Psychiatrie*, 36:1 (1917), pp.86-145; Brody, Eugene B., 'Freud's theory of psychosis and the role of the psychotherapist' – *Journal of Nervous and Mental Disease*, 133:1 (1961), pp.36-45.
14 Jaspers, *Allgemeine Psychopathologie*, pp.323-324. Author's translation.
15 Historisches Psychiatriearchiv Charité M228/1916: Krankenakten.

By 1916, Alfred's wish for a speedy peace, for which he invoked God's endorsement, was probably shared by the majority of men on both sides: the Christian themes of his psychosis also reflect the wish to instill meaning into the meaningless suffering. Of course, it took another two and a half years for peace finally to arrive – and Alfred did not live to see this. Tragically, he died a few days later from the tetanus infection he had contracted with his wounds.

Extreme hardship and religious revival

Medicine regards the Angels of Mons and other hallucinatory phenomena that are shared by many people as part of a 'collective psychosis'. Collective psychosis can develop in closely-knit groups particularly during periods of hardship, and accounts of this phenomenon go back to time immemorial: the most recent British example before the war was the religious revival in North Wales in 1904-1905. Quarrymen and their wives, who had attended religious meetings called by the Chapel movement, developed states of excitement, agitation and confusion; reported visions and epiphanies; and communicated with spirits. Religious awakenings often develop under conditions of crisis and social upheaval: the revival in North West Wales followed a failed three-year strike by quarry workers for better pay and safer working conditions and is commonly seen as a response to this crisis. A large proportion of the population was suffering severe economic hardship, and the future was uncertain; such situations are breeding grounds for collective delusions and hallucinations. During periods of religious revival, delusions were frequently of a religious nature – and thus, related to the triggering situation; the delusional content was understandable in the context of the situation, and had a wish-fulfilling purpose. The experience of the religious revival also showed that these psychotic reactions to extraordinary life events did not result in long-term mental illness, but resolved completely without any special intervention.[16] Today, a similar phenomenon is occasionally encountered in pilgrims who develop a 'Jerusalem syndrome', which is characterised by prophetic behaviour and visions of the end of time in the intense religious atmosphere of the Holy Land.[17]

16 Linden, Stefanie, Harris, Margaret and Healy, David, 'Religion & Psychosis: The effects of the Welsh Religious Revival in 1904/5' – *Psychological Medicine*, 40:8 (2010), pp.1,317-1,323.
17 Bar-El, Yair, Durst, Rimona, Katz, Gregory, Zislin, Josef, Strauss, Ziva and Knobler, Haim Y., 'Jerusalem syndrome' – *British Journal of Psychiatry*, 176:1 (2000), pp.86-90.

Dream Worlds 145

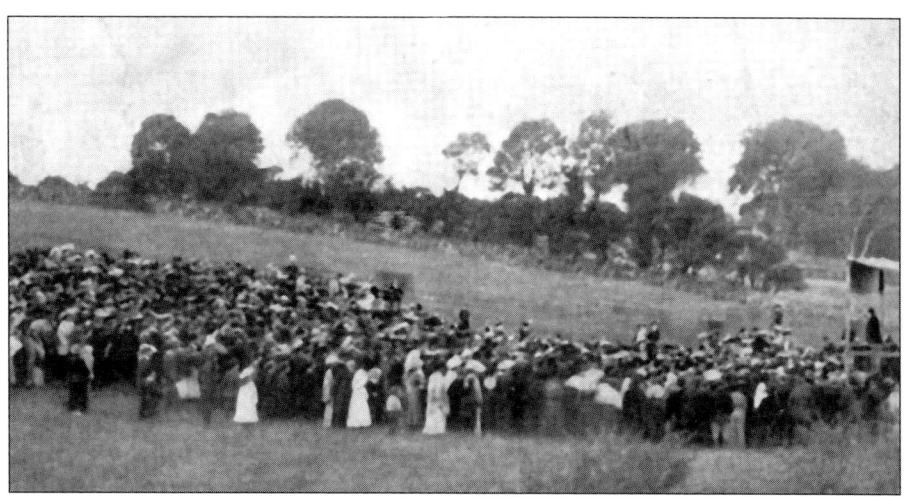
Welsh people during a revival meeting on a field in Anglesey. (Anglesey Archives, Llangefni)

For the military, religion could easily turn into a double-edged sword: belief in a just war and heavenly support was good for morale. Military leaders on both sides availed themselves of the support of the religious authorities, and the latter were eager to proclaim that God surely had to be on their respective side; however, if visions overwhelmed rational decisions, they could seriously undermine the war effort – and any uncontrolled religious movement (especially if it endorsed pacifist tendencies) was regarded as danger. It was easy to see the madness in poor Alfred's visions; yet, others who were not obviously ill specfically had to be declared mad if their religious convictions brought them into conflict with the official doctrine of a justified war (see Chapter 10).

9

The Ultimate Way Out: Suicide in the Trenches

Max K. was born in 1892 in Santomischel, Posen – a Province of Prussia – which in 1919, was to become part of the newly-established Second Polish Republic.[1] When he was 11, Max's family moved into the outskirts of Berlin, where the boy spent a happy childhood. On leaving school, Max trained as a waiter in Berlin for two years – and over the next few years, he worked in Hamburg, Geneva and Cologne, and also in London, where German waiters made up a big part of the hospitality industry.[2] He then joined the *Compagnie Internationale des Wagons-Lits* and worked on the luxury train lines that connected Berlin with other European capitals, and took a steady stream of well-heeled British tourists south to Switzerland. He also worked as a steward on luxury ocean liners travelling on the North Atlantic route.

On 15 December 1914, at the age of 22, Max was drafted into the army and served with the Leib-Grenadier-Regiment Nr. 8; however, his dispatch to the front was delayed because he slipped on ice and broke his right clavicle during his training. He was treated in a military hospital for three weeks and received electrotherapy, physiotherapy and massages. On 17 February 1915, he was finally sent with the 207th Reserve Infantry Regiment to Nieuwpoort in Flanders and fought in several battles; however, he had to go back to hospital in April 1915 after suffering from mental shock after a shell explosion. He was treated in a base hospital that had been established at the Benedictine Abbey of Saint-André in Bruges, Belgium. On his return, Max joined the 208th Reserve Infantry Regiment – and in June 1915, his regiment was sent more than 1,000 miles east to relieve Russian pressure on the Austro-Hungarians on the Eastern Front. The Gorlice–Tarnów offensive, which lasted until September 1915, resulted in the total collapse of the Russian lines and the retreat of the Czar's troops far into Russia. Max was promoted to deputy officer and moved on to participate in

---

1   Historisches Psychiatriearchiv Charité M7596/1917: Krankenakten.
2   Hawes, James, *Englanders and Huns: How five decades of enmity led to the First World War* (London: Simon & Schuster, 2014); White, Jerry, *Zeppelin Nights: London in the First World War* (London: Vintage Books, 2014).

The Ultimate Way Out: Suicide in the Trenches   147

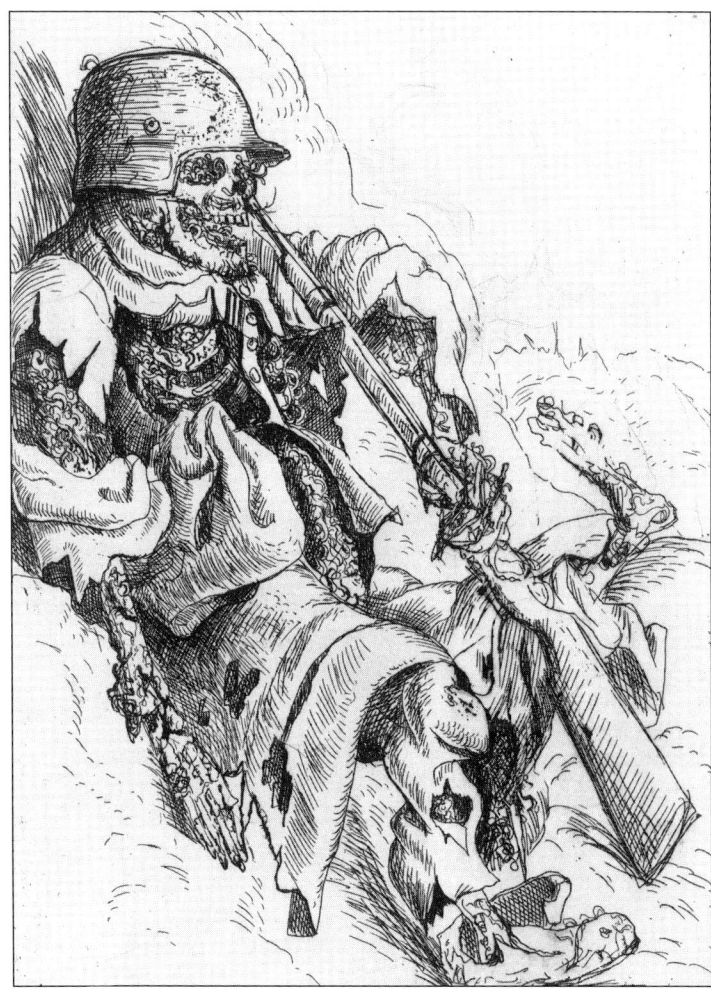

Otto Dix, '*Toter Sappenposten*' ('Dead Sentry'), from 'Der Krieg'; etching, 1924. (British Museum, Artists' Rights Society)

the Serbian campaign; however, his military career was disrupted again (this time for good), when on 6 January 1916, he suffered a gunshot wound at Stara Pazova, which was 35 km north-west of Belgrade. The bullet passed right through his brain – entering his head at the left and exiting at the right temple. According to comrades who witnessed the injury, Max continued running for about 800 metres until he collapsed. He was unconscious for six days and regained consciousness in a field hospital in Batajnica, in the environs of Belgrade. The bleeding caused a massive swelling of Max's brain and made his eyes protrude dramatically. Because Max's optic nerves had been severed by the bullet, he was completely blind. Doctors at Batajnica had to relieve the increased pressure inside Max's skull in an emergency operation: on re-opening the wound, where the bullet had entered the skull, large quantities of

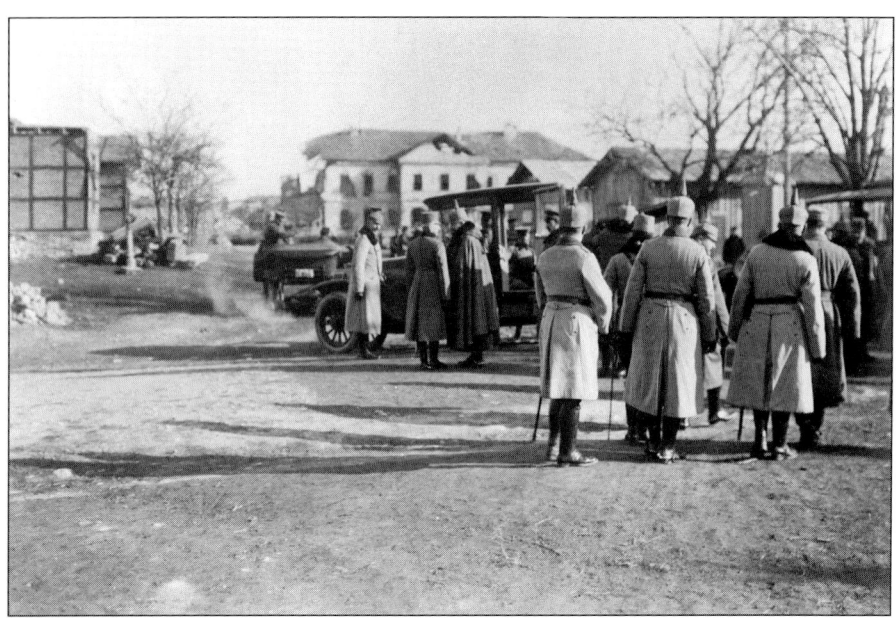

A visit of the Kaiser to the Citadel in Belgrade – the first German Emperor to do so since Friedrich Barbarossa (12th century), 19 January 1916; photograph, Q 27202. (Imperial War Museum, London)

cerebrospinal fluid shot out under high pressure – indicating a life-threatening situation. While Max was fighting for his life, he missed the opportunity to shake hands with the German Kaiser, who was in Belgrade at the time to visit his troops.

Max was still lucky: he survived his injury; however, because his optic nerves were irreversibly damaged, he would never regain his vision. On 12 February 1916, he was stable enough to be transferred to a military hospital in Munich, but he could not remember the circumstances of his injury. In March 1916, his treatment was continued in a military hospital in the centre of Berlin. Although it was relatively far from any of the front lines, Berlin was the most important centre for the treatment of military cases in Germany; Berlin hospitals accommodated 253,000 wounded men during the course of the war.[3]

By the time of his arrival in Berlin, Max was exhausted and in low spirits. He was upset because he had been kept in the dark about the circumstances of his injury; naturally, he wanted to know who had fired the shot. Slowly, his memory seemed to recover, and vague images of the life-changing incident formed in his mind. It slowly dawned on him that he had not actually been a victim of enemy fire: Max started

---

3   Winter, Jay and Robert, Jean-Louis, *Capital cities at war: Paris, London, Berlin 1914-1919* (Cambridge: Cambridge University Press, 1999).

to remember that a German officer had fired the shot at him, out of jealousy. Both men had been wooing the same woman, and Max had eventually won her heart. The officer, jealous and humiliated by the rejection, had intended to kill his rival. Max also remembered that shortly after the injury, a comrade had confirmed every detail of this story; Max enquired about the officer's name. Meanwhile, Max learned to read Braille and was taught to play the piano by another long-term patient, who was a professional musician. Between January and April 1917, he also had a job making hand-rolled cigarettes in a Berlin-based tobacco factory, while still being an inpatient at the military hospital; however, from early April 1917, he started experiencing problems with his right arm: the right hand felt numb, and he occasionally had pins and needles in his whole arm; he also suffered from pain in his right shoulder. On 7 May 1917, Max – now aged 25 – was admitted to the psychiatric department of the Charité. Like the National Hospital at Queen Square, the Berlin Charité was an academic institution with extensive research facilities, which also served as a training unit for military doctors. During the war, approximately 1,043 servicemen were admitted to the psychiatric wing of the Charité – and the head of the department was Karl Bonhoeffer, who was one of the most influential psychiatrists of his time.

On admission, Max was in good spirits and very talkative. He seemed to be completely absorbed in his music – playing the piano and various other instruments. He had learned to play the mandolin and violin from an early age, Max explained, and added that he was now capable of playing any instrument, including the harmonica and flute. His disability would not prevent him from enjoying his music: he could 'still play the harmonica in the dark'. Max also spent much time reading Braille and talking to other patients. He claimed that he did not care about his injury – and he did not seem to worry about his future either: Max talked about his plans of opening a tobacco shop with his friend, Karl F., who was still serving at the Western Front. Alternatively, they could open a beer tavern or hotel, where he could entertain their guests on the piano or violin. As regards his gunshot wound, Max still believed that a jealous officer had tried to kill him. Max insisted that comrades on the same transport from Belgrade to Munich had told him that a lieutenant had fired the shot at him; however, doctors noted that Max's speech was circumstantial and lacking in focus. He often repeated single words or phrases, such as 'isn't it', or 'as a matter of fact'. Was his account credible? Had a lieutenant of the Prussian Army really shot one of his subalterns in a fight over a woman?

A short note attached to Max's medical record proves that his memory had fooled him: on that fateful 5 January 1916, when Deputy Officer Max K. lost his sight and almost his life, he had written the following letter to his comrades:

> To my dear comrades! Because of my weak nerves and my inablity to fullfil my duties any longer, I have decided to end my life. My dear comrades, keep up your courage and faithfulness. I would have preferred to be hit by an enemy bullet rather than my own. I can't bear it any longer. Dear Schad, please send my belongings to my family. … With comradely wishes, Deputy-Officer K.

This note changed the whole story: Max's family found the thought that Max had tried to end his own life very upsetting and incomprehensible; in particular, Max's mother could not make sense of her son's suicide attempt: Max had spent Christmas 1915 with her in Berlin, and her son had not appeared in any way unusual. Before returning to the front line, only days before his self-inflicted injury, Max had been optimistic and courageous, and had tried to comfort his mother by saying: "No bullet will hit me." The only change his mother had noticed was that he was more talkative than usual, and also slightly agitated and distracted.

When Max returned to Berlin after his injury, his mother found him dramatically changed. He was irritable, agitated, aggressive and quarrelsome. His decisions were erratic and inconsistent, he frequently changed his mind and goals, and was restless and unapproachable; this was not the son she had left on the train heading for the Eastern Front after Christmas. On a visit to the hospital, Max's cousin confirmed these changes: Max used to be a considerate, delightful and optimistic boy, and he had been looking forward to returning to his regiment after Christmas.

Max denied that he had written the suicide note, although his brother identified his handwriting. His credibility was further undermined when Bonhoeffer's senior staff psychiatrist, Professor Edmund Forster, provided an expert opinion on Max's mental state and concluded that the young man lacked judgement and insight into his current situation. Forster, a navy physician, and later, head of the psychiatry department at Greifswald University until he was forced out of office by the National Socialist regime in 1933 (committing suicide shortly afterwards), is today mainly famous for another case of war-related blindness: that of Adolf Hitler, although it is unclear whether the professor actually treated him. Hitler was admitted to a military hospital in Pasewalk (near Greifswald) in 1918 for blindness after a gas attack. His medical records are lost, but later secondary sources suggested that he was suffering from hysterical blindness and had been treated by Forster.

When he was examined by Forster, Max could not remember the circumstances of the injury and did not entertain the possibility that he had fired the shot himself: he had a tendency to fill the obvious gap in his memory with fantastic stories, which he believed to be true. These 'confabulations' were familiar from patients with severe memory loss after long-term alcohol consumption – first described by Russian psychiatrist Sergei Korsakoff in the 19th century. Patients with 'Korsakoff syndrome' often have damaged mammillary bodies, small – but important – nodes in the brain's memory networks, which lie very close to the optic pathways; the bullet could have cut through those as well. Max's tendency to confabulate was coupled with an emotional blunting, talkativeness and lack of focus in the interview situation. With hindsight, it was impossible to establish the reason or trigger for Max's suicide attempt: it was not thought to be likely that a further judicial hearing would shed more light on Max's motives to end his life, nor that he would benefit from further psychiatric treatment, and he was discharged from the Charité on 23 May 1917 to another military hospital.

Max's story is interesting in many respects: first, Max survived a usually 'safe' method of committing suicide, against all odds. Max's case record provides a unique account of the time preceding his serious suicide attempt, his lasting disabilities and his coping mechanisms. For obvious reasons, cases like Max's were not discussed in the medical press of the time; secondly, the suicide attempt erased Max's memory of this fateful day, and also the time preceding the event, when he decided to end his life and wrote the suicide note. This could be a mere psychological reaction to the trauma, or a result of the destruction of brain tissue caused by the bullet; thirdly, the nature of the injury changed Max's character – bringing out completely different personality traits in him. From a medical point of view, Max's change in character and other symptoms following his gunshot wound could be attributed to the loss of function in that part of his brain, which had been severed by the bullet. The bullet had travelled through his frontal lobes – the part of the brain which plays a key role in higher mental functions such as planning, motivation, interacting with other people and self-control. Interestingly, this change in his character seemed to have helped him cope with his disability: Max was able to adjust to this new challenge within a short period of time; finally, reading Max's detailed case record, there is one striking issue: the fact that Max had shot himself, with the intention of ending his life, is only briefly mentioned towards the end of the record. Indeed, the reader is largely left in the dark about the circumstances of Max's injury, and the issues of suicide and self-harm – and Max's possible motives – are not discussed. Like Max, everybody else seemed to prefer the alternative version of the story, in which a jealous officer had tried to shoot his rival.

The stigma of mental symptoms, or the 'taunt of having nothing to show'

Neither his comrades nor his close family had noticed any obvious change in Max's mental state before his suicide attempt. In his letter, Max mentioned his 'weak nerves' and the inability to discharge his duties; the fact that Max had written a suicide note proved that his act was pre-meditated. He had decided to end his life and even wanted to make sure that his belongings were sent back to his family. Max could not think of another way out of his situation; he obviously experienced his vulnerability and struggle to cope as shameful.

Soldiers on both sides experienced mental symptoms as stigma and a threat to their reputation and peer group status: a soldier who had been fighting for his country and, all of a sudden, could not fulfill his duties, was seen as suspicious – and the inability to fight was always tainted with the stigma of cowardice, dereliction of duty and moral failure. Smith and Pear described the general public's attitude towards mental illness as 'a mixture of ignorant superstition and exaggerated fear'.[4] The shame of suffering from a mental illness forced 'a person to hide any troubles of a mental nature not only from his friends, but even from his doctor'.[5] Soldiers with mental troubles like Max were in a particularly difficult situation: because their bodies were unscathed and they

---

4 Smith and Pear, *Shell Shock and its Lessons*, p.78.
5 Smith and Pear, *Shell Shock and its Lessons*, pp.102-103.

had 'nothing to show', everybody was expecting them to function; conversely, physical disabilities were widely accepted as a reason to take a break from frontline service – and the 'taunt of having nothing to show' encouraged soldiers without obvious wounds to express their trauma through physical symptoms.[6] The stigma of mental illness possibly explains the large number of soldiers with functional paralyses, bizarre gaits, shaking, deafness or functional seizures. The physical symptoms were the result of a compromise; they were a way to escape the pressures of military life without carrying the stigma of cowardice or weakness – a legitimate 'escape route' for the traumatised or war-weary soldier, which was equally accepted among medical doctors and among the troops.[7]

Many modern commentators have overlooked how widely accepted the validity of neurological symptoms was in that period of war medicine: for example, the historian Jay Winter – editor of the authoritative *Cambridge History of the First World War* – argues that 'most physicians and serving officers believed that the entire category of psychogenic disability was a cover for fraud' and that physical symptoms without detectable injuries were seen as signs of 'cowardice or dissimulation', or 'a tactic to avoid facing the enemy'.[8] The literature of the time and medical case records, however, paint a different picture: although some of the more suspicious doctors thought that soldiers were fabricating many of these symptoms, the general agreement of the medical profession was that conscious malingering was rare; the stigma and ostracism associated with purely mental symptoms might have driven soldiers – subconsciously – to develop physical ailments.

Not only the expression of mental suffering through physical symptoms, but also the labels attached to those traumatic reactions, were relevant: medical diagnoses often became moral judgements and determined the fate of the soldier.[9] The psychopathy concept of constitutional inferiority, which was particularly popular among German academic psychiatrists, replaced concepts that suggested a causal link between traumatic experiences and psychological reactions, such as 'traumatic neurosis'. This constitutional model blamed the individual soldier rather than the terrors of war for the development of symptoms – and it was only with the introduction of PTSD as a new diagnostic category to the standard psychiatric classification systems in 1980 that the aetiological focus shifted, and the trauma of combat was officially recognised as the cause of breakdown – absolving the affected individual from blame and responsibility (see Chapter 14).[10] However, a century ago, patients would have accepted more

---

6   Smith and Pear, *Shell Shock and its Lessons*, p.14.
7   Jones, 'Shell Shock at Maghull and the Maudsley', p.384.
8   Winter, Jay, 'Shell Shock' in Winter, Jay (ed.), *The Cambridge History of the First World War: Volume III: Civil Society* (Cambridge: Cambridge University Press, 2014), p.310.
9   Leese, *Shell Shock*, pp.33-34.
10 Gersons, Berthold P. and Carlier, Ingrid V., 'Post-traumatic stress disorder: the history of a recent concept' – *British Journal of Psychiatry*, 161:6 (1992), pp.742-748.; Jones, Edgar, Hodgins Vermaas, Robert, McCartney, Helen, Beech, Charlotte, Palmer, Ian, Hyams,

easily that they were suffering from a physical disturbance, which could be cured by a physical treatment method, rather than a psychological or mental problem – and to some extent, this is still the case today.[11]

The healing powers of the war?

The history of Max K. also brings up another crucial question: how many patients sought to escape from the horrors of war by killing or injuring themselves? Did suicide figures go up during the war years? Alternatively, the stresses of war may have protected the majority of soldiers and civilians against the comparatively petty worries and concerns that contribute to suicide risk during more peaceful times.

Many members of the psychiatric profession indeed believed that war could be the great healer for all kinds of mental troubles that had been domesticated in the industrialised world: modern life, with its temptations and distractions, had led to a gradual – but steady – decline in mental and moral health. Neurasthenia, hysteria and traumatic neurosis had spread among the urban population. Jena psychiatrist Otto Binswanger, who had treated the philosopher Friedrich Nietzsche and many other celebrities, hailed the war as a great purifier and claimed a positive effect on the health of the nervously-strained youth. According to Binswanger, young men without perspective and aspirations in life, who had drifted into nervous troubles, recovered instantaneously to report to their divisions.[12] Some members of the psychiatric profession reported a decrease in admissions to mental hospitals – and this, again, was taken as proof for the invigorating powers of warfare. Similar opinions were expressed in Britain, as we have already seen in Chapter 3.[13]

One article in the German medical press aroused intense interest in the international medical community: Adolf Gottstein, a social hygienist, had compared the mortality from various causes – such as tuberculosis, cancer and suicide – during the time of peace with that of the first few months of the war.[14] One important observation was an increased mortality from cardio-vascular diseases in men and women over the age of 60; the stresses of war had taken a heavy toll among elderly patients with a pre-existing heart condition. However the most striking observation was a marked decline

---

Kenneth and Wessely, Simon, 'Flashbacks and post-traumatic stress disorder: the genesis of a 20th-century diagnosis' – *British Journal of Psychiatry*, 182:2 (2003), pp.158-163.
11 Yealland, Lewis R. and Adrian, Edgar D., 'The treatment of some common war neuroses' – *The Lancet*, 189:4893 (1917), pp.867-872.
12 Binswanger, Otto, *Der deutsche Krieg. Die seelischen Wirkungen des Krieges. Politische Flugschriften, zwölftes Heft* (Stuttgart, Berlin: Deutsche Verlags-Anstalt, 1914); Sichel, Max, 'Der Selbstmord im Felde' – *Zeitschrift für die gesamte Neurologie und Psychiatrie*, 49:1 (1919), pp.385-392.
13 'Insanity and the War', pp.553-554.
14 Gottstein, 'Die Sterblichkeit in Berlin während des ersten Kriegshalbjahres' – *Deutsche Medizinische Wochenschrift*, 41:25 (1915), p.740.

in suicide rates in Berlin during the first six months of the war. This, surely, was proof of the positive influence of war on the mental well-being of an urban population. On 21 August 1915, the *British Medical Journal* reported on these 'curious facts', which were matched by similarly promising statistics from Britain: the registrar-general's Annual Report of the vital statistics of England and Wales revealed 'some remarkable decrease of male suicides'.[15]

In 1920, the *British Medical Journal* provided a more detailed analysis of suicide rates in England and Wales towards the end of the war, and also in the time after the armistice:[16] while suicide rates had been 'unusually low' until 1917 for both sexes, the deaths allocated to suicide showed an increase in 1918 – especially in the female population. This increase in female suicides was particularly marked in the fourth quarter of 1918, which included a period of national rejoicing and relief from fears and uncertainties of wartime. The rise of suicide mortality in the last quarter of 1918 appeared all the more remarkable because the final months of a year had previously been associated with low suicide rates. The analysis of changing suicide rates over time also revealed that the increase in suicides mainly occurred in the female population of child-bearing age – and the authors had an obvious explanation for these figures: at the time of the armistice, many women 'were greatly disturbed at the prospect of the return of husbands who were likely to discover children – born or unborn – whose existence had been concealed from them during their absence on military service'.

The article not only discussed the motives, but also the different modes of suicide: while there was a remarkable decline in suicide by poison in both sexes over the war years (which could not be explained by a change in availability of these substances), mortality from coal-gas poisoning increased during the war. As would have been expected, suicides committed by civilians by means of firearms and cutting or piercing instruments also increased during the war.

Apart from these statistics, suicide – in particular, in the military – was not a topic that was openly discussed in medical journals of the war years. After the war, short notices about suicides of formerly shell-shocked soldiers sprung up in local and national newspapers, but did not gain much public attention. A small number of publications in the medical press after the armistice analysed motives and modes of suicide, and suicide attempts of soldiers during active service. Of course, the stigma associated with suicide was even bigger than that of mental illness, and we may suspect that the true figures were much higher than those reported in official statistics.

---

15 'The death-rate in Berlin during the first six months of the War' – *British Medical Journal*, 2:2851 (1915), pp.302-303.
16 'Vital statistics of England and Wales' – *British Medical Journal*, 2:3107 (1920), pp.79-80.

Why and how did soldiers attempt suicide?

An article printed in the *British Medical Journal* after the war, which had originally been published in an Italian journal in 1917, discussed methods of suicide employed by soldiers of the First World War;[17] sixty cases of attempted suicide in the military were analysed by the author. Surprisingly, most soldiers attempted suicide by drowning [15] and self-poisoning [14] – methods usually preferred by women – followed by jumps from high buildings or cliffs [11], hanging [9], cutting weapons [6], firearms [4] and suffocation [1]. It is remarkable that only four of the soliders used firearms – the method generally adopted by men in peacetime. The author tried to find an explanation for this unexpected finding: he concluded that military rifles were most inconvenient for self-destruction, 'especially when it is necessary to elude the observation of numerous comrades'. Furthermore, most soldiers who tried to kill themselves had previously exhibited signs of mental disturbance and were, therefore, under observation and deprived of dangerous weapons.

The Italian author also discussed potential motives behind the suicides: in his opinion, the vast majority of soldiers who ended their lives did so in a state of impaired judgement, of 'cloudy consciousness'. Although the suicide could be pre-meditated and was a genuine attempt to end one's life, the suicidal act was not based on a conscious informed decision, but the result of an altered state of mind. The remaining cases were 'degenerates with a bad heredity, morally insensible, inamenable to discipline [and] a prey to passionate crises', who acted impulsively, overwhelmed by strong emotions. Often, the attempt was made after a simple reprimand or punishment, or after a quarrel with a comrade, or the denial of a desired reward, such as leave or a medal, or unrequited love. We can only speculate about Max's motives, but perhaps his obsession with the rival of officer rank had a basis in reality and indicates that he, too, was led to this desperate act by an unhappy love affair.

In another article published after the war, Captain W.D. Chambers of the RAMC analysed all cases of soldiers with self-inflicted wounds treated in the Boulogne area between 1 March 1918 and 11 January 1919.[18] Chambers had been appointed 'Mental Specialist' to the Boulogne and Calais areas and was in charge of the mental wards at No.8 Stationary Hospital at Wimereux. Of the 22 cases with 'self-inflicted' wounds, he identified only three without genuine suicidal intent: 'one being deliberate to avoid duty, one the result of a drunken fight, and one following the attempt of a general paretic to kill rats with a Mills bomb'. Clearly, the last soldier – afflicted with GPI (another term for dementia caused by syphilis, as covered in Chapter 3) – had acted in a confused rage. The majority of the 19 men who had genuinely wanted to

---

17   Adams, Barfield J., 'Attempted Suicide among Soldiers' ['Il Tentato Suicidio nei Militari'] – *Journal of Mental Science*, 66:273 (1920), pp.164-165.
18   Chambers, W.D., 'Mental Wards with the British Expeditionary Force: A Review of Ten Months' Experience' – *Journal of Mental Science*, 65:270 (1919), pp.152-180.

kill themselves had tried to cut their throats [14]; two had shot themselves, one had injured himself with his bayonet, one had thrown himself under a lorry, and one had jumped off a train. Because soldiers who attempted suicide by shooting were 'almost invariably successful', they were rarely admitted to mental health units, which may explain the small proportion of recorded cases in which firearms were used. According to Chambers, the choice of suicide method was not a conscious process, but influenced by various unconscious factors: because firearms and war were inextricably linked, soldiers might have unconsciously chosen a different way of killing themselves; conversely, the daily contact of the razor with the throat might have exerted an 'unconscious but cumulative suggestion on a mind torn asunder by hidden conflict' so that this method was preferably chosen in this group of soldiers. Suicidal behaviour, like functional disorders, was also prone to suggestion – and this might have led to the imitation of suicidal methods reported in Chambers's patients.

The notion that suicides and the particular methods used can be triggered by reported suicides, or suicides in the closer community, has long been discussed: two-hundred and forty years ago, a spate of suicides followed the publication of Johann Wolfgang von Goethe's partly autobiographical novel *The Sorrows of the Young Werther*, in which the hero committed suicide. Although widespread imitation of Werther's suicide was never conclusively demonstrated, authorities in several European countries banned the book out of concern about the suicidal tendencies of Goethe's young readers. Similar phenomena were reported in the second half of the 20th century: press reports on suicides of popular figures led to widespread increases in the number of suicides – and the most remarkable in this respect was perhaps the case of Marilyn Monroe, whose suicide in 1962 resulted in a 12 percent increase in suicide rates across the United States.[19] Many people still think that the term 'epidemic' is a misnomer for the spreading of psychological disorders because they are not caused by an infectious microbe – and yet, one of the most stunning features of psychological stress reactions (including suicide and shell shock) is how readily and unwittingly they are imitated by others.

The blessing of psychiatry

Undoubtedly, suicide and self-harm in the armed forces were delicate topics; after all, attempted suicide was a military offence. Dependants of soldiers who committed suicide were not entitled to a grant or pension under the terms of the Royal Warrant; however, if the soldier's mental condition that caused him to commit suicide could be related to his war service, a full pension could be granted to the dependants. Many suicides, therefore, went unnoticed, or were not officially reported.

---

19 Ziegler, Walther and Hegerl, Ulrich, 'Der Werther-Effekt: Bedeutung, Mechanismen, Konsequenzen', *Nervenarzt*, 73:1 (2002), pp.41-49.

Did Max K. make a conscious decision to end his life, or was he mentally ill? The young man did not suffer from severe mental illness: if he had suffered from delusions, hallucinations or deep melancholia, his family, friends and comrades would surely have noticed and called for help; a state of altered consciousness, or hysterical dissociation, does not fit the whole picture either: Max had been functioning well, he was organised and his suicide attempt was premeditated; the young man had left a note for his comrades and taken care of his belongings. According to the contemporary publications discussed earlier, this degree of preparation was unusual. We get to know from his suicide letter that Max had felt nervous and 'could not take it any longer'. He had obviously hidden his struggle to cope from his family and comrades, but what was the verdict of the psychiatric specialists? The Charité doctors certified that Max had not been responsible for his actions, and therefore should not be tried. This seems to have been a common outcome: prosecutions for attempted suicide during the war were exceedingly rare, and the medical profession seems to have concluded that most cases were down to states of mental disturbance.[20] Hence, psychiatry served a very useful purpose for all concerned: a psychiatric diagnosis absolved the soldier from his responsibility for an unlawful act; yet, it also protected the military system against the major challenge to its moral authority, which would have arisen from large numbers of perfectly sane soldiers choosing suicide as the ultimate escape from the horrors of the battlefield.

---

20   Chambers, 'Mental Wards with the British Expeditionary Force', pp.152-180.

10

Desertion

Musketeer Wilhelm B. of the 161st German Infantry Regiment

This story started like many others: Wilhelm B., a boy on the verge of manhood – and not quite sure what to do with his young life – heard and answered the call.[1] Swept away by the tidal wave of patriotism, Wilhelm was among the first to volunteer, willing to give his life for his *Vaterland*; however, to his utter disappointment, the 16-year-old officer cadet from Neuss, in the Rhineland, was turned away because of his age. In January 1915, a few days after his 17th birthday, he tried his luck again: this time, they were willing to take him on – and Wilhelm jumped at the chance of making a real impact for his country.

And so he jumped in at the deep end: Wilhelm was sent to the Western Front straight away with the 161st Infantry Regiment. Life in the trenches was hard, but Wilhelm soon got used to the relentless firing of the guns, the shell explosions, cold nights and constant starvation; however, in March 1915, he was buried alive in a shell explosion. When his comrades dug him out, he was choking. Blood was coming from his mouth and nose, and he was unable to move his right arm. Wilhelm's torso had been crushed by tonnes of earth and debris; three ribs were broken – and Wilhelm was taken back to Germany. In a military hospital in Munich, his wounds healed and he regained his physical strength. At the end of April 1915, he was discharged to his reserve battalion. Once recovered, Wilhelm was itching to go back to the firing line. He did not have to wait long until he was taken to the Champagne region of France; however, a bout of typhoid fever, with severe diarrhoea, forced him to take another break of three months, but he recovered just in time to take part in the Somme offensive from July until September 1916. After a serious leg injury, Wilhelm was sent to Germany again for a two-month hospital treatment in Fulda; afterwards, he was granted 14 days' leave to stay with his parents in Neuss.

1   Historisches Psychiatriearchiv Charité M9423/1918: Krankenakten.

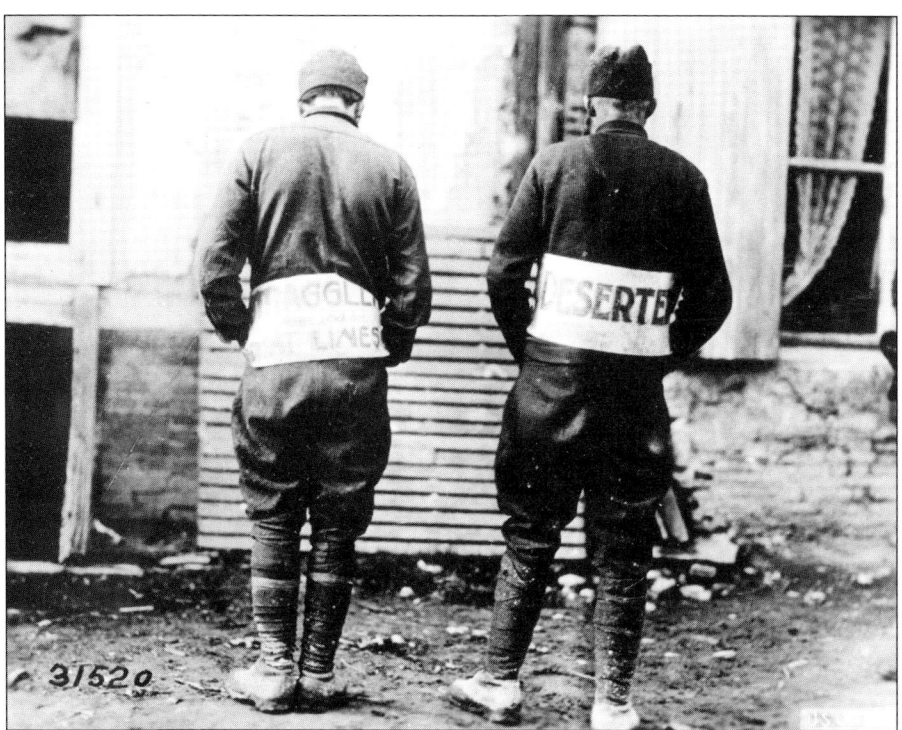
Methods used by Americans to mark stragglers and deserters; photograph, Q 70742. (Imperial War Museum, London)

From then on, Wilhelm's story of unbroken enthusiasm and dedication to fight for his country took a peculiar turn: we do not know what happened during his enforced home leave, but afterwards, Wilhelm seemed to have turned into a different person. Although the young man duly returned to his reserve base in Coblenz, he left the barracks two days later, went to the train station and set out on a northward journey, along the shores of the River Rhine. He changed trains at Cologne and returned to his parents' home. His father soon found out that his son had left his regiment against orders and called the police; it was, after all, a criminal offence to accommodate deserters, and civilians were obliged to report a soldier who absented himself from his regiment, even if this soldier happened to be their own son. Wilhelm was taken back to his unit; however, he did not stay there for long: the next day, he changed into civilian clothes and embarked on another journey home. His father, obviously surprised by this unexpected reunion, alerted the police again. Wilhelm was arrested and taken into custody.

Wilhelm was court martialed for desertion and fraud – the latter because he had travelled on the train without a ticket. The young man was sentenced to seven weeks in prison; however, the prison sentence was 'indefinitely postponed' and Wilhelm

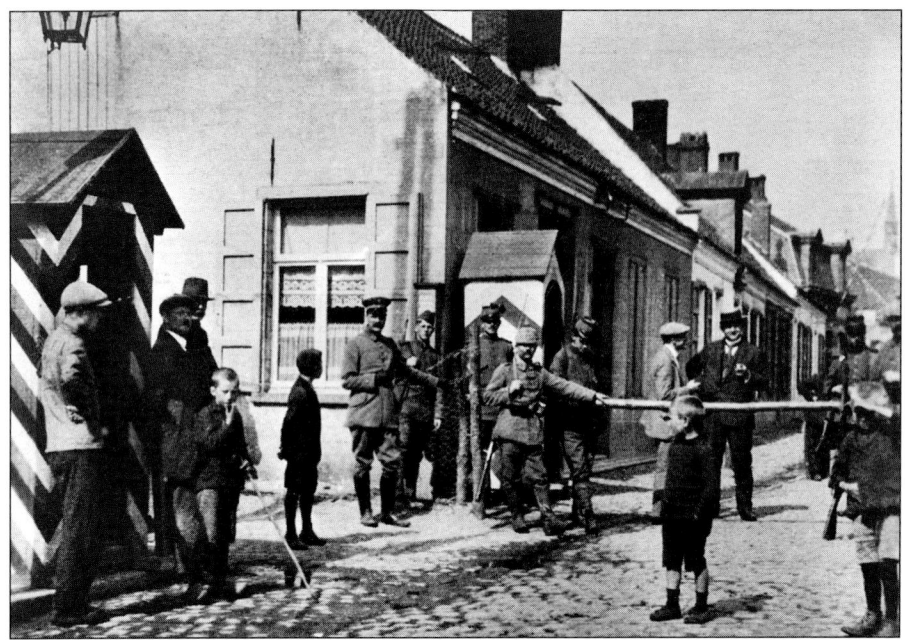

German and Dutch guards at a frontier post on the border between both countries, Q 88209. (Imperial War Museum, London)

was sent back to his regiment in January 1917 to carry out fortification work at the Dutch border. He was still in bad shape and suffered from a persistent facial rash. Because he asked for an extended period of leave, his sergeant accused him of trying to 'duck out of his duty' and punished him with extra military drill. Yet, instead of doing his exercises, Wilhelm went on a drinking spree in the local pubs, then to the train station in Cleve (close to the Dutch border) and travelled to München-Gladbach (present-day Mönchengladbach), where a friend provided him with civilian clothes. He then walked about 30 km north-west – disposing of his uniform on his way – to Kaldenkirchen, a little village on the Dutch border. At dawn, he passed the Dutch border, unrecognised by the border guards, marched through a forest and arrived at Venlo on 29 May 1917.

At Venlo, he encountered a large community of German deserters. Until July 1918, an estimated 100,000 soldiers (approximately 0.75 percent of all men drafted into the German Army) would have sought refuge in the Netherlands.[2] Although Wilhelm was welcomed with open arms by his compatriots, who, as a matter of course, provided him with accommodation and work in a grocery store, he decided to return

---

2   Gröbe, Benjamin, *Desertion im deutschen Weltkriegsheer 1914-1918* (Norderstedt: GRIN Verlag, 2005).

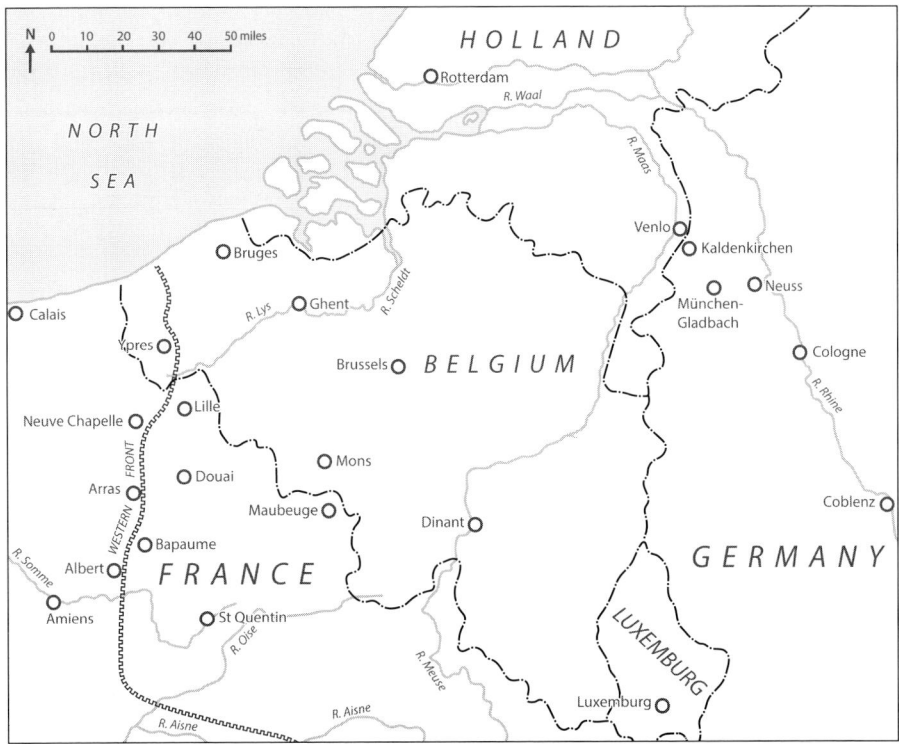

Map 4 The Western Front and the Dutch/Belgian/German border area; remarkably, Musketeer Wilhelm B. moved relatively freely back and forth between the three countries [Coblenz reserve base; Venlo, where Wilhelm lived in a big community of German deserters; Dinant, where Wilhelm was arrested by German military police; Neuss (parents' house), on the west bank of the Rhine; München-Gladbach (modern Mönchengladbach), where Wilhelm met his friend, is located west of the Rhine – halfway between Düsseldorf and the Dutch border]. (Map drawn by George Anderson)

to Germany after only two days. He reported to the German consulate in Venlo, was handed a written document and sent to the German border guards. Wilhelm was then brought back to Kaldenkirchen, where an officer from his company picked him up and took him into custody. This time, Wilhelm was sentenced to five years in prison for desertion. He was also downgraded into second-class military status – by which he lost his medals and forfeited his right to a pension. However, after serving a few weeks of his sentence, he was pardoned and sent back to his reserve regiment in May 1917 – and Wilhelm soon settled back into his routines. He had been incredibly lucky and should have learned his lesson; however, two weeks later, when marching with his unit towards the front line in France, he complained about right-sided chest pain and reported to his officer. The officer, understanding and concerned about Wilhelm's physical health, told him to stay behind and catch up later.

Wilhelm never caught up with his comrades: he shared a lift with two other soldiers who had also stayed behind; yet, instead of returning to their regiments, they crossed the French-Belgian border with their army vehicle the next day. Most of Belgium was, of course, still occupied by German troops, but some local civilians must have been happy to provide enemy soldiers who absconded from their units with food and shelter. Wilhelm and his new friends managed in this way for about one week, but were then arrested by German military police in the town of Dinant, which had been the site of major German atrocities against the civilian population in August 1914.

Once arrested, they were stripped of their medals and Wilhelm was taken into custody in Bonn. Because his behaviour had truly been odd and mental problems were suspected, he was referred to a local psychiatric unit, where he was treated between July and September 1917. Wilhelm was diagnosed with a 'psychopathic predisposition', with 'emotional blunting and shallowness'. According to the medical expert, he could not be held responsible for his repeated desertion and was sent back to his regiment. Again, he left the barracks on the same night and found himself in a Dutch camp for deserters and absconded prisoners of war (he was still in his uniform, and had, obviously, crossed the Dutch border without much difficulty). This time, Wilhelm stayed in the Netherlands for two months. He and other German deserters were taken to a British espionage agency and questioned about military issues, under the pretext of receiving a work permit. Wilhelm was also approached by a Frenchman, who enquired about military affairs. Like him, several thousand German deserters in the Netherlands were targeted by Allied Intelligence, which caused German authorities particular concern, because they feared that Allied propaganda would call the morale of German forces into question.[3]

Wilhelm then decided to return to Germany again. This decision seemed to be random and rushed; however, his move came at a time of an amnesty for German deserters: in an official letter, the Prussian War Ministry had emphasised that desertion was not necessarily the result of a 'bad character', but could be caused by 'strong emotional upheaval, possibly combined with opportunity and external manipulation'.[4]

This announcement marked a shift in the attitude towards deserters: they turned from dishonourable subjects who needed harsh punishment into 'lost sons' who had not been able to resist opportunity and temptation. Of course, the German military administration was keen to get experienced soldiers back from the neutral countries to which they had fled – mainly the Netherlands, Denmark and Switzerland – to return them to the front line. This was the motivation behind these more lenient pronouncements, and the amnesty offered in May 1917 through adverts in the national press: deserters who returned within six weeks could expect their punishment to be deferred, or if they returned to frontline service, even annulled.

---

3   Jahr, Christoph, *Gewöhnliche Soldaten: Desertion und Deserteure im deutschen und britischen Heer 1914-1918* (Göttingen: Vandenhoek & Rupprecht, 1998), p.122.
4   Jahr, *Gewöhnliche Soldaten*, p.192.

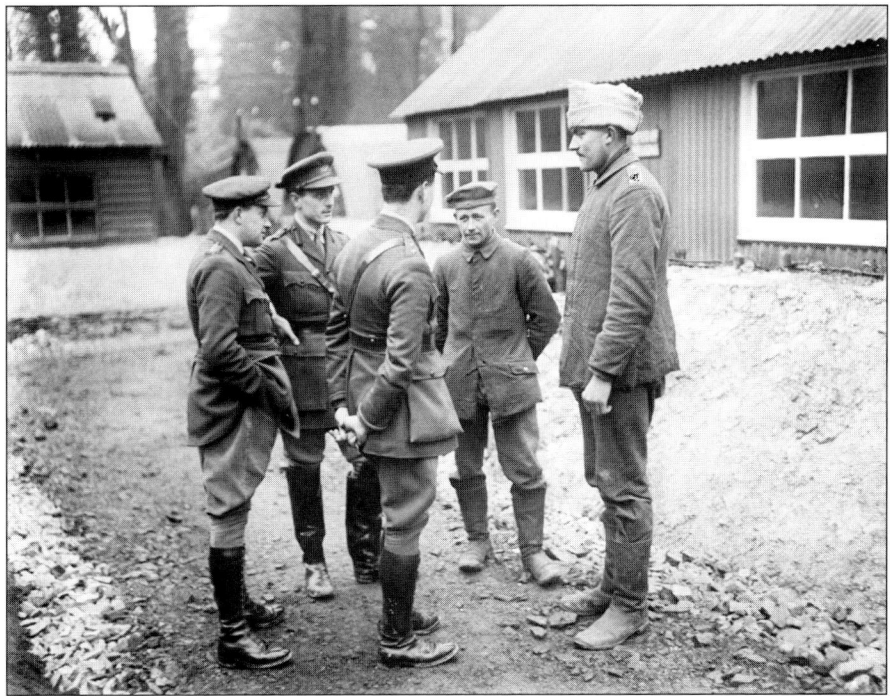

Two German deserters being questioned by an intelligence staff officer at First Army Headquarters, Ranchicourt, 5 March 1918; Q 10715. (Imperial War Museum, London)

Detention centres for deserters were established close to the relevant borders, where returning soldiers were registered and interviewed. At these centres, it was carefully established if they had committed other crimes (in particular, treason), or if they had fought for the Allies – in which cases, the amnesty did not apply. After this vetting process, most returning soldiers were repatriated to their army units; however, because German military authorities could never be sure whether returning deserters had turned into foreign spies, the German War Ministry did not allow them to work in munitions factories and other highly sensitive areas.

Wilhelm had to sign a form to certify that he had not been forced by the Dutch Government to return to Germany. Back on German territory, he had to carry out light duty with about 200 other returned deserters; however, because Wilhelm did not obey orders and threatened his superiors, he was arrested and held in custody pending trial for insubordination. In the meantime, the lawsuit against Wilhelm for desertion to the Netherlands had been abandoned because he had voluntarily returned to his regiment. Wilhelm's repeated offences against the law – and his reluctance or inability to act according to military rules – finally led to his referral to the psychiatric department of the Berlin Charité; we have already encountered this department as the capital's main clinical referral centre for German shell shock cases (Chapter 4).

Its wartime director, Karl Bonhoeffer, was also one of the most sought-after forensic experts in desertion cases where criminal insanity was suspected.

Desertion: A challenge for military and medical authorities

During the war years, desertion was a delicate issue, which was not openly discussed in medical journals; after all, the enemy should not be given the impression that morale and discipline were crumbling. Reports about desertion would also stoke fears among the own ranks and cause uncertainty and moral ambiguities – and it was only after the war that desertion, insubordination and other military offences became a topic of discussion in medical journals. One of the most comprehensive surveys of German deserters was reported by Alfred Storch, a trainee psychiatrist with interests in theology and psychoanalysis, who – during the war years – was based in military hospitals in Hamburg and at the front line. After the war, he worked in the psychiatric departments at Tübingen and Giessen Universities until he was forced out of office in 1933 because of his Jewish descent – having to emigrate to Switzerland.[5]

Storch concluded that the vast majority of deserters were honourable people who had turned into criminal offenders under the exceptional circumstances of war – and he identified three main groups of deserters: the first group were soldiers with psychopathic traits, whose abnormal personalities predisposed them to criminal acts under certain circumstances; the majority had not come into conflict with the law in times of peace. Among them were men with anti-social and unstable personalities who were functioning well within a multi-faceted and relatively tolerant pre-war society, but war had forced them out of their niche – had imposed tightened rules, discipline and conformity upon these individuals – and many of them cracked under these newly-imposed pressures. This group also included anxious and dependent individuals with separation anxiety, who left their regiment without permission to return to the safety of their home. According to Storch, these soldiers who escaped duty as a result of their constitutional weakness formed by far the largest group of deserters.

Storch's second group consisted of deserters who were going through transient episodes of severe mental disturbance; they suffered from post-traumatic reactions triggered by the stresses of war. Often these reactions, which were termed 'terror psychoses' by German psychiatrist Karl Kleist in the same year (see Chapter 8), developed after soldiers had been blown up by shells or buried alive, or after they had witnessed the violent death or injury of a comrade. Many of these soldiers appeared to be detached from their surroundings and acted as if they were in a dream-like state; these twilight states were typically transient and reversible, and patients later had no memory of them. Because such twilight states were commonly triggered by

---

5   Storch, Alfred, 'Beiträge zur Psychopathologie der unerlaubten Entfernung und Fahnenflucht im Felde' – *Zeitschrift für die gesamte Neurologie und Psychiatrie*, 46:1 (1919), pp.348-367.

active fighting, those who left their duty during such a state of reduced consciousness committed the particularly serious offence of desertion during active battle. The psychiatrist's expert opinion could, therefore, decide over life or death of the soldier. German psychiatrists of the time, including the Charité doctors, did not hold acutely traumatised soldiers who had deserted their units during such twilight states responsible for their actions, but it is unknown what proportion of them actually came to the attention of psychiatrists who recognised their condition.[6]

Storch's third group of deserters suffered from frank psychosis. This last group was least controversial in forensic terms: the provisions for diminished responsibility set down in paragraph 51 of the German Penal Code of 1871 stipulated that an offence was not punishable if 'during the commission of the act the perpetrator was unconscious or in a state of pathological disturbance of the mind that ruled out his free will'.[7] This clearly applied to states of psychosis – and psychiatrists unanimously held that perpetrators who were under the acute influence of hallucinations or delusions were not responsible for their acts. The same reasoning could be applied to the twilight states that were characterised by confusion and clouding of consciousness; however, the situation was more complicated for the commonest group – the soldiers who fulfilled Storch's and Bonhoeffer's criteria for a psychopathic constitution – which was not explicitly covered in paragraph 51. If soldiers developed other psychiatric symptoms as a result of their supposed psychopathic personality traits (for example, a low or abnormally elated mood), the Charité doctors were likely to conclude that they could not be made fully responsible for their actions. Other drifters and deserters, however, were judged to be fully accountable for their actions, such as 40-year-old Grenadier Hermann G., who was admitted to the Charité with Ganser syndrome (Chapter 7).

Hermann, who had suffered a head injury in France and, subsequently, underwent a long hospital treatment, had left his regiment to return to his civilian job as a bricklayer in Düsseldorf.[8] It took the military authorities nearly two years to track him down, arrest him and take him into custody in Le Cateau, Northern France; however, Hermann's strange behaviour brought him to Berlin, where the Charité doctors were asked to assess his mental state and accountability for his desertion. The specialists diagnosed a 'psychopathic predisposition', but judged Hermann to have been fully accountable for his actions. This is rather surprising, because Ganser syndrome was usually seen as a serious condition leading to diminished power of judgement.

6   For example, Historisches Psychiatriearchiv Charité M2942/1915: Krankenakten.
7   *Gesetz, betreffend die Redaktion des Strafgesetzbuches für den Norddeutschen Bund als Strafgesetzbuch für das Deutsche Reich*, Deutsches Reichsgesetzblatt Band 1871, Nr.24, pp.127-205, 15 May 1871, § 51: "Eine strafbare Handlung ist nicht vorhanden, wenn der Thäter zur Zeit der Begehung der Handlung sich in einem Zustande von Bewusstlosigkeit oder krankhafter Störung der Geistesthätigkeit befand, durch welchen seine freie Willensbestimmung ausgeschlossen war." Author's translation.
8   Historisches Psychiatriearchiv Charité M9424/1918: Krankenakten.

Wilhelm, the serial deserter encountered previously in this chapter, was unlucky enough to find himself amongst the same category: his medical records tell us that, after the shell explosion of March 1915 that had left him with three broken ribs, Wilhelm suffered from headaches, dizziness and irritability. Although he continued fighting on the Western Front, his mood changed over time: he was frustrated by his lack of advancement in the military hierarchy; his father had repeatedly expressed his disappointment and reproached him for not being promoted (and thus, it is perhaps not surprising that the same father turned him in for desertion twice); Wilhelm was angry and disheartened. Following his second injury on 12 September 1916, his mood deteriorated further: when his superior eventually told him that he could not hope for a promotion, he surrendered to a feeling of helplessness and despair; however, during his hospital stay, the Charité doctors did not detect anything abnormal in Wilhelm's behaviour: they did not find any evidence for a mental disorder, and Wilhelm was willing to answer all their questions; he did not try to downplay or justify his offences.

Ultimately, the Charité doctors overturned the view of their colleagues in Bonn. Karl Bonhoeffer, who carried out the psychiatric examination for the court martial dealing with his insubordination, concluded that Wilhelm's behaviour could be attributed to the disappointment resulting from the denied promotion. Although Wilhelm did have a 'psychopathic predisposition with a tendency towards heightened emotionality', this diagnosis on its own did not fulfil the criteria for a pathological disturbance of the mind. Dysphoria and irritability during the period leading up to the offences were not accepted as causes of diminished responsibility – and Bonhoeffer thus concluded that Wilhelm had not been affected by a relevant mental illness while committing these offences, and that he was fit to stand trial.

Musketeer Adolf S. of the 166th Infantry Regiment

However, in other cases, the Charité doctors acknowledged that soldiers with psychopathic traits had difficulties coping with the immense stresses of active service. These young men were prone to mental breakdown and stress reactions – and if there was evidence of a profound emotional disturbance, they were often judged as having diminished responsibility, as in the case of 23-year-old Musketeer Adolf S.[9]

Adolf was born in Saargemuend in Alsace-Lorraine – formerly French territory which had been annexed by the German Empire following victory in the Franco-Prussian War of 1870-1871. Like Wilhelm, Adolf had started out as a commendable soldier: an actor and musician in civilian life, he was drafted into the army on 18 May 1915 and served with the 166th Infantry Regiment. He fought on the Eastern Front from October 1915 until June 1916, when he was wounded: while on patrol, Adolf had climbed a tree to observe the enemy lines. A bullet from a machine gun grazed his head; at the same time, a shell exploded and Adolf – shocked by the sudden blast

9   Historisches Psychiatriearchiv Charité M9517/1918: Krankenakten.

– fell off the tree and onto his head. He was unconscious for 14 hours and was taken to a base hospital at Schiradow, close to Warsaw. He recovered within two months and was sent back to the front line, but like Wilhelm, he seemed to have changed during his injury break: the feisty and boisterous showman had turned into a fragile and vulnerable individual – prone to headaches, hot flushes and fatigue. When he asked for leave, his request was turned down by the medical officer. Adolf was furious – and on the same evening, left for the next base hospital in Kowel, where he claimed to have lost his letter of referral. He stayed there for two weeks, but was then taken into custody in Drosny. Adolf absconded again, bought a uniform of a NCO and went for long walks during the day. He spent the nights drinking in pubs – sleeping rough for four weeks. On 12 December 1916, he was arrested again and taken into custody; on 20 January 1917, he was sentenced to three months in prison, but was granted amnesty one week later.

In early February, Adolf was transferred to the 203rd Reserve Infantry Regiment in Tegel/Berlin. After a few days there, he was asked to sell tickets for a charity concert in Berlin. He sold 11 tickets and then visited several pubs, drank beer and brandy, and went off with a prostitute. When he woke up, the woman had taken all the money he had raised. Adolf could not face returning to his company: he forged a leave form and, because he was bankrupt, worked in a shell factory for 10 days – but then, things got completely out of hand: Adolf – like before – put on an officer's uniform and rented five different rooms spread over the city. From one landlady, he stole a pair of leather boots; from the others, he took money – pretending that he could supply them with food. Adolf indulged in Berlin's nightlife and spent his time in pubs and at the theatre. This dissolute lifestyle was only made possible by the Germans' deeply entrenched respect for military paraphernalia – famously ridiculed in Carl Zuckmayer's play 'The Captain of Koepenick' about the impostor Wilhelm Voigt, who in 1906 donned a military uniform and brought a group of soldiers under his command.

However, Adolf's high life found its sudden end when he was arrested by a patrol on the night of 21 March 1917: he was taken into custody – and on 12 April 1917, was sentenced to eight and a half months in prison; however, he only spent two weeks in Spandau prison and was then sent to a labour corps in Schleswig in Northern Germany, where he built trenches at the Danish border. In the meantime, Adolf's other criminal acts – the theft and fraud committed in Berlin – came to light, and he was taken into custody again (this time in Schleswig). He was sentenced by a military court in Altona (near Hamburg) to one year in prison, and – like Wilhelm – downgraded to second-class military status. Very soon, he was transferred to a penal company in the Rhineland, where he worked in a shell factory. Because of his good conduct, he was discharged from there on 8 May 1918 and sent back to his unit in Berlin.

The story does not end here: over Whitsuntide, Adolf was granted leave. He rented a flat in the centre of Berlin and enjoyed himself in amusement parks, pubs and on the beach of Lake Wannsee. He pulled off his old trick again – dressing up as an NCO – and engaged in more fraudulent behaviour, until he was finally arrested. The police

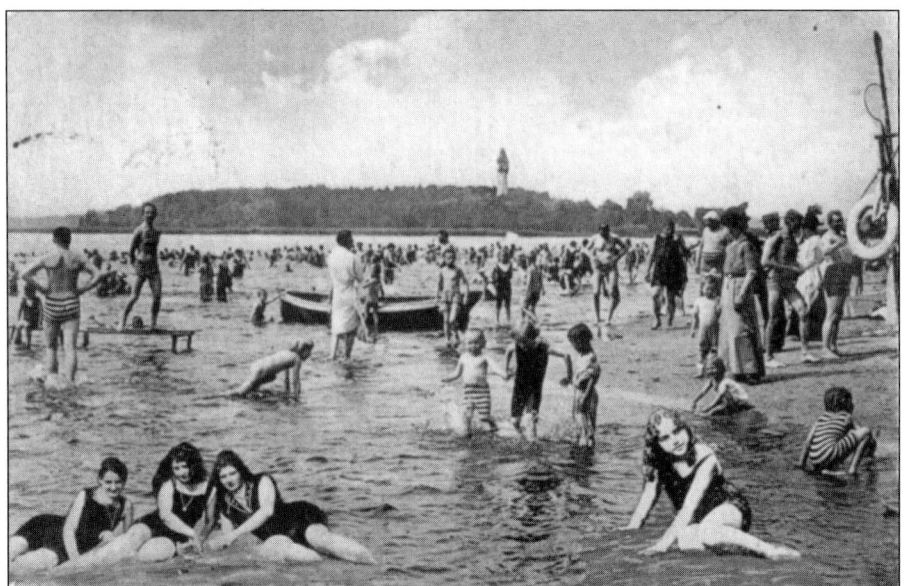

Familien-Freibad Wannsee/Berlin; postcard, 1916. (Author's own archive)

officer had followed Adolf for some time, because he looked suspiciously young in his NCO's uniform. On 25 May, he was taken into custody again and transferred to the psychiatric unit of the Berlin Charité.

At the Charité, Adolf's state of mind and body were put under the microscope – and his personal history was on the agenda as well: he had left school at the age of 14, and then stayed with his parents to help out in the family business. At his father's distillery, he had been exposed to alcohol from an early age and had started drinking wine, brandy and schnapps from the age of 10. At the age of 16, he had moved to Cologne to study at the Academy of Music and Dance. He studied piano, violin and mandolin, and also ballet and acting. At the age of 19, Adolf had his first engagement at the Metropol-Theatre in Cologne; he started with a salary of 35 Marks per month. With his increasing popularity, his salary rose to 1,200 Marks per month in August 1914 (equivalent to the average annual salary of the German workforce) until he was drafted into the army on 18 May 1915. As a tenor and comedian, he played leading parts in operettas and cabaret shows. Adolf enjoyed his lavish lifestyle, indulged in champagne and frequent affairs, and never saved any money. According to his own report, he had 20 glasses of beer every day – and on some evenings, three to four bottles of wine. On one occasion, he had been arrested and sentenced to two weeks in prison because of the indecent assault of a girl, whom he had kissed in the street. Although Adolf had never suffered from serious mental symptoms – neither had anybody in his extended family – his lifestyle was excessive, self-indulgent and unstable. Adolf was highly suggestible and often changed his mind and plans; he was unreliable and could not handle his finances. The Charité doctors also noted that he had always liked to play tricks on others and had been cruel to animals as a child – arousing their suspicion of a psychopathic disposition.

Adolf was also subjected to extensive cognitive testing: his general knowledge, attention, memory, common sense and cognitive flexibility were tested, rated and analysed; his reasoning turned out to be intact. Adolf had no difficulty in finding the absurdity in the following story: 'Recently, a dead body, which had been cut into 18 pieces, was found in a forest. Suicide was suspected'. Adolf demonstrated a deep knowledge of politics, history and geography; to the examiner's surprise, however, he was not able to answer basic questions about music theory and musical genres: for example, he could not name the operas of Richard Wagner and claimed that this high priest of serious German music had composed several operettas; the way he answered these questions bears striking resemblance to the Ganser syndrome. Adolf also had difficulties with musical scales and keys. As regards his practical skills, Adolf was asked to play a piece of his choice on the piano. He sat on the piano stool, and – in virtuoso's style – put his hands on the keys and started playing; however, he did not strike the right chords and claimed that the piano was out of tune.

Although Adolf's case is very similar to that of Wilhelm – and both men had committed equally serious criminal offences according to the military law of the time – Bonhoeffer's final conclusions were fundamentally different: like Wilhelm, Adolf obtained a diagnosis of 'psychopathic predisposition'; like Wilhelm, he belonged to the group of unstable psychopaths described by Storch. In civilian life, Adolf had found his niche in the music and dance world; however, his psychiatrists accepted that military life posed too much of a challenge for this excitable young man. Unable to comply with military rules – and lacking an aim and purpose in life – Adolf had given in to the impulse to run away and had also committed other offences. Bonhoeffer accepted Adolf's inborn psychopathic traits as causes of a diminished responsibility.

Wilhelm's and Adolf's cases were not straightforward for the Charité psychiatrists, even after several years of experience with shell-shocked soldiers: both men did not actually suffer from serious mental illness, or obvious symptoms of shell shock; both men had had a clear intention to escape their duties. For that very reason, it is striking that they had not been subjected to harsher punishments before being sent to the Charité. The legal framework in Germany was provided by the *Militärstrafgesetzbuch* (MStGB – military penal code) of 20 June 1872, which – subject to minor amendmends and changes – was in place until 1918. This law distinguished between 'absence without leave' (§ 64) and 'desertion' (§69), when a soldier abandoned his unit with the intent to permanently escape his duties. Absence without leave and desertion both counted as serious military offences: in the German Army, absence without leave of more than three days could be punished with up to two years in prison, and absence without leave exceeding seven days with up to five years in prison (§§ 64, 66 MStGB). Those who deserted during active service risked prison sentences of five to 10 years, but for repeat offenders, even a life sentence or the death penalty were possible outcomes (§ 71 MStGB). One problem was that, when the First World War had started, many soldiers would have found most of these punishments more appealing than frontline service: imprisonment at home was clearly less stressful than fighting in the trenches – and this is why many soldiers were sentenced to hard physical labour instead (often close to the front line).

Families of deserters were denied financial support, to put moral pressure on those who had breached (or were thinking about breaching) military laws. In addition to a prison sentence, desertion could also result in downgrading into second-class military status, as illustrated in Wilhelm's and Adolf's cases (§§ 39, 74 MStGB). Later in the war, on 25 April 1917, the minimum punishment for desertion during frontline service was reduced from five years to one year in prison; in cases of repeated desertion during frontline service, the death penalty could be abandoned in favour of a lifelong prison sentence; even old sentences could be revised, according to the new law. These changes, and the amnesty of May 1917, may have reflected the insight that no degree of punishment was going to prevent desertion. Desertion increased towards the end of the war – showing the increasing disintegration of the German Army; however, even according to the highest estimates, the overall number of deserters remained below one percent of the total military manpower – and thus never reached real military significance.[10]

Deserters in the British Army

The British military penal law that was in force in 1914 was composed of two major sources: its centrepiece was the 'Army (Annual) Act' (AA) of 1881, which was supplemented by the 'King's (Queen's) Regulations' of 1912. The 'Manual of Military Law' (MML) served as a general reference for legal military issues, and explained and illustrated all offences, their corresponding punishments and instructions on how to run a court martial. Like in Germany, British military law also distinguished between absence without leave and desertion: 'The criterion between desertion and absence without leave is Intention. The offence of desertion … implies an intention on the part of the offender either not to return to His Majesty's Service at all, or to escape some particular important Service« (MML III. 13)'.

'To escape some particular important service' meant that a soldier who stayed behind during an offensive was classified as a deserter, even if he did not have the intention to permanently escape his duties. According to German military law, this would have been absence without leave or cowardice, which was punished with up to five years in prison (§ 85 MSGB).[11]

---

10   Jahr, *Gewöhnliche Soldaten*, p. 150 ff.
11   Jahr, *Gewöhnliche Soldaten*, p.88 ff.

The British military justice system seems to have imposed much harsher and arbitrary punishments on deserters than its German equivalent:[12] the Army Act stipulated that every soldier on active service who deserted, or intended to do so, was sentenced to death 'or any other less severe legal punishment'. This left much scope for interpretation: because there was so much room for interpretation, the court could sentence a deserter to a few weeks in custody, but also to death – even if he had only been absent for a few hours. This policy of uncertainty and deterrence seems to have fulfilled its purpose: even soldiers who were at the brink of nervous breakdown – physically worn out and mentally shaken – kept fighting.

Particular difficulties arose when soldiers were torn between their military duties and home commitments: Daniel T., a 45-year-old private of the East Lancashires, 'A' Company, received official notification of his wife's death and burial during Christmas 1914, when he was serving in the trenches at 'Plug Street' – a small Belgian village close to the French border (about eight miles south of Ypres), whose actual name was Ploegsteert.[13] Naturally, the news rather upset him. He applied for furlough in order to look after his affairs at home and to take care of his wife's effects, but his application was refused. From this time on, Daniel was restless, nervous and absent-minded. Every missile or detonation made him jump and triggered violent shaking of his body; however, leaving his regiment without official permission was not an option; Daniel would have risked his life. When it came to desertion, exceptional circumstances did not count, so Daniel continued his front-line duties. On 8 February 1915, a bullet passed very close to his face – clipping off a piece of skin from his neck. This gave him a great shock and left him in a rather dazed condition; then the exhaustion set in – and the tormenting headaches. The next day, he was ordered to march to the reserve billets, which were about six miles to the rear. Daniel could not keep up with his comrades: 'Slowly and with great effort', he made his way to the hospital in Armentières – a distance of five miles – where he was diagnosed with shell shock; he was eventually sent to England, to be treated at the National Hospital. Back home, he recovered quickly and 'a letter from his sisters had a soothing influence on him'.

Stragglers and deserters who did not enjoy the protection of the medical system were at real danger of suffering severe punishments: between 1914 and 1918, 269 British deserters were executed; in the same period, only 18 German soldiers (out of 49 who had been sentenced to death) were executed for desertion in an army twice the size of the British Army. However, although British military law was harsh and did not tolerate deviant behaviour, punishments for desertion in the British Army became more lenient in the course of the war: although the proportion of death penalties (to

---

12   Oram, Gerard, '"The administration of discipline by the English is very rigid": British Military Law and the Death Penalty (1868 – 1918)' – *Crime, Histoire et Sociétés/Crime, History and Societies*, 5:1 (2001), pp.93-110.
13   QSA: Queen Square Records, Dr Turner, 1915, male L-Z: case record Private Daniel T.

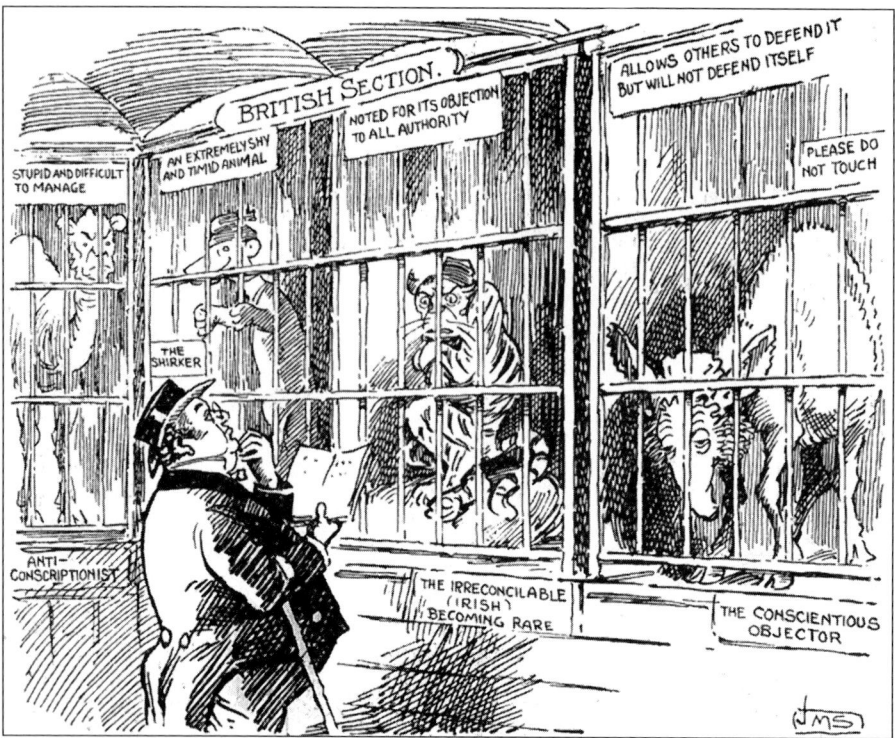

'John Bull: "What extraordinary creatures! And to think that they are British, too!"' – *Western Mail*, 21 January 1916; cartoon by Joseph Morewood Staniforth, Cartooning the First World War Project. (Cardiff University)

all punishments for desertion) increased from 40 to between 60 and 70 percent during periods of intensive fighting – such as the British spring and autumn offensives in 1915, and the Battle of the Somme from July until November 1916 – fewer deserters were sentenced to death towards the end of the war. Moreover, of those sentenced to death, fewer were actually executed: while during the first few months of the war all British deserters sentenced to death were shot, in later years of the war this proportion decreased to around 20 percent.

In the course of the war, British military law also started recognising 'shell shock' as a cause for military offences: the new edition of § 595 of the King's Regulations of September 1916 explicitly stated that shell shock had to be considered in cases of desertion or other criminal behaviour; the Queen Square doctors had followed this rule all along and, generally, did not force soldiers back into battle – even if the diagnosis of shell shock was questionable.

Pacifists and prophets

Shell shock may have saved the life of 24-year-old Private Albert W. of the 5th Northamptons: although Albert, a shoe factory worker in civilian life, never actually deserted the army, he openly admitted that he had always 'hated war and killing people' and that, in his opinion, the war was wrong.[14]

Albert was sent to France in May 1915 and served in the trenches at Ypres and Armentières. With his strong objection to violence and killing, he soon experienced 'an attack of nerves'; he started feeling unwell when one of his comrades shot himself 'on account of some love affair'. After three weeks of treatment at the Royal Victoria Hospital near Southampton, he was sent back to duty at the Western Front. When he witnessed a party of three wounded men – carried by stretcher bearers – being blown up by a shell, he started shaking violently with his whole body; he was also lost for words and could only say 'yes' or 'no'. When Albert was admitted to the National Hospital, he was still paralysed with fear and unable to give an account of his breakdown; however, very soon, he regained his composure: he admitted that he had always been 'horrified at the sight of dead or wounded'; he did not want to hear about the war and was reluctant to talk about his experiences. The doctors diagnosed a 'phobia' – an 'inherent dread of killing people and seeing dead men'. They did not try to treat Albert's fear, and neither did they threaten to send him back to his regiment. Albert was recommended for discharge from the army; he was lucky to escape the machinery of war and military justice.

The medical approach to deserters had to take into account the expectation of the authorities (and the innate belief of most doctors) that desertion could not be the outcome of a rational decision about an irrational war, but had to reflect the collapse of willpower in the face of overwhelming stress. The constitutional model of the Berlin psychiatrists largely fulfilled this expectation; psychiatry had an even more central role to play when it came to people who actively opposed the war, especially when their bravery was not in doubt: there were quite a few war resisters on both sides – most of them motivated by political or religious reasons, or combinations of them – and very few, if any of them, suffered from mental illness. However, it was highly expedient to give them a psychiatric label.

The most prominent such case was that of Siegfried Sassoon, the highly decorated British officer from a wealthy Jewish merchant dynasty who, in July 1917, published a manifesto against the war that contained the lines:

> I believe that the war upon which I entered as a war of defence and liberation has now become a war of agression and conquest. I believe that the purposes for which I and my fellow soldiers entered upon this war should have been so clearly

---

14 QSA: Queen Square Records, Dr Tooth, 1916, male L-Z: case record Private Albert W.

stated as to have made it impossible to change them and that had this been done the objects which actuated us would now be attainable by negotiation.

This was an entirely rational political argument, but one that – proferred by an active member of the British Army – could be construed as amounting to high treason. Court martialling one of its most respected officers was not a prospect that the British Government relished – and it was, therefore, easily persuaded by Sassoon's well-connected friends to accept a diagnosis of neurasthenia and send Sassoon into the care of W.H.R. Rivers at Craiglockhart near Edinburgh (the famous officers' convalescence home).

Sassoon was influenced by intellectual pacifists with no interest in religion – most notably, the leading Cambridge philosopher Bertrand Russell. Their appeal to the wider population was limited: those who questioned the morality of the war on religious grounds were potentially much more dangerous to the war effort; after all, the religious revival movements just before the war (for example, amongst the Welsh quarrymen in 1904-1905, or the rise of pentecostalism and various new sects in Germany), were reminders that religion could still be an all-absorbing force.

In early 1918, Bonhoeffer was asked to assess a soldier who had been influenced by these new religious ideas: Karl E., then aged 43, had lost his parents when he was three and grew up with a childless aunt.[15] Although he trained to be a metalworker, his main interests lay more in the areas of music, literature and philosophy. Karl had always been a loner and felt somewhat special – and from the age of 30, became interested in the ideas of Charles Taze Russell (the founder of the International Bible Students Association, which was the forerunner of Jehovah's Witnesses, who had predicted the end of the world for October 1914). The Bible studies were Karl's epiphany: he developed the conviction that he was chosen by God to be Christ's messenger; he wanted to be among the '144,000 chosen by God from the Book of Revelation' and believed that 'on the day of judgement he would be called to sit on Christ's throne in paradise'. When the Berlin psychiatrists asked him in detail about these experiences, he denied hearing voices, but stated that much in the Bible related to him personally; however, the author of the Bible stories had not written the stories just for him, but for the 144,000 chosen. Karl acknowledged feeling estranged from his country. He reckoned that if everybody complied with Christ's message, the earth would be paradise; whereas everybody else was hypnotised by Satan, he was one of the few people to resist his evil force.

Karl gave up his job in 1914 to study the Bible, but was drafted on 18 August; however, when he was supposed to go into action, he refused to fight. He went to his commanding officer straight away, who actually tried to accommodate his request, by organising for him to work in the laundry and construction of trenches. Karl still felt guilty – in particular, about building trenches – but at the same time, he was

---

15 Historisches Psychiatriearchiv Charité M9716/1918: Krankenakten.

eager to emphasise that he did not want to be perceived as a slacker or agitator, or give a bad example for others. When in enemy fire, he refused to shoot. He had told his comrades before the battle that he was not going to use his weapons; he would rather be shot than shoot another human being. Some of his comrades became angry, but others understood his objections – and various officers spent considerable time trying to change his views. As a compromise, Karl was sent to a carrier pigeon unit; somehow, he managed to get through several years of the war without having to fight. Finally, he decided that he had to actively renounce his duty: he refused to sing on a march and on 28 May 1917 disobeyed orders in front of the whole company, which led to his arrest. Karl was sentenced to four years and four months and sent to prison in Huy, Belgium. Because of his continuing disobedience, he was sent to several military hospitals – and finally, when his case was reopened by a military court, to the Charité.

The doctors at the military hospitals had already suspected a case of disturbance of the mind; Bonhoeffer concurred. Although this was not a case of a classical psychotic disorder such as schizophrenia or manic depression, where patients sometimes developed grandiose delusions of religious content (for example, of being Jesus or a major prophet), he recognised Karl's condition as 'one of the rare psychoses of overvalued ideas'. For Bonhoeffer, Karl's belief in his special status had reached such a degree that it could only amount to a serious mental illness; the stern Lutheran religion of the Prussian State did not allow for any new prophets.

Why were some of the soldiers assessed in Berlin found to be suffering from disturbance of the mind, and others not, when really none of them was affected by any of the classical mental disorders (such as frank psychosis, or syphilitic brain degeneration) to which commonly the meaning of 'criminal insanity' was confined? Wilhelm B., for example, could easily have been classified as 'twilight state', with reduced consciousness, and thus been spared his court martial. Many of his movements in 1916 and 1917 had been erratic and aimless – certainly not the actions of a man with a clear plan to escape duty or danger – and neither those of someone who was merely out to maximise his personal pleasure: his frequent border crossings are much more suggestive of the fugue-like journeys of patients in the typical twilight states. Bonhoeffer may have failed to recognise that such erratic behaviour could indicate a persistent dissociative state, although in other cases, he was quite prepared to accept twilight states as causes of criminal insanity (for example, in that of Adolf S. who, in many respects, had acted in a much more goal-driven way than Wilhelm).

The reasons why the psychiatric verdict could easily go in one direction or the other are complex: psychiatry is hardly an exact science, and psychiatrists themselves often did not agree amongst each other on their patients' diagnoses, which is why a service that specialised in second forensic opinions – like that of Bonhoeffer – became necessary in the first place; secondly, although psychiatrists were legally independent, the assessment of a patient's mental state is never fully independent of the assessor's attitude to the particular offence and the wider societal implications of the psychiatric opinion. The opinions issued by Bonhoeffer's department were all well-balanced and carefully weighed the different diagnostic possibilities; yet, at the end of the day, he was the head of the most important psychiatric department of a country in the middle of an existential war. In this position, it was hardly possible for him to approach the actions of soldiers exclusively, with the objective eye of a forensic examiner – and without regard for the implications of his decisions for the war effort. In this context, the verdict on Karl E. mattered much more than the fates of individual deserters: if, in a still very religious country, true religion could hold that fighting was a sin, the collapse of the holy alliance of throne and altar – the backbone of the Prussian State and its military machine – was nigh; like Sassoon, Karl E. had to be mentally ill.

11

Madness on the Streets of London and Berlin

Minor triggers – major consequences

In June 1916 *[27-year-old Devitt O.]*, was flying over Armentieres in the Lafayette Squadron. He was piloting, scouting at the time and encountered a German who turned his machine gun on him. He was met by a second German and then four more came along. His machine stopped as his petrol was exhausted and he crashed into his own lines. He was unconscious for 4 days. He does not remember crashing but recollects looking at the voltage, the altitude was 2000 ft. He came to at the 9th General Hospital Rouen where he had a terrible headache and found himself in a plaster cast. He had fractured his spine. When he regained consciousness he was unable to use his legs and he was incontinent.[1]

Although America only entered the war in 1917, many Americans had offered their volunteer services to the Allied nations earlier in the conflict: Devitt O., whose Scottish family had settled in America when he was only two years old, was one of them. He had trained as a mechanic and pilot with the American Aircraft Experimental Department and, like other American volunteers, he enlisted with the French Air Service as part of the so-called 'Lafayette Squadron', or *'Escadrille Lafayette'* in French – named after the French general who served alongside George Washington in the American War of Independence.

It was a miracle that Devitt had survived the plane crash; however, the 27-year-old pilot had to go through a tedious recovery: Devitt was confined to bed for nearly a year – nine months of which he had to spend in plaster and two months in a celluloid cast. When he was eventually taken out of the celluloid sheath, the use of his legs completely returned; Devitt had been incredibly lucky. He was subsequently

---

1   QSA: Queen Square Records, Dr Tooth, 1919, male L-Z: case record Private Devitt O.

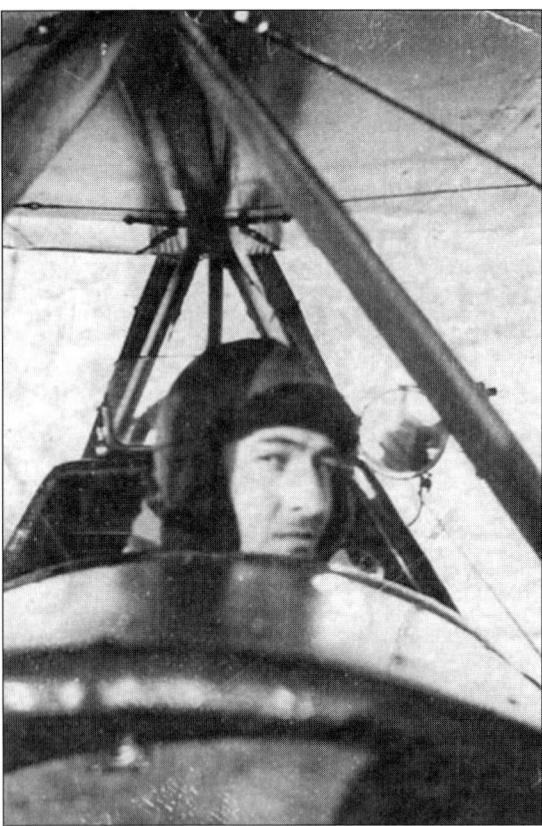

A photograph of an RFC pilot, which was taken by Lieutenant William George Dundas – a reconnaissance photographer of the 82nd Squadron, Royal Flying Corps; photograph kindly contributed by Louisa Cantwell. (The Great War Archive, University of Oxford)

discharged from hospital in Rouen and from the army in September 1917 – returning to the United States.

In February 1918, 10 months after America's formal entry into the war, the Lafayette Squadron passed into American hands. Devitt, feeling fit and healthy, immediately enlisted in Philadelphia and started flying again. In September 1918, he entered the Royal Air Force; he was unfazed by the extreme dangers to which pilots – the group of servicemen with the highest death rate – were exposed. Devitt had survived a plane crash and fully recovered physically and mentally. Ironically, it was not the constant threats, horrors and atrocities of war that finally broke down his mental resistance – not a fall from 2,000 feet, but a minor slip on the transport to England on 12 October 1918, which eventually triggered his breakdown: it started with pain in the back and a terrible headache – upon which his legs got weaker and weaker and started shaking, so that he was unable to walk; he also lost control of his bladder. Was this a return of his previous spinal troubles? The doctors had no doubt that these symptoms were unrelated to the injuries he had obtained during his plane crash: Devitt's symptoms recurred because he had developed shell shock.

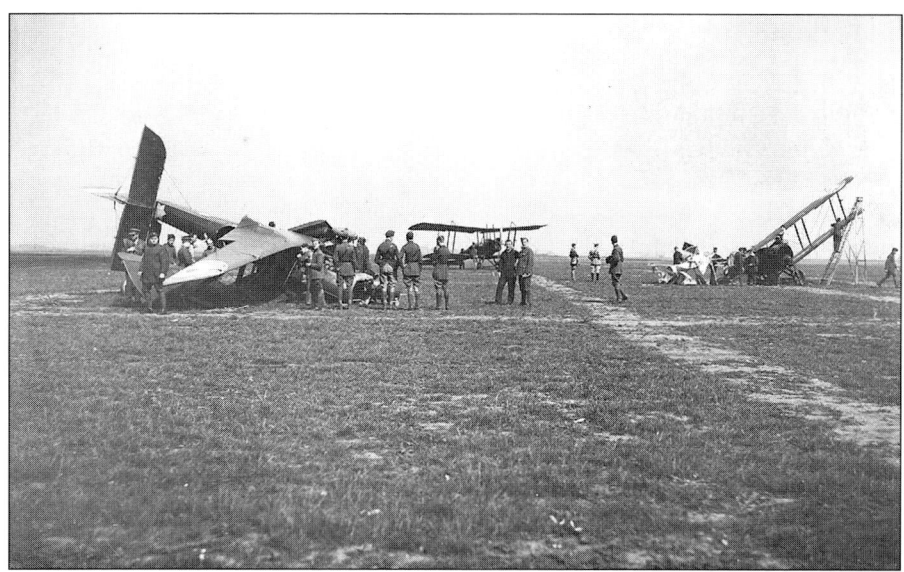

Results of an aerial collision: the aircraft to the far right appears to be a Bristol F2b; that to the far left, a de Havilland DH4, which were introduced respectively in March and April 1917; photograph taken by Lieutenant William George Dundas – image kindly contributed by Louisa Cantwell. (The Great War Archive, University of Oxford)

Devitt was treated at different military hospitals: at Kinmel Park in North Wales, Hounslow in London and in Staffordshire; his symptoms did not improve. Finally, his doctor's wife advised him to seek treatment at the National Hospital in London. It is not clear how the Queen Square doctors managed to cure Devitt, because the last page of his case record – documenting all the treatments – is missing. Whatever they did, it must have been successful, because after four weeks of inpatient care, Devitt was discharged as 'cured'.

A similar British case, in which the trigger seemed to be irrelevant against the backdrop of wartime hazards, was Cornelius B., a 40-year-old private from the 162nd Labour Company.[2] Cornelius, a farm labourer from Oxford, had been granted a well-deserved leave from frontline service, which he spent at home with his wife. On 7 December 1917, he was on his way back to France, when walking down the stairs at Victoria Station, he fell down 'two or three steps' – landing on his back. The police picked him up and brought him to the 4th London General Hospital at Denmark Hill. Cornelius could not remember how he ended up at the 'King's College Infirmary': he was 'feeling bad' and his back was 'tingling'. During his 15-week hospital stay

---

2   QSA: Queen Square Records, Dr Collier, 1919, male A-K: case record Private Cornelius B.

in South London, his physical health deteriorated dramatically: he could not keep down his food, wet his pants several times a day and was unable to move his legs; the paralysis of his legs was interpreted as a 'recurrence of railway spine'. Apparently, weeks before the outbreak of the war, a sack of corn had fallen on Cornelius's back when he was working on a farm – leaving him temporarily incontinent and paralysed from his waist down.

Although the 4th London General Hospital was one of the epicentres of shell shock treatment, the doctors there gave up on Cornelius – and on 5 June 1918, he was transferred to the National Hospital.

At this time, Cornelius was bedridden and still could not retain his urine. His legs were:

> ... extended in a spasm and it [took] several minutes to flex (bend) the legs at the knees passively. To overcome this spasm straps were placed on the middle of the thighs and the limbs flexed at the hip and fastened to the end of his bed. ... When his legs were in this position he groaned continuously and insisted that they should be released.

Cornelius still complained of an aching pain in the lumbar region. He brought up all food fed to him and claimed that he had not eaten anything for a long time; however, the Queen Square doctors observed that 'after being fed by the nasal tube he vomited orange peel. He had evidently hidden the oranges in his bed'. Because Cornelius could not feel his legs, strong electric currents were applied – and although there was no plausible medical explanation for the loss of power and feeling in his legs, he did not feel any pain (even 'when lighted matches were applied to his legs').

When Cornelius was discharged from the National Hospital after nine months of intensive treatment, his condition was unchanged: even Lewis Ralph Yealland, the Queen Square doctor who claimed the highest success rates in the treatment of shell shock (and did not shrink back from the more radical measures), was unable to cure him. This case is also notable for the application of intentionally painful treatment: although I will argue in Chapter 12 that the shell shock doctors at Queen Square and elsewhere did not primarily use electrotherapy as a means of torture, we have to remember that some of the treatments were inhumane. Clearly, Yealland and his superiors – faced with a stubborn case – overstepped the boundaries of what was acceptable even then.

Triggers of shell shock

Physicians involved in the treatment of traumatised soldiers documented the circumstances surrounding their patients' breakdown as potential clues to the aetiology of these disorders. In both the German and the British records, physical trauma (for example, accidental burial after shell explosions in the trenches) accounted for about a third of shell shock cases – and another third was triggered by psychological stress without direct physical injury (for example, witnessing a comrade's violent death). The majority of soldier-patients had been involved in heavy fighting, but some – almost a quarter of the cases at the Charité – had not seen action (and presumably, had never been exposed to any serious hazard). In these cases, an anticipated or feared traumatic experience was sufficient to trigger persistent shell shock symptoms.

The physicians' view on the role of shell explosions in a soldier's mental breakdown evolved as the war unfolded: W.H.R. Rivers, who had treated traumatised soldiers at Maghull and Craiglockhart, wrote in the foreword to *War Neuroses* by John MacCurdy:

> In the early days of the war the medical profession [...] was inclined to emphasise the physical aspect of the antecedents of a war neurosis. As the war has progressed the physical conception has given way before one which regards the shell explosion or other catastrophe of warfare as, in the vast majority of cases, merely the spark which has released long pent up forces of a psychical kind.[3]

By 1918, as we have learned in Chapter 4, most British doctors had moved away from the idea of an underlying organic lesion caused by the impact of the explosion: the shell explosion was, rather, seen as part of a complex aetiological model, in which physical and psychological triggers interacted.

Even the eminent neuropathologist Frederick Walker Mott, who never abandoned the primacy of the organic in the genesis of shell shock, stated in his Chadwick lecture on 'Mental Hygiene and Shell Shock During and After the War' in the summer of 1917:

> Living in trenches or dug-outs, exposed to wet, cold, and often to hunger and thirst, dazed or almost stunned by the unceasing din of the guns, disgusted by foul stenches, by the rats and by insect tortures of flies, fleas, bugs, and lice, the minor horrors of war, when combined with frequent grim and gruesome spectacles of comrades suddenly struck down, mangled, wounded, or dead, the memories of which are constantly recurring and exciting a dread of impending death or of being blown up by a mine and buried alive, together constitute experiences so depressing to the vital resistance of the nervous system, that a time must come when even the strongest man will succumb, and a shell bursting near may produce a sudden loss of consciousness, not by concussion or commotion, but by acting as the 'last straw' on an utterly exhausted nervous system worn out by this stress of trench warfare and want of sleep.[4]

Mott was right: both the immediate initial horror and the cumulative effects of the atrocities of war could trigger shell shock; however, it was less obvious to the medical

---

3   MacCurdy, *War Neuroses*, p.v.
4   Mott, 'The Chadwick Lecture on Mental Hygiene and Shell Shock', p.39.

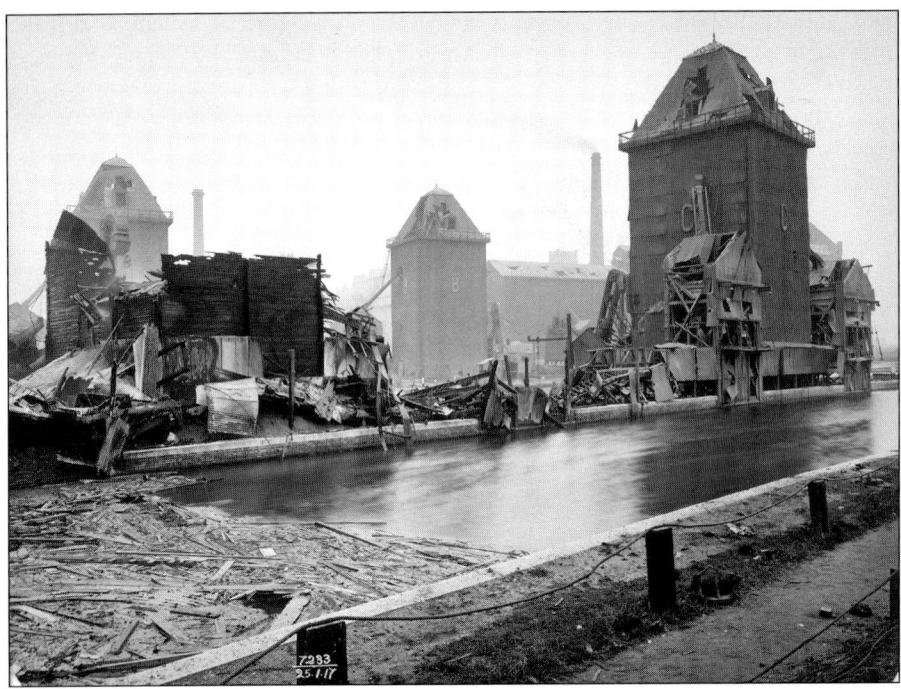

Flourmills after the Silvertown explosion; the grain silos and warehouses of the flourmills were amongst the 17 acres that the Port of London Authority estimated were damaged. John H. Avery photographed the wreckage immediately after and throughout the reconstruction, which was completed in 1921; photograph taken on 25 January 1917 – image ID: 141272. (Museum of London Picture Library)

and military professions – and is still not widely known today – that even minor events after a period of relative calm could kindle the most dramatic symptoms. Similar to Pilot Devitt and Private Cornelius, many soldiers who had coped well with life at the front line broke down during their home leave: Private Edward C., the young electrician whom Dr Farranridge visits on his ward round on 20 May 1917 (see Chapter 6), had coped reasonably well with life in the trenches.[5] After weeks of heavy fighting on the Western Front, he was granted leave and returned to London, but his shell shock symptoms started when, on 19 January 1917, he was 'much upset' by a massive explosion in Silvertown:[6] in Messrs Brunner, Mond and Company's munitions works, 50 tonnes of TNT had been blown up – killing 73 people and damaging up to 70,000 buildings in the eastern part of the capital; the noise of the blast could be heard as far

---

5   QSA: Queen Square Records, Dr Tooth, 1917, male and female A-K: case record Edward C.
6   Silvertown in West Ham, Essex (now part of the London Borough of Newham).

away as Southampton and Norwich. Although physically unscathed, Edward started shaking violently. Edward's symptoms proved to be treatment-resistant and the young electrician was recommended for discharge from the army.

In some cases, even relatively minor incidents during home leave appeared to have triggered a mental breakdown – especially when they reminded soldiers of their frontline experiences (for example, the backfire of a car could be misinterpreted as shell explosion). In all these cases of breakdown during home leave, admission to Queen Square had a potentially life-saving function, preventing the return of the soldier to the trenches.

Another trigger not directly related to combat was marital infidelity: the circumstances of the war, the 'enforced separation of husband and wife and the temptation afforded by bigamy', led to extramarital relationships and the birth of illegitimate children. Women sometimes tried to conceal their pregnancies, or abort the illegitimate child; some women were so desperate that they killed their newborn babies. The national press reported on the increasing number of infanticides, although no actual figures were provided.[7] Marital infidelity was seen as a grave moral offence against husbands risking their life for King and Country: because women who betrayed their husbands were judged undeserving of the separation allowances provided to war wives, the State investigated 41,836 cases of alleged misconduct between 1916 and 1920.[8]

How did men react to these threats to their marital and family life? During frontline service, the prospect of being reunited with their loved ones was often the last straw they hung on to: twenty-three-year-old Private George H., a hospital orderly in France, was devastated when he received 'news from England informing him of conjugal infidelity on the part of his wife'.[9] He stopped eating, was unable to sleep and 'has been crazy with worry and other emotions consequent on these bad news'. George was sent to England, and he must have been in quite an alarming state, because he was directly referred to the National Hospital. The Queen Square doctors showed much sympathy for George, yet, they could not mend his broken heart; after all, they were not in the position to rebuild George's marriage. During his two-week hospital stay in the heart of London, George came to the conclusion that 'this country ha[d] no longer any attraction for him and [that] he wish[ed] to return to France as soon as possible'.

Marital shell shock occurred after the end of the war, too: sixty-year-old clerk John L., a father of three, had been in Egypt for four years without taking any leave.[10] He had been exposed to tough weather conditions, with very long periods of waiting in the desert in the blazing heat of summer. After his long-awaited demobilisation on

7 'Women Police. Government inspector on their help' – *Liverpool ECHO*, 14 March 1918.
8 Pedersen, Susan, 'Gender, welfare, and citizenship in Britain during the Great War' – *The American Historical Review*, 95:4 (1990), p.999.
9 QSA: Queen Square Records, Dr Russell, 1915, male A-K: case record Private George H.
10 QSA: Queen Square Records, Dr Collier, 1920, male L-Z: case record John L.

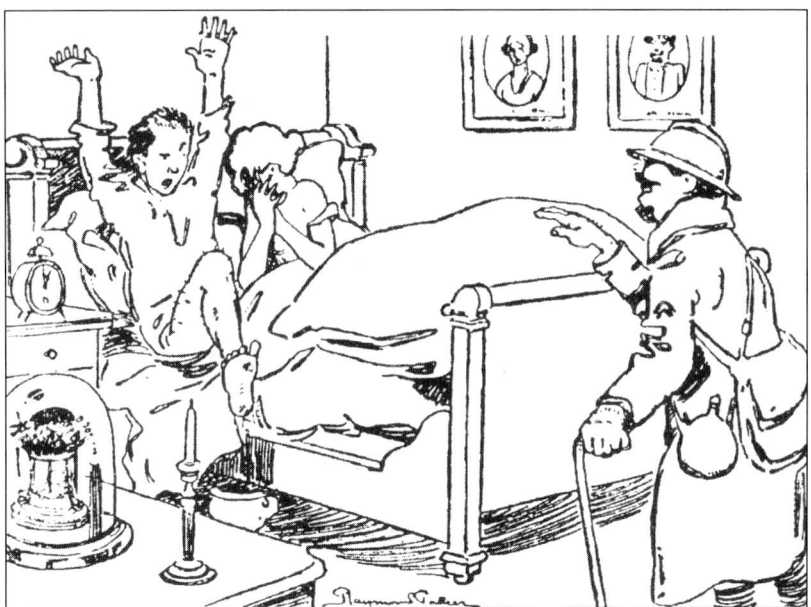

Cartoon, R. Pallier, 'Le Rire rouge', 1917; from Hirschfeld, M. and Gaspar, A., *Sittengeschichte des ersten Weltkrieges* (Hanau: Müller & Kiepenheuer, 1929; re-print of the 2nd revised edition, 1980), p.116.

20 July 1919, he was shipped from Port Said to Taranto in Italy, and thence by cattle truck to the north of Italy.

He arrived in Bologna:

> ... wet through and remained wet through all night, dried in the morning and then got wet again. He then began to feel rheumatic pains for he had just come out of much heat. This was the beginning of the bodily pains at the bottom of the back and in the shins and he couldn't close his hands and had no grip.

Yet, John was tough and his physical health improved steadily; however, when he finally returned to England, he had:

> ... a great mental shock for on arrival home after four years' absence, his wife was out and he found out shortly afterwards that she had been in misalliance with another man. This discovery completely knocked [the] patient out. [He] nearly went mad and his sleeplessness started when he found out his home worries. Lately he has been afraid to cross the street, he was so nervous. He has had no sleep at all and used to get so desperate he took a double draught of sleeping mixture. He has been staying at the Veterans' Club for soldiers and eating practically nothing.

Because John's vision had deteriorated recently and he had developed 'a marked general tremor on voluntary movements, particularly when he was trying to write a letter', he was admitted to the National Hospital. Although John had been relatively sheltered from traumatic war experience through his posting with the Army Pay Corps in Cairo, he found the betrayal at home too stressful to bear: his lack of motivation, difficulty focusing and perceived loss of future prospects were so severe that he failed to apply for a pension and had to be prompted by the Queen Square staff to fill in the necessary forms.[11]

Other soldiers tried to deal with news about marital infidelity in a more pragmatic way, although their legal means were limited, as reported by the *Manchester Evening News* on 24 September 1917:

> ... a private at home from the war on short leave applied to the City Stipendiary for advice as to the steps he should take to secure a judicial separation from his wife on the ground that she had misconducted herself whilst he was abroad. [...] Mr. Brierley [from the City Stipendiary] pointed out that [habitual drunkenness] was the only ground upon which the magistrates could grant a man a separation from his wife. [...]. He expressed regret that he was unable to assist the applicant, whose case, he said, he feared was but one of a substantial number which had arisen during the war.[12]

The Home Front: Berlin

On 15 November 1915, 33-year-old merchant Hans K. was enjoying a day out in Berlin.[13] He had been at the front for over a year, serving as a paramedic in Ypres, Diksmuide and other places in Flanders. After a two-week rest and reunion with his wife, he was feeling well; however, when stepping out of the moving tram, Hans K. tripped and fell on the back of his head. He lost consciousness and woke up sitting on a chair in a pub on Berlin Alexanderplatz, one of the main squares of the capital. He did not have any visible injuries, but felt dizzy and 'funny in his head'; he took a cab home and went straight to bed. From then on, he was suffering from strange episodes: other people told him that he had been behaving inappropriately – and although he could see the results of his actions, he could not remember any of it; on one occasion, he smashed several dishes in his house. Although Hans reported his tram accident and strange episodes to the military authorities, he was sent back to his reserve company on 24 November; however, on his second night back, he had another

---

11 Correspondence between the National Hospital and the London War Pensions Committee, as attached to the clinical record: QSA: Queen Square Records, Dr Collier, 1920, male L-Z: case record John L.
12 'Marital infidelity. City stipendiary and Growing Evil' – *Manchester Evening News*, 24 September 1917.
13 Historisches Psychiatriearchiv Charité M4969/1916: Krankenakten.

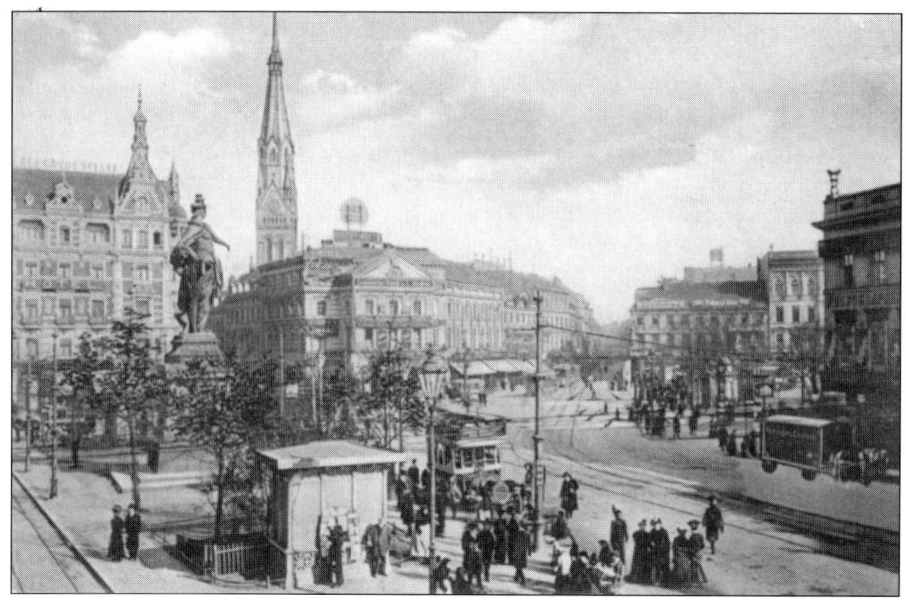

Berlin Alexanderplatz, 1915; postcard. (Author's own archive)

attack, in which he furiously fired his rifle. Afterwards, he felt exhausted and had a headache, but – as before – did not remember any of his actions. Hans continued having these episodes, both during the day – sometimes during ward rounds – and at night. On 20 January 1916, he was eventually admitted to a military hospital at Berlin Hasenheide, and transferred on to the Charité; urgent referral to the foremost psychiatric department was clearly needed to get to the bottom of this bizarre and dangerous behaviour.

The Charité doctors certified that Hans was not suitable for military service – not even for light duties at home; however, in their search for the causes of the breakdown, they followed their usual line of enquiry – digging into the patient's biography and family history in order to exculpate the combat situation. They concluded that the war was not to blame for Hans's mental breakdown: a thorough examination and family history had revealed that Hans's father and uncle had both been treated in mental hospitals. Furthermore, Hans's older brother had recently been discharged from the army because he had developed a paralysis of his left side after a shell explosion; two younger brothers had been exempted from military service because of their nervous character and physical weakness. In addition to this dubious family history, Hans also had his own string of constitutional problems: in childhood, he had suffered from rickets and only learned to walk and talk when he was four years of age; the Charité psychiatrists also suspected that Hans had already suffered similar attacks before the war. All these aspects of his personal and family history clearly pointed towards a diagnosis of a 'psychopathic constitution' – and the diagnosis meant that Hans was not granted a war pension, because his predispostion, rather than the war, was to blame for his breakdown.

A similar case is that of Reservist Benno B., who was in Berlin – on leave from the Western Front – in June 1916:[14] his leave was to end on Saturday, 3 June at 11:00 a.m., but at 10:15 a.m. – when he was travelling on the tram with his *fiancée* – he suddenly experienced an excruciating pain in his stomach. He felt very dizzy, but managed to step out of the tram to ask a policeman to take him back to the barracks. Benno did not remember how he managed to get back: his comrades told him later that he had been very aggressive – lashing about on the barrack yard and inside the buildings. Because he did not calm down, he was taken to the Charité Hospital, where he was admitted to the locked psychiatric ward with a suspected diagnosis of 'alcohol intoxication'; however, this suspicion did not turn out to be true. Although alcohol excesses were widespread, both during tours of duty and home leave, Benno's alcohol consumption had been moderate throughout. On the hospital ward, he appeared to be completely normal, approachable, polite and self-possessed. Eventually, as in Hans's case, doctors suspected some hidden psychopathic traits to be responsible for Benno's abnormal behaviour: they documented that Benno, a printer by trade, had often quarrelled with his parents, and also with his colleagues at work; this was enough evidence to confirm a psychopathic predisposition.

Hans and Benno were, by no means, the only German soldiers who suffered breakdowns on the streets of Berlin, rather than the trenches of France – and understandably, they attracted a great deal of public attention, and were often taken straight to the Charité Hospital. Another such case was that of Walter L. – a 38-year-old soldier of the *Landsturm* (the German militia that was largely drawn from older reservists) who, in the middle of February 1917, was wandering about aimlessly in Berlin;[15] he was feeling extremely anxious and out of control. Sometimes, he paused in one place for a long time – motionless and absent-minded – and at other times, he cried out in extreme fear. Because he was not really aware of what he was doing, he had lunch in several restaurants. He could feel pressure in the back of his skull, 'as if somebody was taking hold of the inside of his head'. Walter was unable to focus his thoughts: when he was taken to the Charité, he admitted that he thought of killing himself; he felt that his life was hopeless and without purpose.

Perhaps Walter should not have been sent to the front line in the first place, because he had a history of depression and anxiety: in 1903, aged 24, he had moved to Amden in Switzerland with his mother, brother and two of his married sisters. They had contributed all their assets towards a religious sect led by a certain Josua Klein, who had acquired property in Switzerland and wanted to establish a Christian community and artists' colony there; however, this '*Grappenhof*' colony was dissolved in 1904 and Walter's family lost everything. At that time, Walter suffered his first mental

---

14   Historisches Psychiatriearchiv Charité M294/1916: Krankenakten.
15   Historisches Psychiatriearchiv Charité M3676/1917: Krankenakten.

breakdown and was treated in a sanatorium. The young man was deeply depressed and tried to kill himself twice (the first time with morphium and the second time with chloroform); it took him years to recover from his deep depression. In 1906, when he was eventually feeling well, he rebuilt his life – establishing a successful career as a merchant and enjoying many interests, such as reading, history, music, theatre and marine life. Everything changed when he was drafted into the army and sent to the Eastern Front in June 1916: it was not so much the physical hardships and adverse weather conditons, but the abuse by one of his superiors that caused his mental breakdown. Walter suffered from incapacitating anxiety, sleeplessness and lethargy, and was incapable of making decisions; he was sent home for a break.

Doctors at the Charité found strong evidence for Walter's constitutional weakness: his mother – an art- and music-loving woman, who had died from cancer in 1907 – had been prone to depression as well. As a child, Walter had been 'more girl than boy': sensitive, anxious and tidy; it is documented in the hospital records that 'he always felt cold and did not tolerate woollen socks'. He was a daydreamer and had a compulsion to count everything. Walter had been engaged once, but never got married, because of his homosexual disposition: he had been convicted of 'homosexual offences' three times and actually spent some time in prison – therefore, it came rather as a surprise to him when after his third sentence of six months, he was drafted into the army straight away. The hospital records clearly reflect the difficult standing of homosexuals in society – and the attitude of medical doctors towards their homosexual patients was overshadowed by irrational fears, prejudice and bigotry. Homosexual soldiers were more likely to be accused of malingering – and although they were denied 'manly qualities', they were, nevertheless, drafted into the army and sent to the front line.

During his stay at the Charité, Walter was extremely anxious and tearful, and showed no interest in his surroundings. After two months, he was eventually discharged in order to contribute to the war effort. According to a new National Service law ('*Gesetz über den vaterländischen Hilfsdienst*'), which became effective on 6 December 1916, all German men between 17 and 60 years of age who had not been drafted into the army, or had not been working in farming or forestry before 1916, were obliged to work in the armaments industry, or in another business relevant to the war effort. Although Walter would have liked to resume his work as a successful merchant, he was not allowed to return to his civilian business.

Many other soldiers were wandering the streets of Berlin in a dazed state: this frequently happened when, after a period of leave, they were on the way back to their unit, or had been asked to return to their military duties. During such episodes – which could last for minutes, hours, or even days – they wandered or travelled away from home. These were unplanned, purposeless journeys, which would be labelled as 'dissociative fugues' by today's psychiatrists. Like Walter, some of them had frequent meals in different restaurants, whereas others forgot to eat for days. What might not have been obvious for strangers was that these soldiers had lost their sense of time, identity and memory for important events in their life. After the episode, previous memories returned, but typically, the person could not remember the fugue episode.

This usually caused confusion and distress, and often led to the admission to a mental hospital, such as the psychiatric department of the Charité.

On 4 June 1918 at 3:30 p.m., another soldier – 25-year-old Otto K. – was spotted by passers-by when he walked down some steps into one of Berlin's inland ports;[16] he was fully dressed and had to be pulled out of the water. Otto had enjoyed a few days of leave in Berlin, while the German Army was losing ground at the Western Front during the spring offensive. On 2 June, Otto had received a message ordering him to return to his regiment the next day; however, on 3 June, his whole body started shaking, so he was referred to a military hospital instead. On 4 June, he was discharged from there and again ordered to return to his regiment straight away, but instead of travelling back to his unit, he went for a long walk and ended up in the canal.

Otto had never seen frontline service: until early April 1918, he had worked as a book keeper in the textile industry – and he was eventually ordered to do garrison service; however, when he was asked to carry shells, he started shaking and lashing about. His comrades could not get through to him; he appeared to be dazed, inapproachable and unaware of what was going on around him. When Otto arrived at the Charité, he was in a state of shock – soaked to the skin and shivering violently. When he regained consciousness, he claimed that he had inadvertently slipped into the water; however, the interview with his wife, Frieda, unearthed a different story: shortly after he had left his home on 3 June, Frieda received a letter from her husband – informing her that he was going to Greifswald (a city approximately 250 km north of Berlin); in the past, Otto had often talked about returning to Greifswald to take his own life at the grave of one of their children. Frieda also reported that she had caught her husband opening the gas tap several times in the middle of the night while on leave at home. The Charité doctors never found out what Otto's intention was when walking along the canal, but in any case, it very soon became clear to them that Otto was a deeply troubled individual: in his childhood, he had had to cope with the loss of his father, and a mother who did not care too much about her children; Otto and his wife had lost two of their three children to meningitis and scarlet fever.

Although Otto survived his own childhood, he had been a weak boy, with frequent chest infections – and this physical weakness had continued into adulthood. Otto's history and symptoms were attributed to a psychopathic constitution; Karl Bonhoeffer made a note in the hospital file. He emphasised that Otto's 'unconscious wish to be ill and to escape military service' was the major reason for his breakdown (but, importantly, Bonhoeffer did not label him as a conscious malingerer). Because Bonhoeffer regarded it as highly likely that Otto would break down again if subjected to military service, the young man was assigned to home service. Escorted by two members of staff, Otto was taken back to his unit.

The cases from the streets of London and Berlin demonstrate the far-reaching consequences of war trauma: even hundreds of miles away from the front line – and

---

16 Historisches Psychiatriearchiv Charité M9510/1918: Krankenakten.

even years after the war – relatively minor tribulations could trigger major mental breakdown. This epidemic of madness in the home countries reinforced the need to develop effective treatments for shell shock; after all, it was even worse for morale to see aimless and confused soldiers on the streets of the capital, than to encounter them in the clearing stations and military hospitals directly behind the front line.

12

Believe Me, He Will Be Cured

'Yards and yards of cable'

> … a fair sized room painted white. In the centre of the room was a white enamelled table, and nearby two dressing trolleys. On the floor were yards and yards of cable, which was strewn all over the place, and connected to a telegraph instrument placed upon an ordinary deal table. The room was crowded with nurses who were in white dresses and white aprons, they were all talking excitedly. A Doctor now enters in a white coat, he walks round the room, stepping over the coils of wire and is also excited and in a great hurry. He has a knife in his hand. … The doctor was an exact representation of Dr. Yealland.[1]

This is a handwritten account of the dream that Frederick O. had on 16 March 1918, while recovering from shell shock at the National Hospital at Queen Square. Frederick had joined the army in June 1916, aged 33, and was sent to France as driver for the Army Service Corps, as part of the 'Mechanical Transport Ammunition Corps'.

In June 1917 – after one year of frontline service – he was knocked out by an explosion while the Germans were shelling a railway depot at Ypres. Frederick was taken to a dressing station at Poperinghe (about eight miles to the west of Ypres). When he regained consciousness, he was unable to move his legs. Over the following seven months, Frederick was treated in different base hospitals: when finally admitted to Queen Square on 4 February 1918, the 'small, poorly nourished man with blue eyes, brown hair and small clean shaven face' was still not able to walk. He lay on his back, with his legs rigidly extended; whenever the doctors approached him, Frederick turned his face away, wrinkled his forehead and closed his eyes tightly; when he was told to bend his knees, the muscles of his legs went into 'violent spasms' – causing excruciating pain.

---

1   QSA: Queen Square Records, Dr Wilson, 1918, male and female L-Z: case record Private Frederick O.

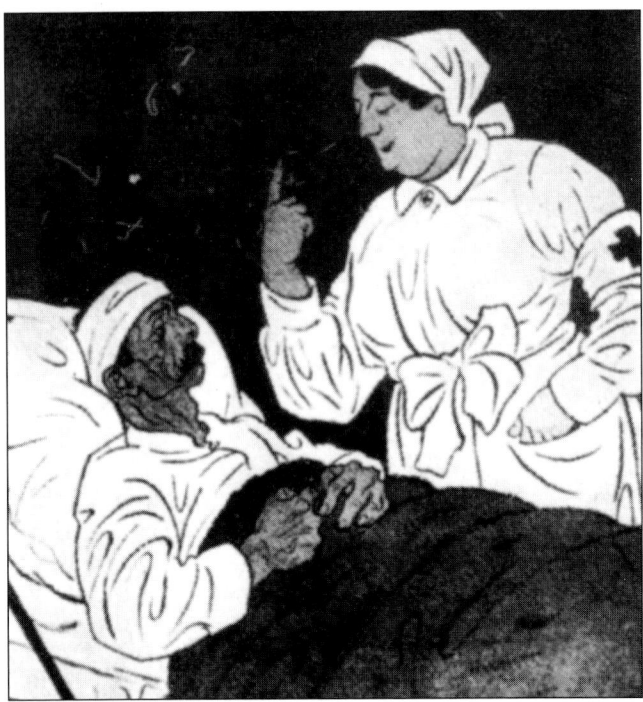

'Cheer up, sweetheart, you will be back at the front in a week's time'; from Hirschfeld, M. and Gaspar, A., *Sittengeschichte des ersten Weltkrieges* (Hanau: Müller & Kiepenheuer, 1929; reprint of the 2nd revised edition, 1980), p.131.

Frederick was also suffering from nightmares; however, unlike many of his comrades on the hospital wards, he did not relive the horrors of war in these terrifying dreams: the nightmares did not restage Fred's battle experiences, but his treatment at Queen Square; yet, was not the safe and caring environment of a hospital in the middle of London the antithesis to the terror of the trenches? Many patients did not feel that way – especially when it came to electrotherapy – and for some, their fears were epitomised by the persona of Lewis Ralph Yealland, who was the most prolific therapist of the National Hospital during the years of the Great War.

Several patients even decided, after having been admitted to the National Hospital, to discharge themselves against medical advice: one of them was 19-year-old paper machine worker James T., who had been wounded and gassed at St Julien (northeast of Ypres) in April 1915.[2] James had to sign a form – which had been handwritten by Yealland – saying that he 'decided to discharge [himself] from the National Hospital because [he was] afraid to undergo treatment which proved beneficial to [him] on a previous occasion' and that he took full responsibility for what might happen to him after he left the hospital. Other patients appear to have recovered – after a long illness history – shortly before Yealland was about to initiate treatment.

---

2   QSA: Queen Square Records, Dr Taylor, 1917, male L-Z: case record James T.

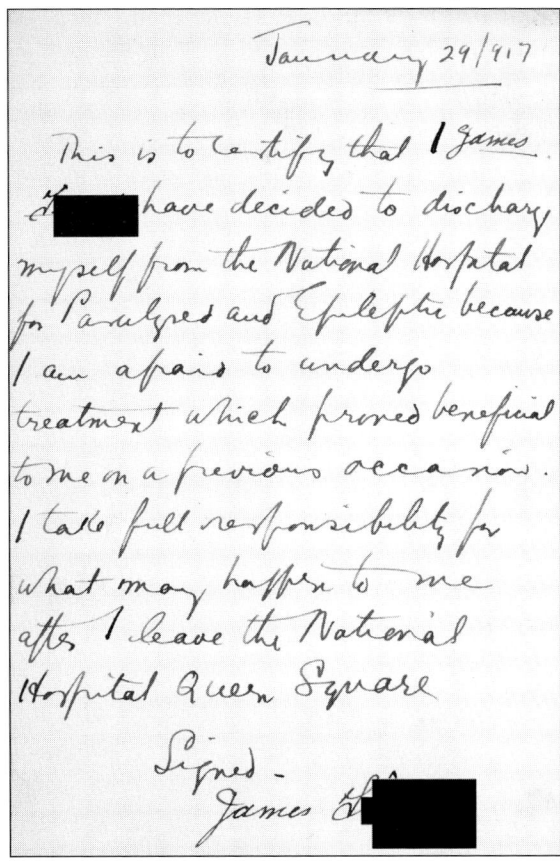

Discharge against medical advice: Dr Yealland's handwriting, patient's signature; Queen Square Records, Dr Taylor, 1917, male L-Z: case record James T. (Queen Square Archives, London)

These drastic reactions on the part of the soldier-patients raise the question: what actually happened to them at the specialist treatment centres? Were the treatments administered by the shell shock doctors on both sides essentially forms of punishment intended to get soldiers back to the front line as quickly as possible, as alleged by later writers? Or were Yealland, Nonne and the other champions of these new therapies right to claim that they were administering the first rational and properly evaluated treatments that had ever been developed for psychological disorders?

How shell shock was treated

When modern readers think of shell shock treatment, they generally have 'electroshocks', or other forms of torture and humiliation, in mind. Lewis Ralph Yealland, who gave detailed evidence of his shell shock treatment in his wartime book *Hysterical Disorders of Warfare*, came under particularly heavy fire for his seemingly unorthodox methods: although he had initially been forgotten by the medical world after his death in 1954, the 1980s saw a revival of interest in the Canadian doctor and his methods, and the 'posthumous disintegration' of his reputation.³ Elaine Showalter, a historian of medicine and a feminist writer, found Yealland's 'Orwellian scenes of mind control [...] painfully embarrassing to contemporary readers'. She contrasted Yealland, the 'worst of the military psychiatrists', with the thoughtful, gentle and empathetic W.H.R. Rivers (Siegfried Sassoon's therapist at Craiglockhart).⁴ This all-too 'convenient dramatic contrast'⁵ between Yealland and Rivers was also adopted by Pat Barker in her widely-read novel *Regeneration* and its later film adaptation.⁶

Pat Barker, whose novel shaped public knowledge and opinion on shell shock treatment, based her Queen Square chapter on two case studies of Yealland's controversial book: the first patient who prominently features in Barker's novel is Yealland's case 'G9'.⁷ Because almost all of the Queen Square Records have survived this patient can be identified as 22-year-old Glaswegian George H. of the Argyll & Sutherland Highlanders;⁸ this young soldier was admitted to Queen Square on 20 October 1916 (in Barker's fictional account, the date of admission is November 1917). In June 1916, George and his comrades had been involved in an attack at Loos – a small town a few miles south-west of Lille in Northern France, where the British had first used poison gas in 1915. At the time, he was with a bombing party, and was just about to 'go over', when a mine exploded and knocked the trench in. George was almost completely buried, and only survived because he managed to keep his head over the ground. He was unconscious for a short time – and when he woke up, he suffered from severe pain in his back and head; on every attempt to stand up, he fell forwards. George was sent to Eastbourne in England, where he learned to walk with a stick, and later was referred to King's College Hospital, where his symptoms did not improve any further. The young man with 'bright red hair and blue eyes' presented at Queen Square with a severely disturbed gait; however, his gait – as recorded by the admitting doctors – was, by far, not as disturbed as described in later (more or less fictional) accounts: George's posture becomes more and more distorted when we compare the original case record with Yealland's report in his book, and then Barker's account in *Regeneration*. In the original case record, George walked 'with a limp bending his back over to the right' and bending his right knee; when he walked in Yealland's *Hysterical Disorders of Warfare*, 'the trunk was flexed at *right angles* [my italics] with the thighs and he

---

3   Duffy, Dennis, 'The Strange Second Death of Lewis Yealland' – *Ontario History*, 103:2 (2011), pp.127-149.
4   Showalter, Elaine, *The Female Malady: Women, Madness and English Culture 1830–1980* (London: Virago, 1987), pp.178 and 181.
5   Duffy, 'The Strange Second Death of Lewis Yealland'.
6   Barker, Pat, *Regeneration* (London: Penguin, 2008).
7   Yealland, *Hysterical Disorders of Warfare*, pp.208-211., Barker, *Regeneration*, pp.223-226.
8   QSA: Queen Square Records, Dr Collier, 1917, male and female A-K: case record Private George H.

supported himself by grasping the anterior surfaces of the thighs with his hands. His body was tilted slightly to the right and the head bent backwards'; Barker finally depicts George as '... a creature – it hardly resembled a man – crawl[ing] through the door..., so bent, so apparently deformed. His head was twisted to one side, and drawn back, the spine bent so that the chest was *parallel* [my italics] with the legs, which themselves were bent at the knees.' Barker here gives fantasy free rein.

The second case on which Barker relied was the first ('A1') of Yealland's book – and certainly his most dramatic:[9] the patient's 'mouth was kept open by means of a tongue depressor; a strong faradic current was applied to the posterior wall of the pharynx, and with this stimulus [the patient] jumped backwards, detaching the wires from the battery'. This treatment scene was vividly recreated in the 1997 film '*Regeneration*', with English-Canadian actor John Neville starring as Yealland and Jonathan Pryce as Rivers (the presence of the latter at Queen Square is owed to dramatic contrast, rather than historical accuracy). Most modern scholars also cite this first 'didactic illustration' of Yealland's *Hysterical Disorders of Warfare*:[10] it certainly is the most brutal case of all – and in many ways, atypical of Yealland's approach. The hospital notes for this case could not be found, and it is possible that this 24-year-old private who fought at the Mons retreat, the Battle of the Marne and Aisne, the First and Second Battles of Ypres, Hill 60, Neuve Chapelle, Loos, Armentières and Salonica never existed; Yealland may have merged details from several of the nearly 200 cases he had treated personally in order to provide a particularly salient illustration of his practice.

A young doctor goes to work

When appointed to Queen Square, Lewis Ralph Yealland was comparatively young and inexperienced: he had completed his basic medical training in Canada and had worked in an asylum for some time when he decided to apply for the post of resident medical officer at the National Hospital. As an ambitious doctor keen to establish his clinical credentials, he jumped at the chance to move to London in order to work at the most famous neurological hospital in the world – the 'temple of British neurology' – at Queen Square; and Yealland thrived in his new position: the young doctor worked relentlessly. During his time at the National Hospital (from 8 December 1915 until 7 March 1919), Yealland treated nearly 200 shell-shocked soldiers – approximately 60 percent of all shell shock cases admitted to Queen Square during this period of time. During the first few months in London, Yealland had Edgar Adrian by his side,

---

9   Yealland, *Hysterical Disorders of Warfare*, pp.7-15., Barker, *Regeneration*, pp.226-233.
10   Binneveld, Hans, *From Shell Shock to Combat Stress: A Comparative History of Military Psychiatry* (Amsterdam: Amsterdam University Press, 1997), p.111.; Leed, Eric J., *No Man's Land: Combat & Identity in World War I* (Cambridge: Cambridge University Press, 1981), pp.174-175., Scull, *Hysteria*, p.171.; Shephard, Ben, *A War of Nerves: Soldiers and Psychiatrists 1914-1994* (Cambridge, MA: Harvard University Press, 2001), p.77; Showalter, *The Female Malady*, pp.176-177.

who in 1932, would receive the Nobel Prize in Physiology or Medicine for his work on the physiology of nerve cells. The two colleagues developed an ambitious treatment programme for shell shock, which they described in a paper published in *The Lancet* on 9 June 1917; electrotherapy was an essential part of their protocol.[11]

What was the rationale behind Yealland's and Adrian's use of electricity in the treatment of shell shock? – The two young scientists mainly used electric currents to stimulate peripheral nerves in paralysed limbs; the electric stimulus produced feeling and movement in limbs that had previously lacked normal functioning and sensation; the muscle contraction and body movement reminded the soldier of how to use the paralysed body part, and it also demonstrated intact nerve and muscle function. While applying electrical currents, Yealland and Adrian encouraged the shell-shocked soldier with a running commentary to move the affected body part.

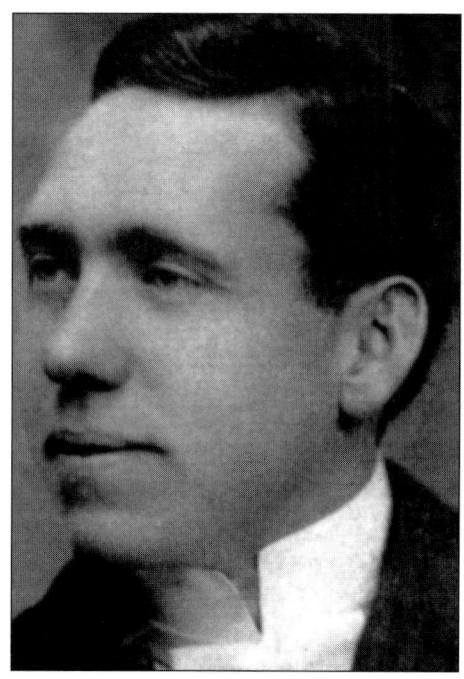

A graduation photograph of Lewis Ralph Yealland, 1912. (With kind permission of Dr Susan Yealland, family archive)

Yealland and Adrian not only applied electrical currents to peripheral nerves, but also – as in the case of a 26-year-old private with a paralysed right arm – directly to the scalp overlying the motor cortex.[12] Although this technique did not allow them to induce contraction of the muscles of the paralysed limb directly, it was believed that stimulating below the threshold for a motor response would still facilitate movement. Today's treatment protocols, with transcranial magnetic or electrical stimulation, use more sophisticated neurophysiological tools, but are based on the same principles.

Although Yealland was among the first in Britain to incorporate electrotherapy into a systematic treatment programme, electrical treatment had a long tradition: during its heyday in the 19th century, departments of electrotherapy were opened in leading teaching hospitals, such as the Radcliffe Infirmary in Oxford and Guy's Hospital in

---

11   Yealland and Adrian, 'The treatment of some common war neuroses', pp.867-872.
12   QSA: Queen Square Records, Dr Steward, 1917, male and female L-Z: case record Walter S.

London, where Golding Bird applied faradic currents for the treatment of hysterical paralysis in the 1840s. The main advocate of electrotherapy in France was Guillaume-Benjamin-Amand Duchenne, who used it for the treatment of disorders of peripheral nerve and muscle. His 1855 work, *De l'électrisation localisée*, was translated into English in 1871 by Herbert Tibbits – the medical superintendent of the West End Hospital for Diseases of the Nervous System in Welbeck Street, London. Electrotherapy was also popular with asylum psychiatrists in the late 19th century: they applied it not only to the limbs, but also to the head – and there were occasional reports of inadvertent seizures, which can be regarded as precursors of electroconvulsive treatment; however, because of the generally disappointing results for mental illness, this treatment had largely vanished from the UK by the beginning of the 20th century.[13]

Yealland and Adrian were, by no means, the only shell shock doctors to resurrect the defunct treatment modality of electrotherapy: for example, Frederick Walker Mott (Sir Frederick from 1919) frequently used electrotherapy for soldiers with shell shock at the newly-founded Maudsley Hospital; he also referred patients he had failed to cure to Yealland. In his Chadwick lecture – delivered on 26 April 1917 on 'Mental Hygiene in Shell Shock During and After the War'[14] – Mott reported on one of his patients, who had been deaf and mute for nearly a year. Mott had tried 'strong electric shocks, tuning-forks to the head, and sudden noises and hypnotism, without any result'. He then referred the soldier to Yealland, who managed to cure him. Mott concluded: 'I think the imposing array of electrical machines, coloured lights, and other strong suggestive influences were partly instrumental in accomplishing what I had failed to do, but also I think the knowledge of success in other difficult cases, attending Dr. Yealland's effort, played a very important part in curing by strong suggestion this apparently hopeless case'.

Strikingly, Yealland is almost exclusively cited for his treatment with strong faradic currents and has been depicted as the leading exponent of disciplinary therapy in Britain. Yealland's treatment undoubtedly had a punitive component, but this was only part of a more comprehensive treatment concept: contrary to its literary depiction, faradism for Yealland was not primarily a punishment, but a neurophysiological procedure with a strong suggestive element. As reckoned by Mott, the impressive electrical machinery increased the suggestive power of the whole treatment procedure. Yealland mainly used weak currents and only resorted to painful strong currents if the patient did not respond to first-line treatment: for example, in patients who had lost their voice, tickling the back of their mouth with a mirror or tongue depressor could trigger a 'reflex phonation' – making the application of painful currents through

---

13   Beveridge, Allan W. and Renvoize, Edward B., 'Electricity: a history of its use in the treatment of mental illness in Britain during the second half of the 19th century' – *British Journal of Psychiatry*, 153:2 (1988), pp.157-162.
14   Mott, 'The Chadwick Lecture on Mental Hygiene and Shell Shock'.

a pharyngeal electrode unnecessary.[15] Yealland also described early applications of cross-modal sensory integration, which is the modification of one sensory modality by stimulation of another – in this case, audition and touch. For the treatment of functional deafness – as covered in Chapter 6, in the example of Private John P. – he applied tuning forks of different sizes to the mastoid (the bony protuberance behind the ear), beginning with very large ones (those in which the vibrations were slow enough to be felt, rather than heard) and reducing the size gradually until the fork could be heard. Yealland's treatment methods – which he revised continuously – were not only influenced by the emerging field of neurophysiology, but also by cognitive (persuasion) and behavioural theories (operant conditioning), as we will see later in this chapter.

Yealland's embracing of the science of his day – and adopting innovative treatment approaches – does not diminish the harshness of some of his interventions: the way he addressed his patients was schoolmasterly, authoritarian, sometimes patronising – denying the patient compassion and moral support. Yealland played on the soldier's greatest fear of being accused of malingering: one example is the case of 24-year-old Percy W., whose hands had been frostbitten at Albert in Northern France, when he was driving with the Royal Garrison Artillery.[16] Percy's right hand had become swollen, cyanosed (blue due to lack of oxygen) and later, infected. At Rouen, an operation was performed under general anaesthesia to remove the pus – and as a result, Percy lost power in his right wrist. His right arm became completely useless and trembled continuously; however, Percy showed marked ambivalence regarding his treatment at the National Hospital: he insisted that his condition was due to 'tetanus' – a life-threatening disease caused by the toxins of bacteria and associated with muscle cramps and paralysis.

Percy denied that his symptoms could be psychological in origin and requested to be sent back to 'his former hospital'. Yealland, not happy with Percy's indecision and reluctance to commit to his treatment regime, unambiguously explained:

> If you insist on returning to your former hospital you may do so, but I shall be in a position to accuse you of malingering. In order that you may understand what I mean by malingering I shall speak plainly to you. You are assuming a paralysis of your hand, so that it will be the means of preventing your return to active service. If you do not accept the treatment I shall be in a position to accuse you plainly of a grave military offence.

Percy succumbed to Yealland's arguments and consented to treatment. The use of Percy's hand was completely restored after 10 minutes of electrotherapy; however,

---

15   Yealland and Adrian, 'The treatment of some common war neuroses', pp.867-872.
16   QSA: Queen Square Records, Dr Collier, 1917, male and female L-Z: case record Percy W.

when assessing Yealland's treatment methods, we also have to consider their historical context: the pressure on doctors to return invalid soldiers to active duty and the other treatment options available.[17] Indeed, Yealland was not isolated in his use of electrotherapy: not only his British colleagues, but in particular, the doctors of the Central Powers, used electrotherapy in combination with suggestion on a much larger scale – and with sometimes disastrous consequences.

What the other side did

In Germany, painful electric currents were frequently used for the treatment of shell shock: here, they were explicitly used as a punishment for abnormal behaviour (such as a bizarre gait, stammer or tics) or loss of function (such as paresis of an arm or leg, or an inability to talk). Electrotherapy had been established at the Charité in 1867 by Carl Westphal, but the initial rise of electrotherapy in Berlin – and elsewhere in Germany – was fuelled by organic models of hysteria and neurasthenia, assuming that electrical stimulation could restore the body's depleted nervous energies.[18] Unlike in the UK, where electrotherapy had lost its popularity, it had remained fashionable in Germany in the decade before the First World War as a treatment for a wide range of neurological and psychiatric problems.[19]

The treatment of Joseph M., a 22-year-old soldier from Berlin Charlottenburg, who stayed at the Charité for two months, is typical of this electrotherapeutic approach:[20] Joseph read medicine from Easter 1914 until the summer of 1916, when he passed his preclinical exam. He was a sensitive boy: a committed vegetarian, fluent in several languages, and a gifted musician and painter. In the summer of 1916, he was sent to the Western Front as an infantry soldier; not long into his service, a shell explosion robbed him of his speech. At various military hospitals, Joseph was treated with hypnosis, electric currents, speech therapy, breathing exercises and massages – without much success. The most drastic measure, however, was a form of shock therapy, which had been specifically developed for cases of speech loss: a metal ball was inserted into Joseph's voice box – taking his breath away and leaving him in the fear of suffocating; his voice did not recover.

When Joseph was finally admitted to the Charité in January 1918, he made desperate attempts to speak, but could only manage to make sibilant and aspirate sounds. When

17 Jones, Edgar, 'Doctors and trauma in World War One: The response of British military psychiatrists' in Gray, Peter and Oliver, Kendrick (eds), *The Memory of Catastrophe* (Manchester: Manchester University Press, 2004), pp.91-106.
18 Killen, Andreas, *Berlin Electropolis: Shock, Nerves, and German Modernity* (Berkeley, Los Angeles, London: University of California Press, 2006), p.55.
19 Linden, Stefanie C. and Jones, Edgar, 'German Battle Casualties: The Treatment of functional Somatic Disorders during World War I' – *Journal of the History of Medicine and Allied Sciences*, 68:4 (2013), pp.627-658.
20 Historisches Psychiatriearchiv Charité M8875/1918: Krankenakten.

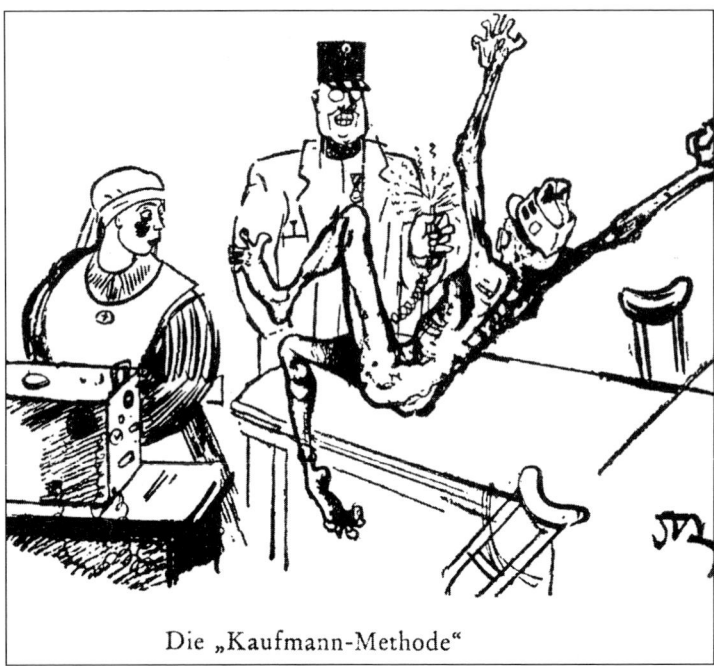

Die „Kaufmann-Methode"

'Kaufmann method'; caricature from Hirschfeld, M. and Gaspar, A., *Sittengeschichte des ersten Weltkrieges* (Hanau: Müller & Kiepenheuer, 1929; re-print of the 2nd revised edition, 1980), p.360.

asked to say 'e', he opened his mouth widely, as if wanting to say 'a'. He grimaced and tried to indicate with gestures that he could not speak; however, there was nothing wrong with Joseph's vocal cords, as confirmed by an ENT surgeon. This was a clear case of shell shock. Under the influence of suggestion – and with the help of a mirror, through which he could observe his facial expression – Joseph was asked to say '*fahne*' ('flag') and '*fahren*' ('drive'). Although he finally managed to say 'fa', the therapist decided to end the session and switch to a more promising treatment method: to accelerate recovery, painful electric currents were applied to the patient's neck. Joseph tried to resist the treatment by lashing about, but was restrained by two male nurses. At first, he only managed to make sibilant sounds, while gesticulating wildly with his hands and moving his head theatrically. The doctors encouraged Joseph, and repeatedly told him that he would be able to speak very soon. After five minutes, Joseph was able to say 'a'; after 10 minutes, he repeated whole words; it did not take long until he could hold a normal conversation. Because Joseph was also dragging his right leg behind, electric shocks were applied, while he was repeatedly cheered on by the physician. After only five minutes of treatment, Joseph was able to walk 'in parade pace'. Following this treatment success, Joseph was allowed to take a rest; however, the young man – obviously glad about his speedy recovery – followed his calling: he read medical books, transcribed patient files and examined other patients' urine. On discharge from the Charité, Joseph was diagnosed with a 'psychopathic constitution'; he was declared 'fit for garrison service'.

It is striking how similar this treatment description is to those documented by Yealland at Queen Square: German shell shock doctors practised this combination of electrotherapy and suggestion, which had been introduced by the Austrian neurologist Fritz Kaufmann, on a wide scale.[21] The *British Medical Journal* published a detailed description of the German 'Kaufmann cure' under the heading of 'disciplinary treatment of shell shock' on 23 December 1916 – attesting to the fact that the war did not stop the exchange of medical ideas across the combatant countries;[22] however, after several reported deaths – and presumably, a considerable number of severe adverse reactions that went undocumented – German resistance against the Kaufmann method grew amongst both patients and doctors, and its use was restricted by the military medical authorities in the final weeks of the war.

Other forms of punishment

Punishments could take a wide range of forms beyond this application of electric currents. In Jena, patients with abnormal body movements, such as tremors or shakes, were immobilised in a cast; for example, soldiers who were shaking with their heads, had their head, neck and shoulders put into plaster for several days. This intervention had mixed results, and symptoms could recur immediately after the plaster was removed. Another common form of punishment, or deterrence, was the confinement to the locked psychiatric ward, where mainly aggressive, agitated and confused patients were treated – and the only way to escape imprisonment was to demonstrate a recovery from symptoms; such cures could occur within a very short period of time (often within hours of admission).

Isolation was another way of punishing patients who did not comply with conventional therapies. Isolation therapy had already been practised before the war in order to remove hysterical patients – mainly women – 'from the noxious influence of both domestic worries and mistaken sympathy'. In Jena, soldiers were confined to their bed in a single room and not allowed to read, write, smoke, talk to the nurses or receive visitors. Otto Binswanger, head of the psychiatric university department (who based this mental deprivation treatment on his view that attending to the patient too much, or showing compassion, resulted in an exacerbation of symptoms), claimed high success rates with this approach. Binswanger himself acknowledged that the ban on reading, writing and receiving visitors was 'harsh and difficult to impose', and thus only applied to severe cases of hysteria.[23] The following history from the Jena case records illustrates that Binswanger's treatment programme could cause suffering, but

21 Raether, 'Neurosen-Heilungen', pp.321-323.
22 'The War. Notes from German and Austrian Medical Journals. Disciplinary Treatment of Shell Shock' – *British Medical Journal*, 2:2921 (1916), p.882.; Binneveld, *From Shell Shock to Combat Stress*, p.111.
23 Binswanger, Otto, *Die Pathologie und Therapie der Neurasthenie: Vorlesungen für Studierende und Aerzte* (Jena: Verlag von Gustav Fischer, 1896), p.395.

at the same time, be very effective – at least from the physicians' perspective: Friedrich S., a 32-year-old nurse, had been at the front line as a stretcher bearer from November 1914 to April 1916.[24] In February 1916, he started suffering from shortness of breath and, in April 1916, he lost his voice.

On admission to the Jena Military Hospital, he was mute and gasping for breath at a continuous rate of 60 per minute – and this alarming behaviour continued for days. Friedrich was referred to the throat clinic and the medical department, which duly ruled out organic disease.[25] Electrical currents were then applied to the patient's larynx, and he also received speech therapy and breathing exercises; however, Friedrich did not regain his voice – and his breathing, which sounded like a 'death rattle', did not slow down. Continued electrotherapy – in combination with verbal suggestions, occupational therapy in the garden, breathing exercises and individual and group speech therapy – made no difference at all, and this had a profound effect on Friedrich's morale. The man who had once cared for the sick and provided encouragement to demoralised troops refused to get up in the morning and clean his room; he did not attend speech therapy and left hospital without permission. As a disciplinary measure, Friedrich was transferred to the locked ward for 'mental deprivation therapy'. Friedrich was isolated, had to stay in bed and received wet packs. Very upset about this enforced isolation, Friedrich cried and sobbed, retched and gasped for breath. He indicated that he wanted to write something down, but was refused pen and paper.

On 23 December, Friedrich still could not utter a single word. He was told that – because of his lack of progress – he would not be allowed to take part in the Christmas celebrations; Friedrich was furious. In his rage, he threw his faeces and some dishes against the wall and threatened a male nurse. The nurse, unimpressed by his outrage, took Friedrich to the observation room, where – all of a sudden – Friedrich regained his voice (just in time to attend the choral service and Christmas celebrations). However, not all patients responded to Binswanger's cures: in some of the unsuccessful cases, Binswanger abandoned his practice of offering them a discharge from military service, as illustrated in the following case of a 27-year-old reservist who had also lost his voice before he could be sent to the front line. After 19 days of unsuccessful treatment with electrotherapy and waking suggestion in Jena, he was sent back to his regiment with the note: 'The absence of speech does not prevent him from doing his service'.[26] This case showed the considerable power that psychiatrists could exercise over their soldier-patients; clearly, failure of the cure was not blamed on the doctor, but on the patient.

---

24 Universitätsarchiv Jena, Bestand S/III Abt. IX, Kriegsarchiv, Nr.710.
25 With laryngoscopy, bacteriological examination of sputum and a chest X-ray.
26 Universitätsarchiv Jena, Bestand S/III Abt. IX, Kriegsarchiv, Nr.360.

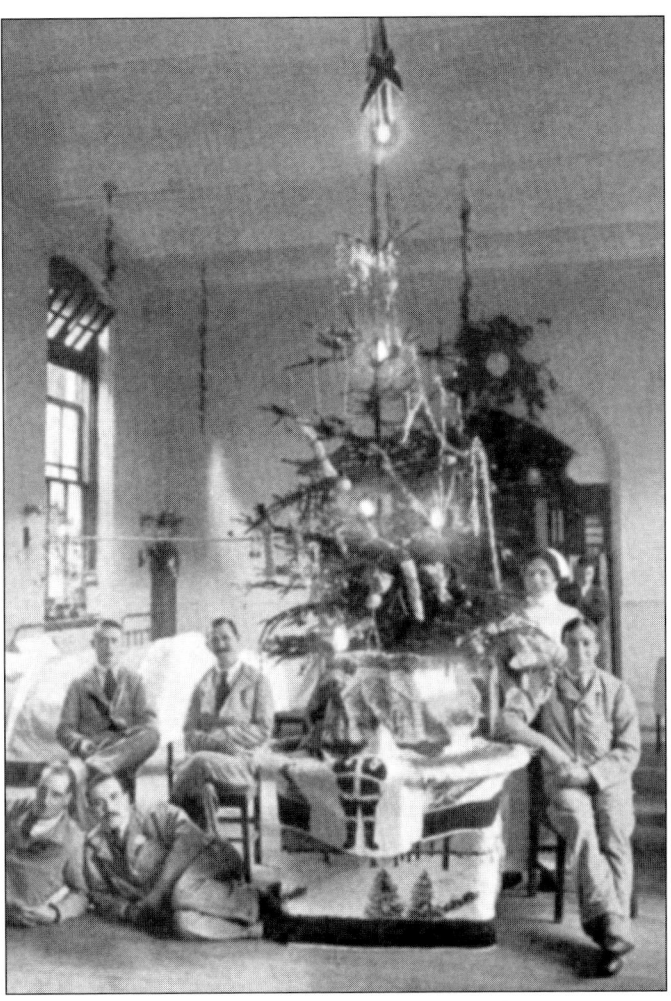

Christmas in a soldiers' ward, 1916; QSA/15491. (Queen Square Archives, London)

Believe your doctor

Suggestion as a powerful therapeutic aid already had a long tradition in European medicine (for example, for the induction of pain relief during surgical interventions).[27] We have already made the acquaintance of the most prominent promoter of suggestive methods in the 19th century – Professor Jean-Martin Charcot (see Chapter 1), who induced hypnotic states ('somnambulism') in hysterical patients from 1878 onwards – thus, First World War physicians could rely on a well-developed arsenal of suggestive

---

27   Linden and Jones, 'German Battle Casualties', p.632.

```
                                    C O P Y
                                    -----
TELE. 3960 Mayfair.                              78 Wimpole Street. W.I.
                                                 11th January 1918.

Dear Sir,
            I saw Private J...........
            I also saw Pte.E...........
            Private ▓▓▓▓▓▓▓▓▓ is suffering from chronic hysterical
hemianaesthesia.  If you will apply for his transference to the
National Hospital as an In-Patient, he will very rapidly be cured.
                           Believe me
                              Your very truly,
                                    (Sgnd) E.FARQUHAR.BUZZARD.
Major.H.W.M.Tims.
    O i/c Bermondsey Military Hospital.

            CERTIFIED that the above is a true copy of the above letter
so far as it relates to Private ▓▓▓▓▓▓▓▓.

                                    [signature]
                                    Major.  R.A.M.C.
                                    Officer in Charge.
```

A referral letter for Private Harry T., which was written by S. Farquhar Buzzard, consultant at Queen Square. (Queen Square Archives, London)

techniques. The most simple and effective way to facilitate recovery was to tell the patient – either when awake ('waking suggestion') or while under hypnosis ('hypnotic suggestion') – that his symptoms would disappear, or had already been cured. Many prominent physicians emphasised the importance of creating an 'atmosphere of unfeigned optimism', in which the patient was made to believe strongly in his own recovery.[28] To John Thomson MacCurdy – the Canadian biologist, neuropathologist and psychiatrist, who had worked at Alois Alzheimer's laboratory in Munich before the war, and was sent to Maghull to learn about shell shock in 1917 – 'the most potent influence in suggestion seem[ed] to be the general morale and attitude of a hospital as a whole'.[29]

Several therapeutic interventions were based on the idea that shell-shocked soldiers would learn healthy behaviour from recovered comrades or their attending doctor; for example, German military doctor Ferdinand Kehrer – who actively participated

28 Myers, *Shell Shock in France*, pp.59 and 61; "Suggestions of recovery".
29 MacCurdy, *War Neuroses*, p.82.

in military exercises with his patients – only allowed them to socialise with successfully-treated comrades. This so-called 'propaganda of the cured' was used as 'suggestive preparation' before the actual treatment was started.[30] At the same time, it was deemed important to minimise the influence of negative role models: in Jena, where military hospital and psychiatric units were separated, Binswanger had introduced a strict policy of separating shell-shocked soldiers with acute symptoms from their comrades in order to avoid 'hysterical infection'.

Fake treatments were another way of using suggestion as a catalyst for cure: a deaf soldier, who was treated at the Royal Victoria Hospital in Netley, was told that he had to undergo an operation in order to cure his deafness; his doctor was the renowned shell shock specialist Arthur Hurst. Hurst made incisions to the patient's scalp and inserted sutures while the patient was in an ether-induced semi-conscious state. The pseudo operation was successful: the patient regained his hearing.[31] On other occasions, a hammer was banged on a sheet of iron while the sham procedure was carried out – adding to the dramatic effect and giving the impression of a major surgical intervention.[32] Another advocate of such *faux* therapeutic interventions was Ninian Bruce, who worked on the neurological wards of the Royal Victoria Hospital in Edinburgh. He told a patient who had developed functional blindness of his left eye after a shell explosion that 'the reason he could not see with this eye was because it had become so weak as the result of the explosion, and that he was going to be given a series of injections into his left temple of a very strong drug, which would so strengthen his eye that the sight would be restored'. The patient then received daily injections of gradually increasing quantities of normal saline solution into the left temple;[33] according to their promoters, these sham procedures resulted in an immediate and complete recovery of symptoms.

Very similar interventions were popular in Germany: a German specialty was the so-called 'wonder drug technique', which entailed making the patient believe that a potent drug was administered while he was under a general anaesthetic.[34] German soldiers who had lost their voice were put under general anaesthesia after being told that they would be able to speak after the procedure. On waking up, they received strong electric currents to their auricle (the pain-sensitive part of the ear's cartilage) and nasal mucosa; simultaneously, the doctor made them believe that they had already talked in their sleep. As soon as the patient started talking – still drowsy from the anaesthesia – he continuously had to recite poetry. Another procedure was implemented by

---

30   Kehrer, Ferdinand, 'Zur Frage der Behandlung der Kriegsneurosen' – *Zeitschrift für die gesamte Neurologie und Psychiatrie*, 36:1 (1917), pp.1-22.
31   Hurst, *Medical Diseases of the War*, pp.27-28.
32   Hurst, *Medical Diseases of the War*, p.120.
33   Bruce, Ninian, 'The treatment of functional blindness and functional loss of voice' – *Review of Neurology and Psychiatry*, 14 (1916), pp.195-198.
34   Rothmann, M., 'Zur Beseitigung psychogener Bewegungsstörungen bei Soldaten in einer Sitzung' – *Münchner Medizinische Wochenschrift*, 63 (1916), pp.1,277-1,278.

German physician D. Dub, who etherised his patients and, on waking, operated an X-ray machine – pretending that something measurable had changed and the patient was cured.[35]

While many physicians took advantage of the fact that patients were highly impressionable and susceptible to verbal suggestions on waking from a general anaesthesia,[36] others achieved this state of high susceptibility with hypnosis: in Germany, the Hamburg physician Max Nonne reached celebrity status for his large-scale application of hypnotic suggestion in shell-shocked soldiers.[37] Nonne, who had first witnessed the therapeutic application of hypnosis in Paris in 1889, enjoyed performing his technique in front of big audiences (like his famous teacher, Jean-Martin Charcot). By the end of the war, Nonne and his Hamburg colleagues – so he claimed – had treated 1,600 cases of shell shock with a response rate of 95 percent; however, despite its reportedly high success rate, many of Nonne's colleagues did not share his enthusiasm for hypnosis (indeed, leading German shell shock doctors were deeply divided on the issue of hypnosis). In his textbook on hysteria, Binswanger mentioned three reasons why he strongly opposed treatment methods involving deep hypnotic states: firstly, he did not believe in its effectiveness and argued that the powers of suggestion were highly overrated; secondly, he had seen cases in which hypnosis had actually triggered hysterical symptoms; and thirdly, he believed it to be too deep an intrusion into an individual's mind.[38]

Binswanger's attitude towards hypnosis was similar to that of many influential British psychiatrists who doubted its long-term efficiency, or believed that psychotherapy should be addressed to the conscious mind: because all suggestive methods at some point replaced the patient's will with that of the doctor, they were hard to reconcile with increasingly popular concepts of patient autonomy and self-efficacy.[39] Although hypnotic suggestion did not become widespread practice in Britain, there were a few enthusiastic therapists who incorporated this technique into a more complex treatment plan: J.A. Hadfield, who worked at Ashurst War Hospital in Oxford, used hypnotic and post-hypnotic (in the waking process) suggestions to help his patients cope with the terrifying experiences which had come to light under hypnosis. These suggestions were aimed at restoring the patient's calmness and self-confidence, and

35   Dub, D., 'Heilung psychogener Taubheit, Stummheit (Taubstummheit)' – *Deutsche Medizinische Wochenschrift*, 42:52 (1916), pp.1,601-1,602.
36   Milligan, E.T.C., 'A method of treatment of "shell shock"' – *British Medical Journal*, 2:2898 (1916), p.73.
37   Nonne, Max, *Funktionell-motorische Reiz- und Lähmungs-Zustände bei Kriegsteilnehmern und deren Heilung durch Suggestion in Hypnose* (Hamburg: Allgemeines Krankenhaus Hamburg-Eppendorf, 1918); Nonne, *Anfang und Ziel meines Lebens*, pp.177-183.
38   Binswanger, Otto, *Die Hysterie* (Wien: A. Hoelder, 1904).
39   Smyly, Cecil P., 'Treatment by Suggestion' – *Dublin Journal of Medical Science*, 139:4 (1915), pp.252-268; Norman, Hubert J., 'Treatment of Insanity: Treatment by Suggestion' – *Journal of Mental Science*, 63:260 (1917), pp.122-123.

reassure him that he would recover from his terrors. Hadfield also practised collective hypnosis, sometimes hypnotising 20-25 patients at once, and then used general suggestions of confidence and reassurance – followed by suggestions adapted to the symptoms of the individual patient.

Psychoanalyst Montague David Eder applied suggestion in the waking state and under hypnosis at a specialised psycho-neurological department in Malta. His approach was more complex, because – true to his Freudian pedigree – he based his suggestions on an in-depth analysis of his patients' conflicts.[40]

The only British physician who publicly considered hypnotic suggestion a universal cure for all functional disorders of wartime was Oxford-trained J. Bennett Tombleson; he reported that all soldiers he treated with hypnosis – most of them suffering from functional disorders – were permanently cured.[41]

Surprise attack

Many British and German doctors also considered shock and surprise to be powerful treatment tools:[42] a very pious German soldier, with functional mutism, was woken up from sleep by shouting at him: "Praise the Lord." The soldier – suddenly alerted and confused – immediately replied: "Now and forever, amen."[43] The most radical shock treatment was that promoted by ENT surgeon Otto Muck from Essen; we have already come across this harsh procedure earlier in this chapter (in the case of medical student Joseph M.): Muck induced an intense fear of suffocation through the insertion of a ball probe into the larynx of the mute soldier, and this terrifying experience commonly led to the patient shouting out in extreme fear – thus recovering his voice within seconds.[44] Along similar lines, spilling boiling tea over a mute soldier, or throwing a bucket of cold water over him when sitting in a hot bath immediately restored the lost voice in the majority of cases.[45]

Similarly dramatic was the sudden recovery of 19-year-old Private Charles A. from the London Scottish Regiment, who had been suffering from a paralysis of one leg. Although this was not a planned intervention, he was 'cured by a fall over hospital

---

40   Eder, *War-Shock*, pp.128-143.
41   Tombleson, J. Bennett, 'A series of military cases treated by hypnotic suggestion' – *The Lancet*, 188: 4860 (1916), pp.707-710.
42   Mott, 'The Chadwick Lecture', p.40.
43   Mann, G., 'Zur Frage der traumatischen Neurose' – *Wiener Klinische Wochenschrift*, 52 (1916), pp.257-261; as cited by Bresler, Johannes, 'Das Kaufmann-Verfahren bei funktionellen Nervenstörungen' – *Psychiatrisch-Neurologische Wochenschrift*, 17/18 (1917-1918), pp.101-105.
44   Muck, Otto, 'Psychologische Betrachtungen bei Heilungen funktionell stimmgestörter Soldaten' – *Münchner Medizinische Wochenschrift*, Feldärztliche Beilage, 63 (1916), p.441.
45   McDowall, Colin, 'Mutism in the Soldier and its Treatment' – *Journal of Mental Science*, 64:264 (1918), pp.54-64; Mott, Frederick W., 'The psychic mechanism of the voice in relation to the emotions' – *British Medical Journal*, 2 (1915), pp.845-847.

steps' on admission to Queen Square in 1915, as documented in the notes.[46] Other anecdotes by influential therapists of the time recounted how the torpedoing of a ship suddenly restored the vision of a functionally blind soldier,[47] or 'the announcement at a picture house of Rumania's entry into the war' had cured two cases of functional mutism simultaneously.[48] After one such event, it became almost impossible for the soldier to maintain his functional symptoms.

A similar surprise cure of functional mutism could be achieved with a sudden squeeze of the abdominal wall. McDowall, the propagator of this treatment, also described another surreptitious treatment for functional deafness:

> The patient is seated in a chair and holds a small mirror in his hand. I stand behind the man and instruct him to look at my eyes reflected in the mirror. After a suitable interview a sudden noise is made without any movement on my part. The patient will blink and the mirror will render him conscious that he has moved his eyelids. He is also conscious that the movement is a proof that he can hear.[49]

MacCurdy used a similar 'trick' on a deaf-mute patient, who was made to see in a mirror that he jumped when a sudden sound occurred behind his back.[50] These procedures, whose success was based on unconscious reflexes in reaction to unexpected stimuli, were strikingly similar to Robert Sommer's treatment method for functional deafness in Germany: Sommer exposed mute patients to unexpected auditory stimuli (usually, a bell ringing behind the patient); the patient was startled and moved his hand, which was recorded on a graph – and this record served as prove of intact hearing.[51]

Early behavioural therapy

Not all behavioural approaches to functional neurological symptoms were quite as drastic as the surprise attack; doctors knew that more gradual changes could shape a patient's behaviour as well: a few years before the First World War, the American psychologist Edward Thorndike had developed animal learning theory – and one of its basic tenets was that a particular behaviour increased in frequency if it produced a positive outcome, such as a food reward, and that it decreased if coupled with an

46 QSA: Queen Square Records, Dr Batten, 1915, male A-K: case record Private Charles A.
47 Hurst, *Medical Diseases of the War*, pp.127-128.
48 Smith and Pear, *Shell Shock and its Lessons*, p.12.
49 McDowall, 'Mutism in the Soldier and its Treatment', p.64.
50 MacCurdy, *War Neuroses*, p.94.
51 Sommer, Robert, 'Beseitigung funktioneller Taubheit, besonders bei Soldaten, durch eine experimental-psychologische Methode' – *Archiv für Psychiatrie und Nervenkrankheiten*, 57:2 (1917), pp.574-575.

unpleasant consequence.⁵² Such links between rewards and desirable behaviours, or between punishments and undesirable behaviours, could also be adapted for behaviour modification in humans. The analogies between animal learning experiments and wartime treatment programmes for functional disorders are striking – and indeed, the treatment of war neurotics was frequently compared to the taming of a wild animal. Nonne applied electric stimuli 'like the spur of a rider used for a lazy or stubborn horse' and Kehrer compared the treatment of bed-wetting in his soldier patients to the 'house training of a young dog'.⁵³ German psychiatrists were familiar with concepts of reinforcement and model learning, and also gradual exposure, which later assumed a central role in behavioural therapy.

Most physicians tried to consolidate progressive treatment successes with rewards, such as baths, massages and garden walks. Repeated praise and reassurance accompanied most therapies – and some programmes even included performance-related pay; some physicians granted their patients home leave when a certain treatment goal had been achieved.⁵⁴ In the latter stages of the war, successfully-treated soldiers were even rewarded with discharge from military service (probably the most potent reinforcement for the traumatised serviceman).⁵⁵ Nonne told soldiers who were discharged from his wards as 'unfit for military service' that they would not have to return to active duty if they worked efficiently in their civilian occupations; alternatively, they would have to undergo more therapy in a military treatment unit – a procedure approved by the War Ministry.⁵⁶ A number of British soldiers, with apparently chronic disorders, recovered in 1918 when regulations changed to allow their discharge from the armed forces (provided their symptoms had remitted).⁵⁷

Motherly pampering and tea parties

Massages, physiotherapy, baths, exercises and work therapy were an essential part of the treatment of shell-shocked soldiers: at the 4th London General Hospital in South London, Mott advocated continuous warm baths for muscle relaxation and sleep induction; improved nourishment; pain relief; quiet rest in single rooms; simple games; and light occupation.⁵⁸ Under his direction – in the extensive grounds of the Maudsley

52 Thorndike, Edward L., *The Elements of Psychology* (New York: A.G. Seiler, 1912).
53 Nonne, 'Über erfolgreiche Suggestivbehandlung', p.196; Kehrer, 'Zur Frage der Behandlung der Kriegsneurosen', p.6.
54 Hirschfeld, R., 'Zur Behandlung im Kriege erworbener hysterischer Zustände, insbesondere von Sprachstörungen' – *Zeitschrift für die gesamte Neurologie und Psychiatrie*, 34:1 (1916), pp.195-205.
55 Beyer, E., 'Die Heilung des Zitterns und anderer nervöser Bewegungsstörungen' – *Psychiatrisch-Neurologische Wochenschrift*, 35/36 (1917-1918), pp.225-228.
56 Nonne, 'Über erfolgreiche Suggestivbehandlung', pp.207-208.
57 Jones, 'Shell Shock at Maghull and the Maudsley', p.387.
58 Mott, 'The Chadwick Lecture on Mental Hygiene and Shell Shock', pp.482-484.

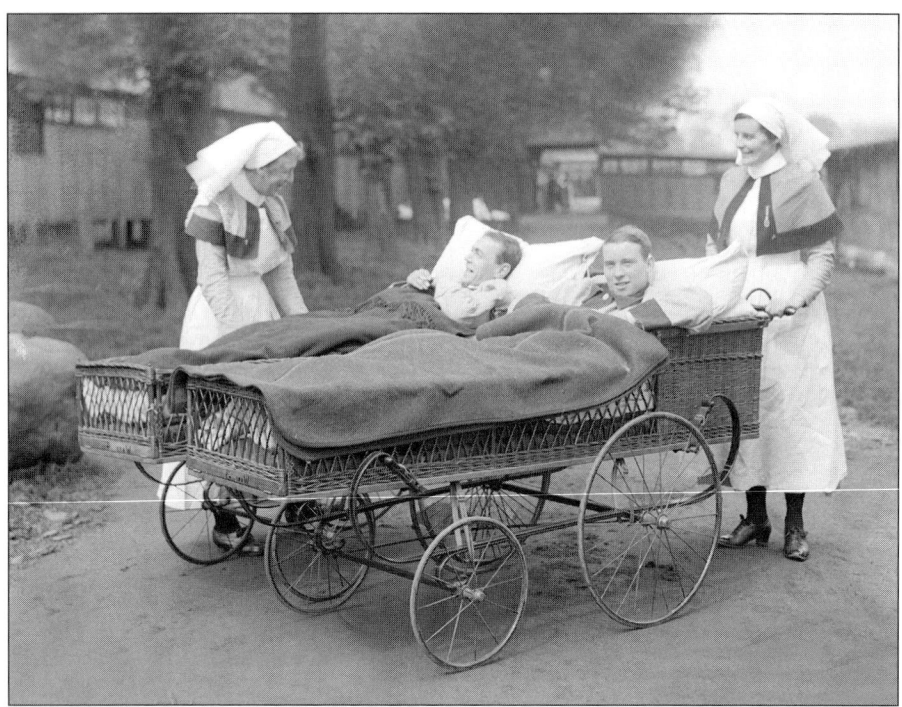

Wounded soldiers in invalid chairs being taken around the grounds of No.4 London General Hospital, Q 27814. (Imperial War Museum, London)

Hospital – reconvalescent shell shock sufferers made 'a fountain and flowerbeds', grew vegetables and kept poultry. Mott also recommended 'choral singing of good music, [...] an uplifting mental diversion, which by promoting cheerfulnesss and healthy recreation could not fail to beget that sense of well-being so essential for mental and bodily recuperation'.[59] Mott's approach resembled that of Silas Weir Mitchell – the American physiologist, who had studied with Claude Bernard in Paris, and had developed his famous rest cure in the 1870s (first applying it in physically exhausted soldiers of the Civil War).[60] Weir Mitchell's cure – which entailed a combination of physical and mental rest, special diet, massages, hydro- and electrotherapy – was eventually introduced to the British medical profession by William Smout Playfair, a professor of Obstetric Medicine at King's College, through a publication in *The Lancet*.[61]

59 Mott, *War Neuroses and Shell Shock*, p.297.
60 Lutz, Tom, 'Varieties of Medical Experience: Doctors and Patients, Psyche and Soma in America' in Gijswijt-Hofstra, Marijke and Porter, Roy (ed.), *Cultures of Neurasthenia: From Beard to the First World War* (New York, Amsterdam: Rodopi, 2001), p.56.
61 Playfair, William S., 'Notes on the systematic treatment of nerve prostration and hysteria connected with uterine disease' – *The Lancet*, 117:3013 (1881), pp.857-859; Marland,

The basket-making class at Lonsdale House; photograph, QSA/15492. (Queen Square Archives, London)

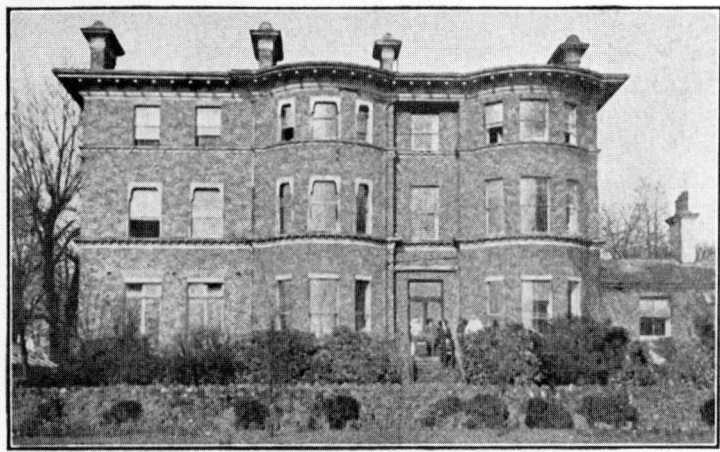

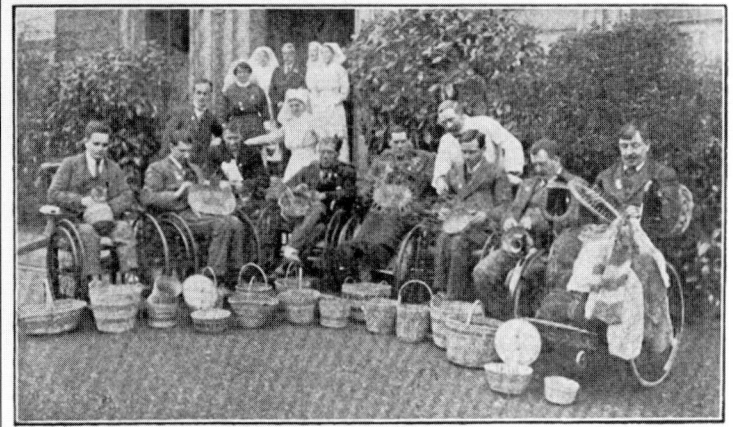

Around the same time (1880s), Weir Mitchell's holistic treatment became known in Germany:[62] Binswanger's deprivation therapy also had its origin in Weir Mitchell's treatment concept, although it was partly reinvented as a behavioural intervention to punish undesired behaviour.[63]

Hilary, '"Uterine Mischief": W.S. Playfair and his Neurasthenic Patients' in Gijswijt-Hofstra, Marijke and Porter, Roy (ed.), *Cultures of Neurasthenia: From Beard to the First World War* (New York, Amsterdam: Rodopi, 2001), pp.120-121.

62 Beard's neurasthenia concept was introduced to German psychiatry in the 1880s; Beard's cure combined the application of electric currents to replenish the nerve force with rest, food, diversion, exercises and medication. Later, Beard also employed suggestion (see Lutz, 'Varieties of Medical Experience', p.54).

63 Linden and Jones, 'German Battle Casualties', p.17.

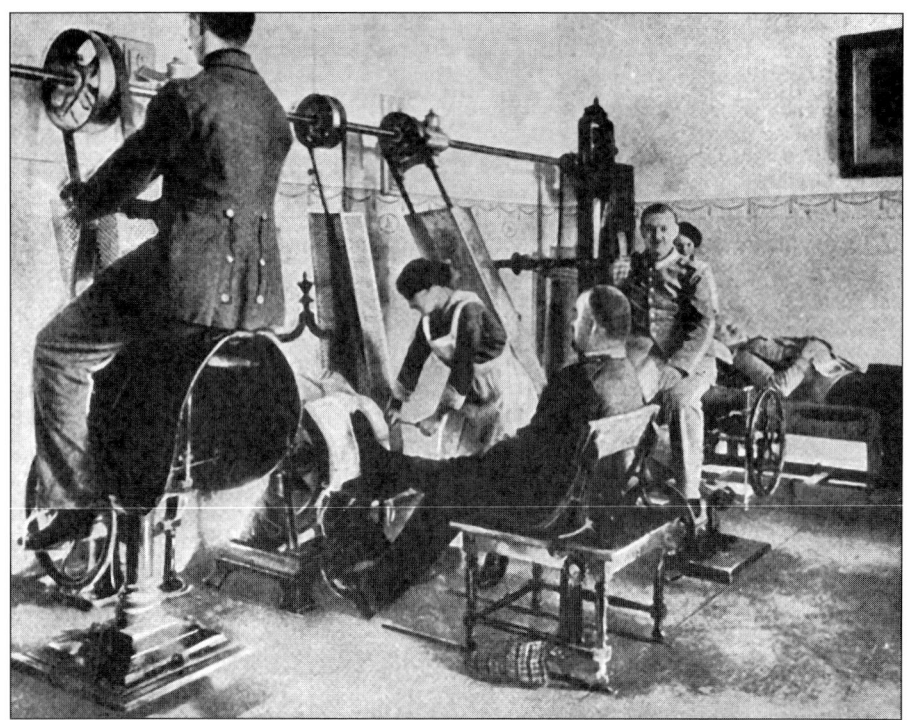

Getting fit to return to the trenches: German wounded undergoing scientific treatment in a Berlin hospital. (From *The Times History and Encyclopaedia of the War*, part 57, Vol 5, Sept 21, 1915, p.197)

Although rest and motherly pampering of acutely traumatised soldiers was promoted by the majority of physicians, others warned against making soldiers feel too comfortable: Mott declared that '[l]axity of discipline, over-sympathy and attention by kind well-meaning ladies giving social tea-parties, drives, joy-rides, with the frequent exclamation of 'poor dear' has done much to perpetuate functional neuroses in soldiers'.[64] Even psychoanalysts thought that an early return to life's duties was important, whereas too much rest could strengthen the motives for remaining ill.[65] To prevent such consolidation of symptoms, treatment had to move slowly, but steadily, from rest to increasing physical and mental exertion; eventually, games and recreational activities were replaced by regular employment (for example, agricultural labour).

64 Mott, 'The Chadwick Lecture on Mental Hygiene and Shell Shock', p.484.
65 Eder, *War-Shock*, p.141.

Talking therapies

A small group of academically-minded doctors in Britain harshly criticised the use of all treatment methods that involved force, pretence or manipulation; they did not approve of the 'stage settings, the drawn curtains and closed shutters', which were all calculated to impress the patient and rob him of his reason.[66] In their opinion, a therapeutic approach which empowered the patient to cure himself, through his own efforts, was not only essential from a moral point of view, but also beneficial for the long-term outcome. The French neurologists Joseph Jules Dejerine – the second successor to Jean-Martin Charcot at the Salpêtrière – and his pupil, Ernest Gauckler, developed a new form of psychotherapy called 'persuasion therapy'. Dejerine's and Gauckler's rationale differed from most other treatment methods, which worked through suggestion or punishment: instead of introducing 'into the consciousness of the subject new ideas, or destroying existing ideas without his consent and judgement', methods of persuasion intended to change thought patterns 'with the consent of the subject, voluntarily after reflection and with full knowledge of the cause'.[67] Dejerine's book was translated into English just before the outbreak of the First World War, and became the 'therapeutic Bible' for many psychologically-minded physicians.[68]

Dejerine's Swiss colleague, Paul Dubois, developed 'rational psychotherapy', which had many similarities with the French approach: rational psychotherapy, which explicitly addressed abnormal thought patterns and was, therefore, based on reasoning and argument, found many supporters among German academic psychiatrists of the time;[69] its application to war trauma entailed the correction of wrong assumptions about the organic origin of symptoms.[70] Persuasion and rational psychotherapy were closely linked to the idea of 'self-efficacy' – a concept which was to become well established in cognitive models of depression in the 1990s, but was already foreshadowed in the thoughts of Dejerine and Gauckler, and their followers.[71]

Although these ideas about more patient-centred treatment approaches were passionately debated, wartime reality – with thousands of shell-shocked soldiers who needed urgent and efficient treatment – required different measures. Persuasion therapy was certainly an exception – reserved for the more privileged soldiers, who

---

66 Dejerine and Gauckler, *The Psychoneuroses and their Treatment by Psychotherapy*, p.283.
67 Dejerine and Gauckler, *The Psychoneuroses and their Treatment by Psychotherapy*, p. 277; translated by Smith Ely Jelliffe.
68 Shephard, Ben, 'The early treatment of Mental Disorder: R.G. Rows and Maghull 1914-1918' in Freeman, Hugh and Berrios, German E. (ed.), *150 Years of British* Psychiatry (London, Atlantic Highlands, NJ: Athlone, 1996), pp.434-464.
69 Dubois, Paul, *Die Psychoneurosen und ihre psychische Behandlung* (Bern, Verlag von A. Francke, 1905); Flatau, Georg, *Kursus der Psychotherapie und des Hypnotismus*, 2nd and 3rd edn (Berlin: S. Karger, 1920), pp.34-40.
70 Flatau, Georg, *Kursus der Psychotherapie und des Hypnotismus* (Berlin: S. Karger, 1920), pp.34-40.
71 Bandura, Albert, *Self-efficacy: The exercise of control* (New York: Freeman, 1997).

were lucky enough to find a dedicated therapist; however, some doctors were adventurous enough to practise individualised talking therapies – and some of them went deep into the unconscious mind to fathom the hidden source of their patients' troubles.

Exploring the unconscious

Hypnosis was not only used to enhance suggestion, but also to access repressed or dissociated traumatic memories.[72] Long before the outbreak of the First World War, the Austrian physician Josef Breuer had been the first to report that hysterical symptoms vanished when hidden memories and emotions associated with the triggering event were brought back into the conscious mind.[73] However, this approach was highly controversial: one central issue of the debate was whether traumatic war experiences should be forced back into the patient's mind. Indeed, most doctors thought that these soldiers should try and forget the horrors of the trenches and move on with their lives.[74] However, this advice was contrary to the principles of psychoanalysis, which held that traumatic memories had to be faced, rather than banished from the mind in order to achieve a permanent cure – and not only a temporary relief from symptoms.[75] Psychodynamic therapies did not only bring war-related traumatic experiences, but also other earlier traumatic events, back into the patient's mind: although Rivers – one of the strongest advocates and, at the same time, one of the sharpest critics of the theories of Sigmund Freud in Britain – considered the reflection of painful experiences as paramount for recovery, he cautioned against focusing too much on the trauma. Rivers, the doctor of Siegfried Sassoon and the other officer-patients at Craiglockhart, also cautioned against paying too much attention to the patients' sexual life. In his view, Freud and his followers had become 'so engrossed with the cruder side of sexual life that their works could often be taken for contributions to pornography rather than to medicine'. Rivers was adamant that he had learnt from his own officer-patients at Craiglockhart that symptoms occurred in persons whose sexual life seemed 'normal and commonplace'.[76]

---

72 Brown, William, 'The treatment of cases of shell shock in an advanced neurological centre' – *The Lancet*, 192:4955 (1918), pp.197-200.
73 Breuer, Josef and Freud, Sigmund, *Studien über Hysterie* (Leipzig, Wien: Franz Deuticke, 1895).
74 Hurst, Arthur F., 'Observations on the etiology and treatment of war neuroses' – *British Medical Journal*, 2:2961 (1917), pp.409-414; Eder, Montague E., 'The Psycho-Pathology of the War Neuroses' – *The Lancet*, 188:4850 (1916), pp.264-268.
75 Bury, Judson S., 'Remarks on the Pathology of War Neuroses: An Address given to the Officers at the Lord Derby War Hospital, Warrington', *The Lancet*, 192:4952 (1918), pp.97-99.
76 Rivers, W.H.R., 'Freud's Psychology of the Unconscious' – *The Lancet*, 189:4894 (1917), pp.912-914.

Although psychodynamic methods gained in authority over the war years – and Maghull provided systematic training in psychoanalysis[77] – classical psychoanalysis was hardly ever practised as a treatment for shell shock in Britain. The constraint on resources was one reason: unlike other treatment methods, such as hypnosis or electrotherapy, psychoanalysis required a long apprenticeship[78] – and although psychoanalysis had originated from the cultural heartland of the Central Powers, psychodynamic treatment of traumatised soldiers was not very common in the German-speaking countries either.[79] Psychoanalysis was still, largely, a procedure employed for outpatients by neurologists and general physicians – and both academic and asylum psychiatry only slowly overcame its hostility to this new treatment philosophy.[80] The military authorities were primarily interested in psychoanalysis because they were hoping for improved recovery rates, with permanent treatment successes, which would facilitate the soldier's return to the front line:[81] on 28 September 1918, members of the International Psychoanalytic Association (among them Freud, as well as high-ranking medical officials from the Austro-Hungarian and German Armies) met in Budapest to discuss the potential of psychoanalysis in the battle against war neurosis. Subsequent plans to establish psychoanalytic treatment units for war neurosis could not be realised though, because of the imminent collapse of the Central Powers.[82]

The treatment revolution

The First World War marked a turning point in the history of neurological treatment:[83] psychiatrists and neurologists were provided with the opportunity – and resources – to evaluate and treat large numbers of patients with similar symptoms.[84] As we have seen in this chapter, treatment approaches for shell shock in Britain and Germany were similar in many respects: suggestive methods (including suggestion under hypnosis and in combination with electrotherapy) were popular and widely practised in several treatment centres in both countries; however, although many treatments were similar – and had already been practised in both countries before the war – there were also notable differences in the preferred treatment approaches: in Germany, behavioural reinforcement – with systematic punishment and reward – was practised in the univer-

---

77   Leese, *Shell Shock*, p.83.
78   Eder, *War-Shock*, pp.139-140.
79   Linden and Jones, 'German Battle Casualties'.
80   Shorter, *A History of Psychiatry*, pp.154-160.
81   Brunner, José, 'Psychiatry, Psychoanalysis, and Politics during the First World War' – *Journal of the History of the Behavioral Sciences*, 27:4 (1991), pp.352-365.
82   Lerner, Paul, *Hysterical Men: War, Psychiatry and the Politics of Trauma in Germany, 1890-1930* (Ithaca, London: Cornell University Press, 2003), p.185.
83   Smith, Grafton E., 'Shock and the soldier' – *The Lancet*, 187:4834 (1916), pp.853-857.
84   Linden and Jones, 'German Battle Casualties', pp.627-658; also Linden, Stefanie C., Jones, Edgar and Lees, Andrew J., 'Shell Shock at Queen Square: Lewis Yealland 100 years on' – *Brain*, 136:6 (2013), pp.1,976-1,988.

sity departments of Berlin and Jena. This approach was also widely described in the contemporary German medical literature, although certain methods of punishment evident from the original case records (such as detention on locked psychiatric wards, or putting body parts into plaster) were not openly discussed.

In Britain, persuasion – in combination with re-education – found much support among academically-minded psychiatrists and neurologists; yet, although British doctors – much more than their German counterparts – promoted patient autonomy and active involvement in the treatment process, the practice at Queen Square followed a different rationale and mainly involved therapies that were clearly based on the doctor's superiority, such as suggestion and electrotherapy. This indicates that the small group of academically-minded doctors who published extensively in medical journals – and were responsible for important theoretical advances in their field – had limited impact on actual treatment practices. This also applied to psychodynamic theories: although we know about several hospitals where these methods were advocated (such as Maghull and Craiglockhart), these time-consuming, elaborate therapies never became common practice.

Treatments developed for war neurotics were diverse and reflected a broad range of theoretical positions. Most of them were forgotten after the armistice, yet, functional neurological disorders remained a major challenge – and thus, some of these techniques (notably electrotherapy and suggestion) made a comeback in the second half of the 20th century, as we will see in Chapter 14. Others, however, such as sham operations, isolation and full-body plaster casts – albeit effective for some soldier-patients – are clearly incompatible with today's ethical standards, and thus not being considered for modern practice.

It has been suggested that the First World War occasioned 'the birth of military psychiatry',[85] but the revolution of psychiatry and neurology during 1914-1918 went beyond the confines of this new discipline: the war years created a new spirit of therapeutic effort and optimism – and in this brief period, neurology and psychiatry claimed treatment successes that had hitherto been unheard of (see Chapter 14). The 1920s and 1930s then saw a quick succession of treatment innovations for the most severe and intractable disorders: several of them were dubious (but nevertheless, attracted Nobel Prizes), such as malaria cure for general paralysis of the insane and leucotomy for melancholic depression and schizophrenia, but others, such as electroconvulsive therapy, constituted transformative treatment innovations. After the war, many psychiatrists would simply not be content largely to administer patients and record their symptoms: they had seen that their discipline could make a real change to the suffering of large numbers of patients, and started subscribing to what Smith and Pear (in their 1917 book) called 'psychiatry as the science of the treatment of mental disorders'.

---

85 Jones, Edgar and Wessely, Simon, 'Battle for the mind: World War 1 and the birth of military psychiatry' – *The Lancet*, 384:9955 (2014), pp.1,708–1,714.

13

The Obsession with the Shell

The organic disease model – the belief that shell shock was a result of micro-lesions in the brain or spinal cord – had fallen from favour by 1916. The mystery of shell shock had been resolved, and psychological theories had won the day (Chapter 4). As a consequence, a wide array of psychological interventions were implemented in rehabilitation units on both sides, which worked surprisingly well – at least, in the short run (Chapter 12); although Yealland's interventions seldom lasted longer than an hour, instantaneous treatment successes were possible. Rapid cures were also promoted in the films produced by charismatic doctors like Max Nonne in Germany, or Arthur Hurst in Britain, who used hypnotic suggestion as their treatment of choice; however, relapses were not uncommon and long-term follow-up studies scarce. Indeed, few shell shock doctors looked into long-term outcomes of those who had been successfully cured.

One of these exceptions was Max Nonne: by the end of the war, Nonne claimed that he and his Hamburg colleagues had treated 1,600 cases of shell shock, with a response rate of 95 percent. Beyond the acute treatment phase, Nonne offered a comprehensive rehabilitation programme at his Hamburg hospital, which included manual labour, various workshops and physical exercises;[1] however, the most effective long-term relapse prevention – so he believed – was to return cured patients into their civilian occupation. Nonne was, by no means, the only shell shock doctor to hold this view, and many German and British doctors followed a similar rationale. What set him apart from his colleagues was his inquisitiveness, which triggered his enquiry into the long-term outcomes of those personally treated by him. Nonne allowed his former shell shock patients to settle back into their civilian routines – and a few months after their discharge from his unit, he sent them a questionnaire to enquire about their symptoms and transition into civilian life (in particular, their occupational functioning). Nonne sent out 60 questionnaires, and 46 patients replied

---

1 Nonne, 'Die erfolgreiche Suggestivbehandlung', p.200; Nonne, *Anfang Und Ziel meines Lebens*, p.178.

– a high response rate even by today's standards. According to the written responses, 26 soldiers had returned to their pre-war occupation, 16 worked reduced hours and four had experienced a relapse of symptoms.[2] Nonne also systematically compared the 'Kaufmann cure' – a combination of suggestion and electrotherapy – to his signature treatment, hypnotic suggestion; naturally, his method turned out to be superior, with 80 percent of patients cured versus 74 percent with the Kaufmann method.[3] His study even found recognition in the British medical press of the time;[4] however, considering the fact that Nonne treated 1,600 patients and only chose 60 for his long-term follow-up study, the evidence of his long-lasting success seems inconclusive.

Some British shell shock doctors also evaluated their long-term treatment success: R. Eager, of the mental section of the Lord Derby War Hospital, documented treatment outcomes for all patients admitted to the hospital between 17 June 1916 and 16 June 1917.[5] His study was noteworthy in two respects: firstly, with 2,429 military admissions within 12 months, the number of cases was impressive;[6] secondly, Eager followed up discharged soldiers by sending a standardised letter to close relations of 170 of his patients some months after their discharge, 'inquiring into their progress'. Replies were received from 123 – a similarly high return rate as in Nonne's follow-up study. According to the replies, 68 (55 percent) 'were keeping fit and well' – and in this group, 28 soldiers had already returned to active service in France. Twenty-seven cases (22 percent of replies) were mentally unstable and 19 (15 percent) had required re-admission to hospital; ten (eight percent) soldiers had been discharged from service.

Another British physician who followed up on his patients' progress was J.A. Hadfield, who had been based at Ashurst War Hospital in Oxford from 1917. Eighteen months after their discharge, Hadfield sent out a questionnaire to the first 100 soldiers he had treated with suggestion and abreaction under hypnosis ('hypno-analysis') – and the treatment success was impressive: 90 percent of his former patients were working full-time in their pre-war employment, and only 10 percent had received a war pension.[7] Other studies with high numbers of patients with functional disorders that provided

2   Nonne, 'Die erfolgreiche Suggestivbehandlung', pp.204-206.
3   Nonne, 'Die erfolgreiche Suggestivbehandlung', pp.197-199.
4   For example, Eder, *War-Shock*, pp.133-134.
5   Eager, R., 'A Record of Admissions to the Mental Section of the Lord Derby War Hospital, Warrington, from June 17th, 1916, to June 16th, 1917' – *Journal of Mental Science*, 64:266 (1918), pp.272-295; for another diagnostic study on cases of the mental section of the Lord Derby War Hospital, see Henderson, D.K., 'War Psychoses: An Analysis of 202 Cases of Mental Disorder occurring in Home Troops' – *Journal of Mental Science*, 64:265 (1918), pp.165-189.
6   The most common diagnoses were melancholia, followed by delusional insanity, and then mental deficiency; very few cases were diagnosed with hysteria – and over half of the cases were discharged to their civilian occupation within a year. Treatment combined physical therapies, rest and occupational programmes.
7   Hadfield, James A., 'Treatment by Suggestion and Hypno-Analysis' in Miller, Emanuel (ed.), *The Neuroses in War* (London: Macmillan & Co., 1940), pp.146-148.

treatment outcomes were conducted by Superintendent Robert D. Hotchkis at the Dykebar War Hospital[8] and by Dudley William Carmalt-Jones at a specialised shell shock centre at No.4 Stationary Hospital in France.[9] Eighteen percent of Hotchkis's patients with predominantly mental disorders – such as depression, alcohol-related disorders and psychoses – eventually returned to duty.[10] Carmalt-Jones, whose report was not published until after the war, had studied the medical records of a stunning number of patients – 4,700 – (of whom he had examined and treated the first 1,300 himself) and analysed clinical features and military outcomes. Of the soldiers he treated himself, 946 (73 percent) suffered from non-organic disorders – and of these shell shock cases, 40 percent were sent back to duty, 40 percent to light duty or prolonged rest previous to duty, and about 20 percent to base hospitals. Carmalt-Jones, who promoted a rest cure and gradual exercises, concluded that cases of shell shock had a good prognosis if they were given sufficient time to recover. Although these studies are impressive, neither Jones, nor Hotchkis, developed a comprehensive treatment concept, or compared outcomes for different therapies.[11]

The only British physician who recorded outcomes for *different* treatment approaches for shell shock was psychoanalyst David Montague Eder: he provided detailed data on symptoms, family and personal history, physical status and treatment outcomes for 100 shell shock cases he treated in Malta; he also compared treatment outcomes for soldiers with or without a personal or family history of mental problems. Eder treated the vast majority of his patients with suggestion under hypnosis (79/100), some with suggestion in the waking state (5/100) or under anaesthetic (6/100), and only five cases with psychoanalysis. Because Eder believed that psychoanalysis was only necessary and successful in patients with a personal or family history of mental problems, he only chose this group of soldiers for this more time-consuming treatment method. At the end of his treatment trial, Eder recorded an 80 percent recovery rate – and four out of five patients with 'a strong neuropathic history', who were treated with psychoanalysis, 'improved';[12] however, Eder's study would not withhold the scrutiny of present-day proponents of evidence-based medicine because his assessments were subjective, and he obviously knew in which group the patients were.

8   Formerly the Renfrew District Lunatic Asylum, where certifiable mental disorders had been treated before the war; Hotchkis, Robert D., 'Renfrew District Asylum as a War Hospital for Mental Invalids: Some Contrasts in Administration. With an Analysis of Cases admitted during the First Year' – *Journal of Mental Science*, 63:261 (1917), pp.238-249.
9   Carmalt-Jones, Dudley W., 'War-Neurasthenia, Acute and Chronic' – *Brain*, 42:3 (1919), pp.171-213.
10 Hotchkis, 'Renfrew District Asylum as a War Hospital for Mental Invalids', p.249.
11 Jones promoted gradual mobilisation with encouragement, gradual exercise, occupation and education (sometimes faradisation).
12 Eder, *War-Shock*, pp.131-132.

The study that came closest to a modern controlled design was Edith Green's treatment study carried out at the Maudsley Hospital: Green, a co-researcher to Mott and an MRC research fellow (see Chapter 4), not only measured physiological changes in shell-shocked soldiers, but also treated 20 of these patients with extract of the pituitary gland (one of the body's main centres of hormone secretion and production). Green tried to eliminate suggestion as a factor contributing to the improvement of symptoms, and to prove the specific effect of the gland extract by introducing a placebo condition: she gave three of the most marked cases 'other pills instead of pituitrin for two to three days'.[13] These outcome studies attest to the level of organisation of the medical systems of both Germany and Britain, and the considerable interest in dependable data on the most effective treatment. The need of the military apparatus to find the most efficient cure for shell shock thus led to some of the first systematic follow-up studies in the entire history of medicine.

Recharging the nerves

Psychological therapies proved successful in the treatment of shell shock symptoms; however, for many traumatised soldiers, the label of a 'psychological deficit' was a heavy burden: as we have learned from many individual stories, British and German soldiers experienced mental symptoms as stigma and a threat to their reputation and dignity. How could they explain to their families, their wives, brothers and children, that they were suffering from a mental breakdown, rather than a 'genuine' combat injury? Even the expression of traumatic experiences through physical symptoms – such as seizures, tremors or paralyses – could not beguile their doctors into thinking that these men suffered from a physical illness. 'War neurosis', 'functional disorder' or 'hysteria' were not only medical diagnoses: they became moral judgements and character references which determined the fate of the individual soldier.

Many doctors realised that pure psychological explanations for the wide range of shell shock symptoms were neither beneficial for the doctor-patient relationship, nor useful for the recovery process. If the patient wanted to believe that he suffered from a physical problem, why aim for a compromise on the illness model? Yealland must have had these arguments in mind when he devised his treament rationale – and although he believed that the symptoms of shell shock were psychological in origin, Yealland communicated a physiological illness model to his patients, which is documented in the description of one of his treatment cases in his 1918 book: this 24-year-old telegraph operator had been rendered unconscious by a shell explosion while working in a signal office on the Somme. Following this incident, he developed a persistent shaking and numbing in his right hand. The shaking got worse every time he moved his hand, and the young man was not able to hold a cup of tea, nor could he execute any purposeful movements. During the first treatment session, Yealland

---

13   Green, 'Blood pressure and surface temperature in 110 cases of shell shock', p.456.

took the patient's shaking hand and applied electric currents to his own hand – saying: "This spasmodic blocking [of nervous impulses] can be easily overcome if a current of electricity is transmitted through my hand to yours. You can see that my hand is steady, and your hand will also be steady in a few minutes."[14] The young soldier could feel the vibrations; Yealland then directly stimulated the patient's hand with a roller electrode while asking him to squeeze his doctor's hand. When the patient's grasp got weaker, Yealland increased the strength of the electric current. After 10 minutes of continuous treatment, the telegraph operator had regained control over his hand; the shaking had subsided and he could be discharged for Home Service. One can imagine the strong suggestive power behind Yealland's words: laying on his hands like a healer, he miraculously cured the traumatised young man. His 'physiological' model – the idea that energy was transmitted from doctor to patient, and that depleted nerves were recharged – took away a huge burden from the shell-shocked soldier. He was absolved from being a 'mental case', or even worse, a malingerer or shirker; by imparting an organic illness and treatment model, Yealland paved the way for a dignified exit.

An even more impressive case is that of a 26-year-old officer with a functional paralysis of his right arm, following the recovery from a gunshot wound he had received in France.[15] Every possible therapy had been tried – including faradism, mobilisation of the arm under general anaesthesia, hypnosis and even psychoanalysis. The officer explained that it felt as if he had 'forgotten how to use [his arm]' and that 'the limb [did] not seem to be part of [him].' Yealland quickly jumped in with his illness model: he gave the officer a lesson about some basic anatomical facts (for example, that the left side of the brain controlled the right side of the body) and he also drew 'a rough diagram of the brain, marking the left motor area, and printing in large letters the arm area'.

This area was responsible for the movement of the right arm; then he explained to the patient why his right arm was not working:

> There is a break, no doubt due to some chemical disturbance, in the motor pathway from the arm area to the nerves of your arm; a flow of current must be established at the base, which is the cortex. … You understand enough about electricity to know that it will transmit an impulse from the brain to the arm if stimulated in the proper place.[16]

After that, Yealland marked out the arm area on his patient's scalp with a blue pencil, and he then applied repeated weak electric currents to this area – encouraging the patient to move his arm; the officer was cured after 10 minutes and could move his arm again. There is no possibility that Yealland's weak transcranial electrical stimulation

---

14 Yealland, *Hysterical Disorders of Warfare*, p.73.
15 Yealland, *Hysterical Disorders of Warfare*, pp. 92-97.
16 Yealland, *Hysterical Disorders of Warfare*, p.95.

could have caused this through actual physiological mechanisms: this recovery of motor function was brought about by suggestion.

The justifiability of therapeutic lying

Many of Yealland's colleagues did not agree with his treatment methods: some of them criticised his use of electrotherapy; others condemned the illness model he communicated to his patients. One of his harshest critics was Charles Samuel Myers, consultant psychologist to the BEF in France and editor of the *British Journal of Psychology*: in a letter published in *The Lancet* in December 1919, Myers harshly condemned Yealland's strategy of making the patient believe that he suffered from an organic problem.

Although Myers did not mention Yealland's name, he must have referred to Yealland's treatment practice – and the case we have just discussed above – when he wrote:

> During the war there were certain physicians who would explain to a patient suffering from functional hemiplegia that the cortical cells on one side of his brain were out of order, or to one suffering from functional deafness that there was something radically amiss with his ear. And they would proceed to tone up the disordered cells by painful faradism.[17]

Myers found the communication of a somatic illness model 'unnecessary and dangerous': with an organic diagnosis, the patient very much relied on the doctor's intervention; if this intervention failed, the patient was left with an organic disorder – bereft of any hope of being cured. Even if the physical intervention was successful, the patient – believing that he was suffering from an organic illness – would live in constant fear of recurrence; however, Myer's latter argument is not entirely convincing, because such a fear of relapse could equally be induced by psychological illness models.

By contrast, Yealland believed that patients were more amenable to the suggestion that they suffered from a physiological disturbance that could be potentially remedied by a physical treatment, such as faradism;[18] for the same reason, Yealland avoided the term 'hysteria' in clinical notes and instead preferred the term 'functional disorder'. Yealland also feared that by communicating a mere psychological interpretation, the patient would be given the impression that he was suspected of malingering, which would have jeopardised the therapeutic process. It is not clear if Yealland believed in some of the neurophysiological mechanisms he explained to his patients, or if he

---

17 Myers, Charles S., 'The justifiability of therapeutic lying: Correspondence' – *The Lancet*, 194:5026 (1919), pp.1,213-1,214.
18 Yealland and Adrian, 'The treatment of some common war neuroses', pp.867-872.

purely used them as a suggestive means; however, by acknowledging the important contribution of suggestion and other psychological techniques, Yealland recognised the interaction of psychological and physiological processes, both in the aetiology and in the treatment of functional neurological syndromes. He came close to contemporary models, which assume that physiological changes can induce functional impairment even in the absence of gross 'organic' lesions.[19]

The revival of organic models

The illness model really mattered to patients: by attributing symptoms of shell shock to a physiological dysregulation or a 'biochemical imbalance', doctors could absolve their patients from 'blame' and enhance therapeutic outcomes – but what did doctors really believe? As we have learned in Chapter 4, the vast majority of neurologists and psychiatrists had settled on a psychological illness model by the middle of 1916 – and indeed, in the course of the war, the search for macroscopic and microscopic changes in the brain and spinal cord of shell-shocked soldiers lost its popularity. Mott modified his views, and Oppenheim – the major German proponent of an organic illness model – was overruled by his colleagues. However, although the search for visible organic lesions had been abandoned, a new wave of research looked at more subtle physiological changes in shell shock victims: in the summer of 1918, Judson S. Bury, a professor of Clinical Medicine at Manchester University and physician to the Manchester Royal Infirmary, warned against dismissing an organic explanation solely because available methods of investigation were insufficient to detect these changes: 'Visibility is a relative term; it depends on our eyesight and the powers of our microscopes, and to some extent on staining reagents. [...] We must admit the possibility that even an emotion such as fear may produce minute changes in some of the cortical neurons'.[20]

Bury's view had many supporters: organic (or physiological) models had remained particularly strong in Britain – and the enduring search for a biological basis of shell shock can be illustrated by the British epidemic of functional heart disorders (labelled 'Disordered Action of the Heart', or 'DAH').[21] DAH was characterised by exhaustion, headaches, irritability, insomnia, tremors, sweating, shortness of breath on exertion, faintness, palpitations, tachycardia (fast heartbeat), tachypnoea (increased breathing

---

19   Vuilleumier, Patrik, 'Hysterical conversion and brain function' – *Progress in Brain Research*, 150 (2005), pp.309-329.
20   Bury, 'Remarks on the Pathology of War Neuroses', p.97.
21   Also called 'irritable heart'/Da Costa's syndrome (Da Costa's syndrome was named after Jacob Mendes Da Costa, who investigated and described the disorder during the American Civil War; Da Costa introduced the term 'irritable heart'), 'soldier's heart', and later, 'effort syndrome'. Jones, Edgar, 'Historical approaches to post-combat disorders' – *Philosophical Transactions of the Royal Society B: Biological Sciences*, 361:1468 (2006), pp.533-542.

rate) and cardiac pain. This disorder was first recorded by the British in the Crimea and called 'palpitation', and it resurfaced in the American Civil War as 'cardiac muscular exhaustion'[22] – emerging as a common cause for unfitness for military service amongst the British colonial forces. W.C. Maclean, professor of Military Medicine at the Army Medical School in Netley, investigated 5,500 soldiers admitted to the medical division of the Royal Victoria Hospital who had served abroad between 1863 and 1866, and found that eight percent had been invalided with what appeared to be heart disease.[23] Maclean, short of an obvious explanation, considered that the weight and distribution of the soldier's equipment were responsible for these common symptoms: the heavy equipment constricted the soldier's chest and circulation – exhausting the heart muscle, which could not keep up with the demands of rigorous physical exertion. Following a War Office inquiry of 1865, soldiers' equipment was re-designed; however, soldiers with irritable heart still flooded the military treatment centres.

Although most functional disorders would, over time, be unmasked as psychological reactions, heart-related symptoms in soldiers continued to attract organic explanations: although the faulty equipment hypothesis was eventually abandoned, organic explanatory models were developed further and became more elaborate over time. This was particularly true for the First World War, when advances in methods for analysing bodily tissues and fluids enabled more sophisticated investigations, but still left much room for speculation.

Although some British doctors of the Great War considered DAH to be a functional disorder, many continued to explore organic explanations: in his monograph *Medical Diseases of the War*, Arthur Hurst included the 'soldier's heart' into the section 'infective disorders'. Hurst believed that 'toxaemia' – a poisoning of the blood, in combination with physical and mental strain – could damage the heart of an otherwise healthy individual without any congenital weakness.[24] Along similar lines, Dublin-born Florence A. Stoney – first female radiologist in the UK and head of the X-ray department of the Fulham Military Hospital from March 1915 – attributed all symptoms of DAH to an over-secretion of the thyroid gland.[25] Stoney destroyed parts of the thyroid gland through the application of radiation, and promoted this procedure as curative treatment.

DAH was so common among British soldiers in the First World War that several specialist treatment and research units for heart disorders were established both in Britain and in France.[26] Although heart-related functional symptoms also occurred in

---

22 Jones, 'Historical approaches to post-combat disorders', pp.533-542.
23 Maclean, W.C., 'Diseases of the heart in the British Army, the cause and the remedy' – *British Medical Journal*, 1:320 (1867), pp.161-164.
24 Hurst, *Medical Diseases of the War*, p.282.
25 Stoney, Florence A., 'On the connexion between "soldier's heart" and hyperthyroidism' – *The Lancet*, 187:4832 (1916), pp.777-780.
26 Jones, Edgar and Wessely, Simon, *Shell Shock to PTSD: Military Psychiatry from 1900 to the Gulf War* (Hove, New York: Psychology Press, 2005), pp.40-43.

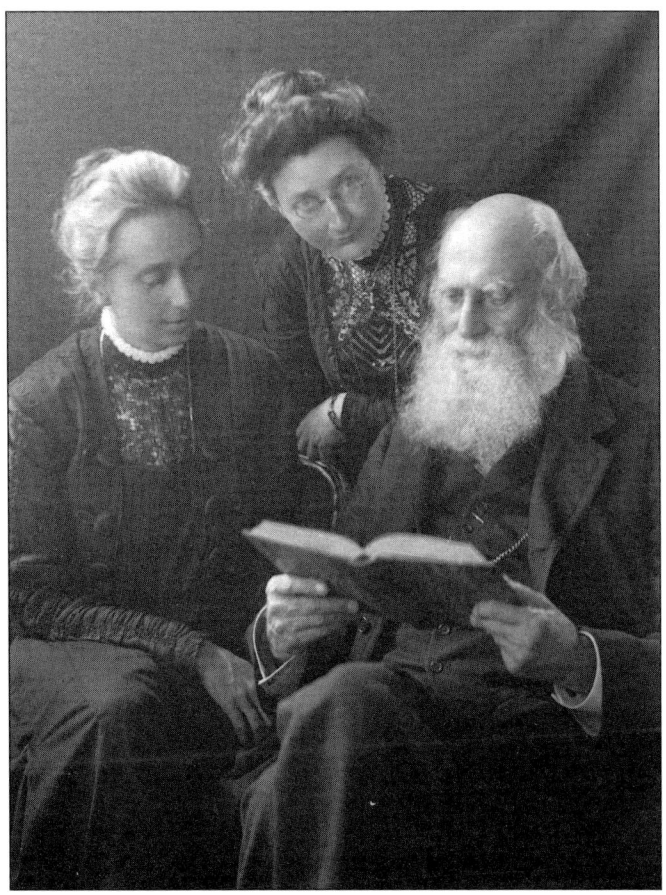

Florence Stoney (centre) with her sister, Edith – a physics lecturer at the London (Royal Free) School of Medicine for Women – in 1899, and their father, G. Johnstone Stoney (the Irish physicist, who coined the word 'electron'). During the war years, Edith left her teaching career to work in field hospitals, in order to provide X-ray and electrotherapy services to wounded soldiers and civilians with the Scottish Women's Hospitals (SWH); PH/10/4 Chrystal album no.2 (Newnham College Archives, Cambridge)

German soldiers, these complaints did not arouse much attention and were generally considered to be part of the complex symptom repertoire of neurasthenia or hysteria; in Germany, no special treatment or research units focused on these disorders.

In Britain, not only heart-related functional symptoms were re-investigated in the light of new scientific advances, but other unexplained medical problems of soldiers became a focus of closer scrutiny as well: the endocrine system, which regulates the release of hormones, seemed to provide the hitherto missing link between mind and body, psychological stress and physical disabilities. D.W. Carmalt-Jones came to the conclusion that all symptoms of shell shock – whether cardiac or neurological – were, at least in part, due to a 'prolonged over-stimulation of the ductless glands, chiefly the adrenal'.[27]

27 Carmalt-Jones, 'War-Neurasthenia, Acute and Chronic', p.212.

Dysfunction of the sympathetic nervous system – the part of the autonomic nervous system that promotes the release of the hormones adrenalin and noradrenalin by the adrenal gland – was also central to another organic concept, which was adopted to explain functional disorders of traumatised soldiers: towards the end of the war, many British neurologists – among them, Mott and Hurst – adopted the concept of 'reflex nervous disorder', which had been introduced by French neurologists Joseph Jules François Félix Babinski and Jules Froment. Like functional motor disorders, reflex paralyses or contractures were not associated with any obvious organic lesions; however – in contrast to mere functional disorders – they showed signs of localised autonomic dysfunction, such as hypothermia (a drop in temperature), cyanosis (blue colouration of the skin – indicative of reduced oxygen supply) and muscular atrophy.[28] Other researchers observed increased skin conductance in shell-shocked soldiers: when electric currents were measured on the surface of their skin with a galvanometer, large currents could be detected in localised areas; this was interpreted as evidence for 'nerve leaks' – an 'escape of nerve energy' from damaged nerve fibres. The loss of nerve insulation and leakage of energy led to neurological deficits, as seen in shell shock patients.[29]

Likewise, German doctors investigated the effects of stress on the endocrine system and believed that some post-traumatic reactions could be related to glandular dysfunction and hormonal imbalance; however, somatic undercurrents proved to be more persistent in the British medical community, which retained organic explanatory models beyond the end of the war. The attempt to ban the term 'shell shock' from official medical terminology did not quite succeed – and even Queen Square neurologists used this term until the end of the war. Although 'shell shock' became a ubiquitous symbol for the horrors of trench warfare, its persistent use also reflected the ethos of a whole generation of British neurologists and psychiatrists who struggled to accept psychological explanatory models for the symptoms exhibited by traumatised servicemen. It was only after the war that medical officers openly admitted that they had frequently attested organic disorders, despite the absence of clear organic signs; after all, the stigma of a psychological diagnosis was highly detrimental to a man's self-respect.[30]

The aftermath

This unofficial practice of attaching an organic label to the various symptoms of shell shock was continued after the armistice: British doctors retained a tendency to provide organic labels wherever possible, and kept searching for physical causes; pension

---

28 Mott, *War Neuroses and Shell Shock*, p.134.
29 Bayliss, William M., 'On the Origin of Electric Currents led off from the Human Body, especially in Relation to "Nerve-Leaks"' – *British Medical Journal*, 1:2934 (1917), pp.387-388.
30 Hargreaves, G. Ronald, Wittkower, Eric and Wilson, A.T.M., 'Psychiatric organisation in the services' in Miller, Emanuel (ed.), *The Neuroses in War* (New York: The Macmillan Company, 1943), pp.169-170.

records reveal how psychological labels were transformed into medical diagnoses – and fits, in particular, left much room for interpretation, because no final proof existed to confirm either a psychological or organic origin.

One example is the case of 19-year-old Private Alfred K. of the 20th County of London Battalion – a bright student with a promising academic career.[31] On 3 September 1914, while preparing for his teacher's diploma, Alfred was drafted into the army. We learn from the notes – and Alfred's pension records – that the young man had suffered a single fit at the age of 16 while he was in the choir at church (a fortnight before he was due to have an operation to be circumcised); Alfred had no further fits until he was sent to France in September 1914. In spring 1915, while serving in France, he fell 30 feet from a ladder and was unconscious for a short time. He was sent to a base hospital, the No.2 Canadian General Hospital at Treport, where he had two fits; he passed urine on one occasion and was told that he had been violent and had hit the attendants. Alfred was given light duty, but after suffering another fit was sent back to England; he was admitted to the newly-opened King George Hospital in London Waterloo. Long tunnels connected Waterloo Station to the hospital buildings so that severely injured men from the Western Front would not arouse public attention – and although Alfred was not one of the badly-wounded cases, his fits could be quite alarming: Alfred – like many of his comrades – was badly shaken by the London Zeppelin raids on 7/8 September 1915. Doctors at King George Hospital – under pressure to treat increasing numbers of severely wounded soldiers from the Western Front – were at a loss to explain Alfred's ever-deteriorating mental health, his fears and violent fits.

Compared to the long tedious journey from the Western Front, the transfer to the National Hospital at Queen Square was just a smooth straightforward trip north: over Waterloo Bridge and Kingsway, and into the beautifully landscaped area of Bloomsbury. When admitted to the National Hospital on 4 November 1915, 'the bright and intelligent' young man was very depressed and 'inclined to be tearful'. He was easily frightened and suffered from night terrors – and his movements appeared to be jerky and artificial. Very detailed seizure protocols provide a valuable picture of Alfred's endless repertoire of fits: in one fit, Alfred was 'throwing [his] head violently from side to side' and passed urine; in another attack, he was very flushed and moved his arms and legs. Many factors clearly pointed towards functional seizures (for example, the fact that these attacks were brought on by fright, the nature of the bodily movements, and the fact that neurological reflexes after the attack were normal). Grainger Steward, a consultant neurologist, and Edgar Adrian, Yealland's senior colleague, ordered rest, sedatives and light exercises. The Medical Board on 3 November 1915 recommended discharge as 'permanently unfit for active war and home service'. The 'epilepsy' was 'not the result of active service, but aggravated by it' – and it is not clear which final diagnosis the Queen Square doctors provided; the notes just document

---

31 QSA: Queen Square Records, Dr Steward, 1915, male A-K: case record Private Alfred K.

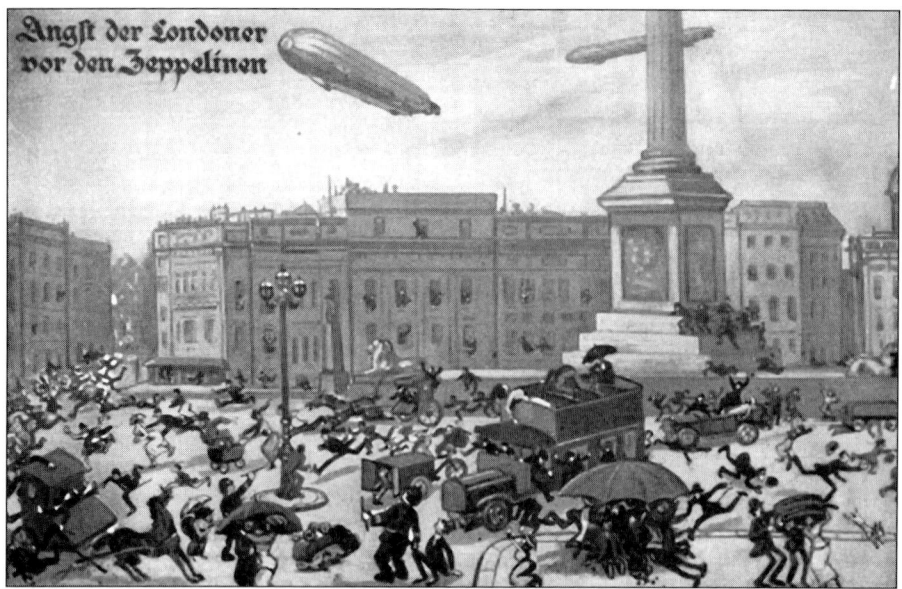

'Angst der Londoner vor den Zeppelinen' ('Londoners in fear of Zeppelin raids'), postcard. (Author's own archive)

'fits', without further specification. The Medical Board noted Alfred's 'excitable disposition' and the fact that he was 'easily upset by rifles'. The whole picture clearly pointed towards shell shock, but against all evidence, the Medical Board diagnosed Alfred with genuine epilepsy.

A similar history is that of 21-year-old Private Randolph S. of the East Lancashire Regiment:[32] Randolph had first developed fits at the age of 13, just before leaving school to work in a paper mill. He enlisted on 11 November 1915 and was sent to Egypt on 13 July 1916. Randolph was in Egypt for nine months, but spent eight months of that time in hospital with an eye infection, which left him blind in his left eye; he also suffered frequent fits. Despite his deteriorating health, he was sent to France in March 1917. Here, he spent most of his time as an inpatient in different base hospitals. Randolph continued to have fits, and he also suffered from heart problems and sore feet. His changing medical problems were identified as 'hysterical' – and on 28 June 1917, the young man arrived at Queen Square for specialist treatment. On admission, Randolph carried a handwritten note: Major C.S. Miller from the RAMC had certified that he was 'satisfied that the man suffers from true epilepsy'. It was not uncommon for soldiers who returned from the battlefields and base hospitals

---

32 QSA: Queen Square Records, Dr Buzzard, 1917, male and female L-Z: case record Private Randolph S.

The Obsession with the Shell 229

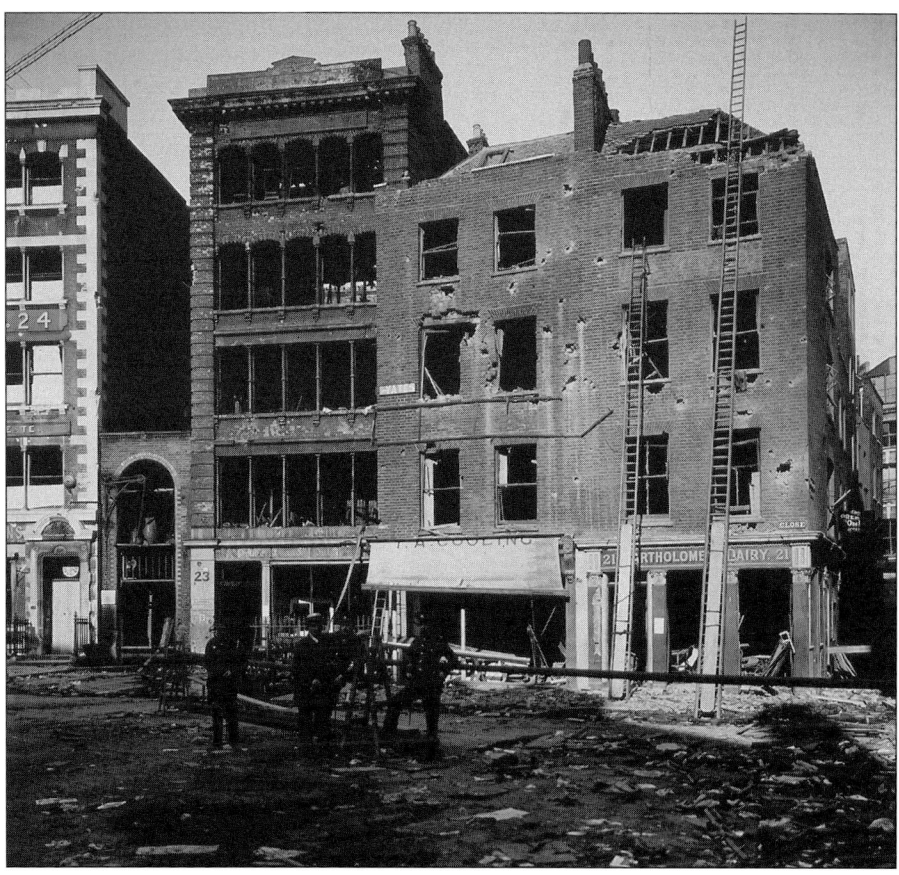

The church of St Bartholomew the Great and the surrounding area (Bartholomew Close) after the Zeppelin air raid on 8 September 1915; photograph, V0029993.
(Wellcome Library, London)

to present these '... treasured notes, which certified that they suffered from some physical malady. All of them had the name of some disease ready on their tongues, which had presumably been endorsed by their doctors.'[33] Patients themselves were amenable to the suggestion that they suffered from an organic illness or physiological disturbance that could be remedied by a physical treatment, such as faradism.[34]

In London, Randolph continued to have fits – initially two per week, but their frequency increased. During these fits, he would lose consciousness and then engage

33 Burton-Fanning, F.W., 'Neurasthenia in soldiers of the home forces' – *The Lancet*, 189:4894 (1917), p.907.
34 Yealland and Adrian, 'The treatment of some common war neuroses', pp.867-872.

in 'violent fighting and kicking'; he also attempted to throw himself out of his bed. On several occasions, Randolph bit the tip of his tongue. Although tongue biting is characteristic of generalised tonic-clonic seizures, it classically affects the lateral aspect of the tongue, and not the tip, as in Randolph's case. Randolph also suffered attacks of shaking during which he did not lose consciousness; he complained about 'throbbing bursting pain in his head'. The fits were identified as 'functional' and Yealland managed to stop some of them by applying painful supraorbital pressure. Randolph's left-sided blindness also responded to the same treatment regime: the young man was told that pressure on the eye would restore sight, which it did after four minutes of treatment – unmasking the blindness as purely functional as well; the successful treatment is described in Yealland's book *Hysterical Disorders of Warfare*. Randolph was discharged from Queen Square on 18 July 1917 – and on 27 August that same year, he was officially discharged from military service as 'being no longer physically fit for War Service'. The cause of discharge is noted as 'epilepsy' which, according to the Medical Board, was 'aggravated by service'. Randolph received a pension of £60 per year.

There were many other cases in which the Pension Board preferred medical diagnoses over psychological explanations: in a driver of the Royal Engineers who suffered from facial pain, Queen Square neurologists diagnosed 'neurosis', a psychological disorder; the Pension Committee discharged this man from service with a diagnosis of 'neuralgia', a neurological condition.[35] A glass blower from York, who presented with severe anxiety, dizziness, confusion and shaking, was diagnosed with 'shell shock' at Queen Square.[36] When his eyesight was tested, the vision in his right eye appeared to be severely impaired, while the visual acuity in his left eye was perfect; during his hospital stay, he was discharged from military service because of 'defective vision' – and the pension records do not mention his severe state of shock and inability to cope with frontline service.

Continuing the search for organic causes

The discussion on the origins of shell shock did not end with the armistice: British doctors, it seems, harboured profound feelings of unease, or even bitterness, when shell shock became just another variation on classical hysteria – and the debate on the aetiology of war-related disorders was re-opened. Captain Alfred Carver of the RAMC and Lieutenant A. Dinsley of the Royal Army Ordnance Corps (RAOC) claimed that 'a purely psychogenic explanation [to account for all the neuroses of war] will not suffice. […] Disease without some underlying physical basis is inconceivable.

---

35 QSA: Queen Square Records, Dr Howell, 1917, male and female L-Z: case record Private Lawrence T.
36 QSA: Queen Square Records, Dr Tooth, 1916, male A-K: case record Private James A.

The lesion may not be visible microscopically; it may be molecular or biochemical'.[37] Like the Swiss scientists of the early war years, Carver and Dinsley conducted animal experiments, in which they exposed fish, mice and rats to shell explosions. Animals very close to the detonation suffered gross physical injury or death. Further away from the explosion, the authors observed a transitory loss of consciousness, stupor and disorientation in the animals, followed by gross disturbances in conduct, posture and gait. Carver and Dinsley attributed these symptoms, which resembled those of shell-shocked soldiers, to strong physical forces causing an indirect concussion – and actual lesions – in the central nervous system. Animals which were even further away from the centre of the explosion showed, at first, diminished activity, but then excitement and disturbed behaviour.

With repeated exposure, these animals developed lasting behavioural changes: they remained in an 'absolutely stuporose condition. When liberated [from their cages], they made no efforts to run away but remained for a long time motionless in a huddled-up posture'.[38] Today – after a century of further research into animal learning – we know that even such profound behavioural changes can be produced by purely psychological manipulation, and without any need for direct impact on the brain. If animals are prevented from escaping in situations of danger, they will ultimately fail to make any effort to escape – a condition termed 'learned helplessness' (and promoted as the animal model for depression since the 1960s).

Although British anatomists like Mott ultimately failed to prove the organic causation of shell shock symptoms, the search for visible lesions in soldiers with post-combat disorders goes on. History repeats itself in the current discussion on mild traumatic brain injury, as stated by Judson S. Bury: 'Visibility is a relative term; it depends on our eyesight and the powers of our microscopes';[39] but can we, with improved methods of investigation – such as brain imaging – detect the biological correlates of symptoms that are strikingly similar to those of First World War soldiers – and if we find these biological imprints of trauma, what difference would this make to the individual? The final chapter of this book will seek answers to these questions and explain why the lessons from the Great War are still important today.

---

37   Carver, Alfred and Dinsley, A., 'Some biological effects due to high explosives' – *Brain*, 42:2 (1919), pp.113-129.
38   Carver and Dinsley, 'Some biological effects due to high explosives', p.122.
39   Bury, 'Remarks on the Pathology of War Neuroses', pp.97-99.

14

Shell Shock and PTSD: The Debate Goes On

Today, we live in the age of genetic medicine: every human being's genetic code can be read out, with relatively little effort and cost – and many abnormalities in our genetic makeup have become detectable. Many mental disorders are highly heritable, and there are high hopes that a better understanding of the exact genetic abnormalities will, ultimately, lead to better treatments; yet, not everyone is convinced that genes are the main factor underlying mental illness: there is a long tradition implicating an individual's biography in the risk of developing mental illness. The Freudian focus on (often inferred) childhood trauma was particularly influential in the development of this line of thought, but the anecdotal evidence adduced by psychoanalysts was not particularly convincing; however, when later therapeutic schools started to actively explore the patients' traumatic life events, it became clear that childhood sexual abuse, in particular, was often associated with mental illness, which could have an immediate onset, or occur with a delay of many years.[1] This increasing awareness of the enduring effects of trauma paved the way for the recognition of PTSD, which occurred in large numbers of Vietnam veterans and entered psychiatric classification systems in the 1980s.

Cases of enduring mental illness that was caused by life events challenged the genetic model in the same way the traumatic reactions of First World War soldiers challenged the degeneracy model that dominated medical debates at the time. Strategies for solving this apparent contradiction have not changed much: we have seen that psychiatrists of the First World War sought to demonstrate an underlying psychopathic disposition in their shell-shocked patients and often argued that constitutional weakness, rather than military deployment, had caused mental breakdown. Along similar lines, today's psychiatrists would seek to determine 'gene x environment interactions' (for example, a genetic predisposition that would make soldiers prone to collapse under stress). Although the methods have become more sophisticated – genotyping and twin studies, rather than accounts of bed-wetting and intolerance of

---

1   Healy, David, *Images of Trauma* (London: Faber and Faber, 1993).

woollen socks – the principal fault lines between constitutional models and psychological reactions have remained the same.

Much of this current debate on the nature and causes of traumatic reactions focuses on present-day military engagements in the context of affluent Western societies; for example, it has been argued that PTSD was as much a product of a culture of trauma that developed in the USA of the 1960s and 1970s, as of the harsh conditions in the jungles of South-East Asia.[2] Looking back over the entire century will enable us to put phenomena such as PTSD into the wider historical context, and ask questions such as:

- Does shell shock still exist today?
- Can trauma cause psychotic illness?
- Did First World War soldiers already suffer from PTSD?
- Are mental illnesses by-products of particular cultures?

The analysis of the medical response to shell shock also brings up interesting parallels to the quest for organic causes in the ever-changing theatres of modern warfare: after the shockwaves of the shells came the cold of the Korean War, the chemicals of Vietnam and the Gulf, and the improvised explosive devices (IED) of recent Middle Eastern deployments. Much time and money has been spent both to investigate these potential causes and compensate their victims, and pressure groups of war veterans have generally favoured organic over psychological explanations. Tracing the history from Carver and Dinsley's animal experiments (Chapter 13) and Mott's post-mortem examinations to today's search of imaging correlates of 'mild traumatic brain injury' will provide interesting insights into the sociology of this quest for physical causes.

Shell shock today

War trauma is still a major problem for military personnel today, but clinical presentations have changed: functional neurological symptoms – such as paralysis of a limb, loss of voice or an abnormal gait – are rarely reported as post-traumatic reactions in today's soldiers. This cannot be explained by their general disappearance; up to a third of patients who attend general neurology clinics have such functional symptoms that are unexplained by organic disease.[3] These – mainly civilian – patients are today's shell shock cases, and although the causes and triggers of their neurological deficits

---

2   Jones, Edgar and Wessely, Simon, 'War Syndromes: The Impact of Culture on Medically Unexplained Symptoms' – *Medical History*, 49:1 (2005), pp.55-78.
3   Stone, Jon, Carson, A., Duncan, R., Coleman, R., Roberts, R., Warlow, C., Hibberd, C., Murray, G., Cull, R., Pelosi, A., Cavanagh, J., Matthews, K., Goldbeck, R., Smyth, R., Walker, J., Macmahon, A.D. and Sharpe, M., 'Symptoms "unexplained by organic disease" in 1144 new neurology out-patients: how often does the diagnosis change at follow-up?' – *Brain*, 132:10 (2009), pp.2,878-2,888.

are very different from those of shell shock (and mostly do not involve war trauma), the clinical presentation often bears a striking resemblance to the case reports of the Great War. Some of today's patients with functional disorders present with a single deficit (for example, inability to speak), whereas others suffer from a broader psychiatric syndrome that may involve symptoms of depression and anxiety as well. Today's patients exhibit the full range of functional syndromes we encountered in the records of the First World War – including paralysis of legs and arms, sensory deficits and pain, shaking and convulsions, deafness, blindness and memory loss. Functional neurological disorders are not only relatively common, but also very hard to treat: a recent survey of the medical literature since the 1950s found that over half of the patients affected by functional motor symptoms had no long-term improvement[4] – and even more concerning was that treatment showed little noticeable effect on the outcome; the outcome data collected by Nonne and his contemporaries looked far more promising.

In today's traumatised servicemen, classical shell shock presentations have been superseded by complaints that are more obviously related to a person's mental state: low mood, anxiety, intrusive imagery and flashbacks of battle scenes, avoidance of potential danger, and states of 'high alert' and suspiciousness; these are all components of today's post-traumatic stress disorder. Historian of psychiatry Edgar Jones has argued that each armed conflict from the late 19th century to today had its own signature functional disorder: rheumatism and heart problems in the Crimea, shell shock in the First World War, bowel problems in the Second World War and PTSD in Vietnam; he also observed that the balance between physical and psychological presentations varied over time.[5] This observation brings out two fascinating facets of reactions to trauma: they seem to be both highly culturally dependent and highly contagious; basic human biology has not changed much over the last couple of centuries – evolution proceeds at much slower timescales – which makes it impossible to explain these dramatic changes of somatic presentations in purely constitutional terms. The importance of contagion had already been observed during the epidemics of functional seizures, as described in Chapters 6 and 8. This was not contagion in the biological sense of a spreading infectious agent, but rather a learning process by which soldiers observed a repertoire of possible stress reactions and unconsciously adopted some of them; it may also have been important for them to learn – again, probably unconsciously – which reactions to trauma were socially acceptable (at least to the extent that they were not immediately punished by a court martial).

---

4   Bass, Christopher, 'Prognosis in patients with psychogenic motor disorders' in Hallett, Mark, Lang, Anthony, Jankovic, Joseph, Fahn, Stanley, Halligan, Peter, Voon, Valerie and Cloninger, Robert (eds), *Psychogenic Movement Disorders and other Conversion Disorders* (Cambridge: Cambridge University Press, 2012), pp.249-253.
5   Jones and Wessely, 'War syndromes', pp.55-78.

Cultural forces and neurological symptoms

Cultural and environmental factors, which can include nutrition, type of weaponry, medical progress, societal expectations and gender stereotypes (amongst many others) thus play a major role in shaping the physical expression of the basic fear and terror mechanisms evoked by combat stress. This cultural dependence of post-traumatic reactions can be traced over time, but also across different cultures at any particular time; even during the First World War, different combatant countries experienced different post-combat reactions: the comparison of post-combat syndromes at the National Hospital in London and the Charité in Berlin showed a much higher proportion of functional seizures among German soldier-patients. Indeed, about one third of German soldiers treated for shell shock at the Charité suffered from seizures, as described in Chapter 1 – and this observation raises more questions about the way culture can shape the expression of trauma and distress. We know that approaches to – and management of – functional seizure disorders were very similar in Britain and Germany; shell shock doctors in both countries found seizures much harder to treat than functional paralyses or gait disorders because they rarely responded to conventional therapies. Electrotherapy – a central element of shell shock treatment in both countries – proved to be without effect for functional seizures (and was, therefore, largely abandoned for this indication). Even Yealland, a strong advocate of electrotherapy, did not apply electric currents in patients with functional seizures; instead, he based his treatment on suggestion, re-education and isolation. Because of the contagious nature of functional seizures – and their tendency to become more prominent with increased attention and compassion – the favoured treatment in Britain and Germany was isolation. So why were seizures such a common presentation in traumatised German soldiers, and why were they more common in German (as compared to British) servicemen? Historian Edgar Jones and psychiatrist Sir Simon Wessely have argued that functional somatic syndromes may be particularly prone to cultural forces: out of a general 'symptom repertoire', individuals tend to 'pick' certain functional symptoms[6] – and these symptoms typically mimic 'genuine' illnesses. At the same time, clinical investigation or scientific experiments fail to determine the aetiology of the symptoms; symptoms cannot be clearly identified as either organic or functional on the basis of objective markers. A striking example is a psychogenic stomach ulcer – a prominent 'psychosomatic' presentation in Second World War servicemen – which all but disappeared after the widespread introduction of gastroscopy and the identification of a bacterium (*helicobacter pylori*) as the prominent cause of the ulcer.[7] The physical expression of distress may also be mediated by cultural forces through popular health fears, which alert patients and doctors to particular areas of the body:

---

6   Shorter, Edward, 'Paralysis: the Rise and Fall of a "Hysterical" Symptom' – *Journal of Social History*, 19:4 (1986), pp.549-582.
7   Jones and Wessely, 'War syndromes', pp.55-78.

because it was impossible to detect potentially life-threatening peptic ulcers in the pre-endoscopy era, doctors and patients were easily alerted towards symptoms related to the gastrointestinal system.

During the First World War, functional seizures were a common presentation in traumatised servicemen – and there was no objective proof that these disturbing symptoms were of a psychological origin. The discovery of the electroencephalogram (EEG), which allowed for the recording of epileptic brain activity through the intact skull (by Binswanger's successor, Hans Berger, in 1924), transformed the field of seizure disorders by providing a tool for objective diagnosis; however, because the EEG can be completely normal between seizures – even in patients with epileptic disorders – this diagnostic technique has not disposed of functional seizures altogether, and the distinction between epileptic and functional (or 'pseudo-epileptic') seizures is still a diagnostic challenge for today's neurologists.

What public opinion considers acceptable or unacceptable, authentic or false, respectable or shameful also influences the expression of distress: popular attitudes towards seizures might have been different in Britain and Germany, which might explain the higher incidence of seizures in German soldiers. As argued in Chapter 1, the British were reluctant to accept the idea that men – in particular, soldiers – could develop symptoms that were so closely linked with the stereotype of female hysteria.

Electricity and seizures

Another potential cause of the greater 'popularity' of seizures in Germany (compared to Britain) is the different role of electricity in the two countries: cultural historian Andreas Killen has demonstrated how the rapid rise of electrical industries in Berlin – and the electrification of many aspects of daily life – transformed thinking not just about technology, but about society and the human mind.[8] The influence of the electrical industry, led by the Siemens conglomerate and the Allgemeine-Elektrizitäts-Gesellschaft (AEG) – two of the corporate giants underpinning the superiority of German industry at the beginning of the 20th century – set Berlin apart from both London and Paris.[9] Several soldiers who had worked in the electrical industries in Berlin actually developed hysterical seizures during their active military service and were treated at the Charité. Frequently, seizures occurred on the electric street railways ('*Elektrische*'), while soldiers were on leave from their frontline service. Conceptual links between electricity and epilepsy had already been proposed in the mid-19th century by the anatomist Jacobus Schroeder van der Kolk (1797-1862) in the Netherlands[10] and by the physician to King's College Hospital, Robert Bentley

---

8   Killen, *Berlin Electropolis*.
9   Winter and Robert, *Capital Cities at War*, p.34.
10 Temkin, Owsei, *The Falling Sickness: The History of Epilepsy from the Greeks to the Beginnings of Modern Neurology* (Baltimore, London: Johns Hopkins University Press, 1945), p.283.

Shell Shock and PTSD: The Debate Goes On 237

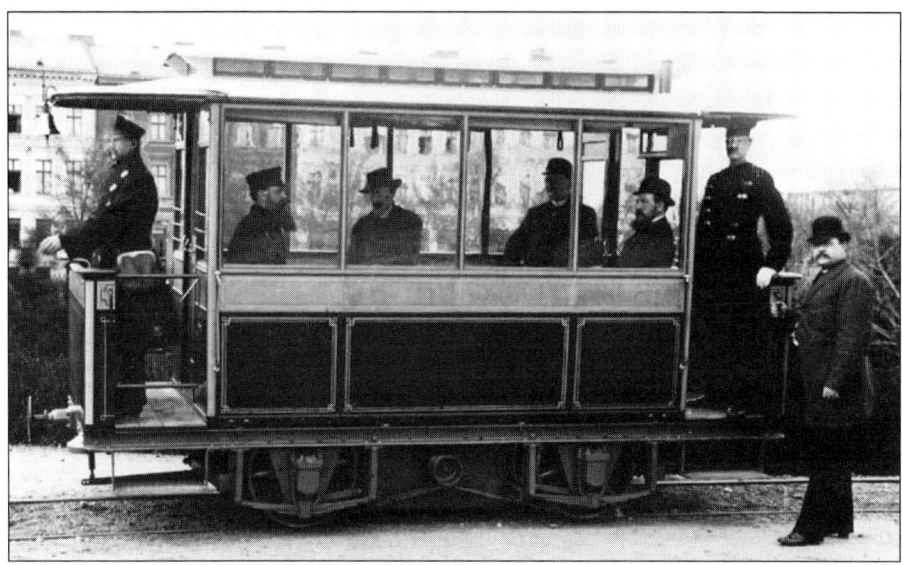

The world's first electric tram – the Groß-Lichterfelde Tramway – began operation in 1881 in the Lichterfelde neighbourhood of Berlin, Germany and was produced by Werner von Siemens; a direct current was supplied through the rails. (Photograph in public domain)

Todd (1809-1860) in Britain.[11] The first experimental demonstration of this link was achieved in 1914 when Polish physiologists Napoleon Cybulski and Sabina Jelenska-Macieszyna published a photographic record of changes in electrical activity in the cerebral cortex of a dog during a seizure[12] – thus, by the time of the war, the link between electricity and seizures was well-established.

The finding that the incidence of functional seizures was significantly lower in British soldiers – compared with their German counterparts – supports the idea that similar traumatic triggers can produce different phenomenological consequences in different cultural settings.[13] Even PTSD and mild traumatic brain injury (mTBI) – signature disorders of more recent military conflicts – seem to be prone to cultural forces; it seems to be a consistent finding that the incidence of PTSD and mTBI in the military appears to be lower in UK than in US personnel. A number of explanations have been put forward – among them differences in combat exposure, demographic

11　Reynolds, Edward H., 'Jackson, Todd, and the Concept of "Discharge" in Epilepsy' – *Epilepsia*, 48:11 (2007), pp.2,016-2,022.
12　Grzybowski, Andrzej and Pietrzak, Krzysztof, 'Napoleon Cybulski (1854-1919)' – *Journal of Neurology*, 260:11 (2013), pp.2,942-2,943.
13　Linden, Stefanie C. and Jones, Edgar, '"Shell Shock" Revisited: An Examination of the Case Records of the National Hospital in London' – *Medical History*, 58:4 (2014), pp.519-545.

differences between UK and US troops, differences in leadership and previous experience, and also cultural perspectives.[14]

The question as to why certain individuals react to traumatic experiences with somatic symptoms, while others develop psychological symptoms, has to remain open: 'How is it that with one person the hysteria bears on the arm, with another on the stomach, and that, with a third, it only reaches a system of ideas?'[15] Janet's question is still very relevant for today's clinicians – not just in relation to combat stress, but for the huge field of medically-unexplained symptoms in general. Future research may unearth some of the individual predisposing factors – genetic or biographical – that make a person more susceptible to one or the other functional syndrome, and collective patterns of behaviour also seem to play a role; for example, although functional neurological symptoms – the hallmark of shell shock in the First World War – do not seem to be acceptable any longer as reactions to war trauma, they can be a legitimate way of expressing distress of civilian patients, which is reflected by their high prevalence in general neurology clinics.

Can trauma lead to psychosis?

If psychological trauma can cause – or, at least, trigger – such a wide range of mental and physical abnormalities, does this also extend to that least accessible of altered mental states, psychosis? Kleist's category of 'terror psychosis' embraces psychotic and dissociative reactions to traumatic experiences and demonstrates how narrow the line between transient psychotic disorders and dissociative states can be. Although he called them 'psychoses', not all of Kleist's different syndromes would be categorised as psychotic disorders in the modern diagnostic systems (the International Classification of Disease (ICD) of the World Health Organisation, or the Diagnostic and Statistical Manual (DSM) of the American Psychiatric Association), which have dominated concepts of mental illness since the 1950s; for example, in the ICD, Kleist's cases of terror psychosis would partly be classified as 'dissociative disorders' (e.g. dissociative stupor, dissociative amnesia) partly as reactions to stress, whereas only a small number would meet the present criteria for a diagnosis of acute and transient psychotic disorder (ATPD). Kleist and other psychiatrists of the pre-ICD/-DSM era have not always tried to separate the subjective and objective manifestations of dissociation and psychosis – and indeed, these states often merge into each other.

Since Jaspers introduced the concept of 'reactive psychosis' and Kleist published his paper on 'terror psychosis', similar reactions to traumatic events which incorporate dissociative, psychotic and affective symptoms have been described under the

---

14   Hunt, Elizabeth J.F., Wessely, Simon, Jones, Norman, Rona, Roberto J. and Greenberg, Neil, 'The mental health of the UK Armed Forces: where facts meet fiction' – *European Journal of Psychotraumatology*, 5 (2014), 23617.
15   Janet, *The Major Symptoms of Hysteria*, pp. 332-333.

headings of 'shock psychoses',[16] 'psychogenic psychoses'[17] and 'hysterical psychoses'.[18] This broad concept of reactive disorders is still widely used in Scandinavia,[19] where up to 30 percent of all psychiatric admissions are diagnosed with 'reactive psychosis'[20] – thus we would have to conclude that the states of hallucinatory experiences, delusional thought systems and bizarre beliefs and behaviours that are subsumed under the term 'psychosis' can, indeed, be the result of a traumatising experience, and not just the result of a genetically-determined process of disturbed brain development; the reactive psychoses thus provide an interesting counterpoint to the currently prevailing genetic model of psychosis.

Did soldiers of the First World War suffer from PTSD?

A core phenomenon of Kleist's terror psychoses – and of similar categories that were proposed by his contemporaries – was the re-living of combat experiences in confusional or dreamlike states, and also in the fully conscious individual (sometimes accompanied by a re-enactment of battle scenes). The resemblance to modern concepts of post-traumatic reactions (in particular, PTSD) is striking: very vivid memories and intrusive images of the traumatising event (called 'flashbacks') are the hallmark of PTSD; a core feature of PTSD was thus described in traumatised soldiers many decades before PTSD was officially recognised as a psychiatric disorder (after the Vietnam War).

Was shell shock then simply another term for PTSD? It is not that straightforward: Edgar Jones was right to point out that the presentations of trauma change from war to war; indeed, things seem to have moved on from PTSD, which today, is probably more frequently encountered in victims of traffic accidents than in war veterans. In today's service personnel, alcohol abuse and depression have become a more prevalent problem than PTSD[21] – thus it seems wrong to be fixated on PTSD, as if this were to be the only possible psychological expression of combat stress after Vietnam. PTSD is just one of a range of historically-developing psychological reactions to the fears and stress associated with combat – and certain aspects of it can already be observed in the victims of shell shock.

16   Wetzel, 'Über Schockpsychosen', pp.288-330.
17   Schioldann, 'Classic Text No. 87', pp.347-367.
18   Hollender and Hirsch, 'Hysterical Psychosis', pp.1,066-1,074.
19   Marneros, Andreas and Pillmann, Frank, *Acute and Transient Psychoses* (Cambridge: Cambridge University Press, 2004).
20   Dahl, A.A., 'The DSM-III classification of the functional psychoses and the Norwegian tradition' – *Acta Psychiatrica Scandinavica Supplement*, 328 (1986), pp.45-53; Opjordsmoen, Stein, 'Reactive psychosis and other brief psychotic episodes' – *Current Psychiatry Reports*, 3:4 (2001), pp.338-341.
21   Murphy, D., Iversen, A. and Greenberg, N., 'The Mental Health of Veterans' – *Journal of the Royal Army Medical Corps*, 154:2 (2008), pp.136-139.

Traumatic reactions as learnt behaviours

The initial reaction of humans – and indeed, many animals – to a frightening situation is fairly schematic; there are really only two options: fight or flight. Both are characterised by the mobilisation of energy from stores in the body to facilitate the essential fast actions of brain and muscles, which is mediated by the activation of the sympathetic nervous system. The psychological concomitants – heightened arousal, vigilance, aggression and increased (but very selective) memory – can all be seen as serving the goal of combating or escaping the immediate threat. If the threat seems overwhelming and there is no means of escape, animals – and humans – may instead enter a state of complete inaction and 'freeze'; the almost motionless and speechless state that was common in the initial phase of shell shock may represent a prolonged freezing reaction.[22]

This initial stress and fear reaction is deeply entrenched in the brain and body, and does not seem to change much with cultural influences; however, the later phase of post-traumatic symptoms, which are then observed and treated by doctors in military hospitals – and sometimes usher into long-term disability – seem to be shaped by history and culture: how is this possible? Through the studies of the behaviourists of the early 20th century on the effects of reward and punishment on human behaviour, we know that much of the more complex human behaviour is learnt, rather than being totally determined by innate physiological processes.

There are two main learning mechanisms: learning by reward (also called 'instrumental' or 'operant' learning) and learning by observation (also called 'social' learning). Let us consider the scenario of a shell-shocked soldier who is just emerging from the initial frozen state after the immediate danger has passed: his ultimate goal is survival. The prospect of further fighting is too frightening for him – and thus flight is the only option. He cannot just run away from the front line; he will likely be shot, or court martialled. He has observed a certain repertoire of protective behaviours in other soldiers who were transported away from the front line to safety in base hospitals: confused, quasi-delirious states carry a high chance of this type of temporary rescue; however, in the long term, they entail the danger of social exclusion and confinement in an asylum. Conversely, a shift of symptoms to a more neurological presentation – seizures, paralysis, loss of sensation – is rewarded by the interest of specialised doctors outside the asylum system and the compassion of the civilian population, which is almost on a par with that conferred upon the physically wounded soldiers. By a combination of social and instrumental learning, the soldier's symptoms have thus developed out of the initial generic stress reaction into the functional neurological disorder that confers the highest chance of survival – and most, if not all, of this process is likely to have happened subconsciously (the doctors of the time were probably right in estimating the rates of conscious malingering as very low).

---

22 Mott, *War Neuroses and Shell Shock*, p.205.

Learning mechanisms can also explain the healing rates: some of the treatments – for example, isolation, plastering and electric shocks – were very unpleasant, and the reduction of symptoms promised relief. In terms of instrumental learning, symptom reduction was 'negatively reinforced' (it led to the cessation of an unpleasant consequence, the treatment); patients also received positive rewards, such as praise and a transfer to more pleasant surroundings, for symptom reduction. Such links between rewards (or positive reinforcers) and desirable behaviours, or between punishments and undesirable behaviours had been suggested by the American psychologist Edward Thorndike – the father of animal learning theory – a few years before the First World War: we have seen in Chapter 12 that these learning principles, derived from animal husbandry, were consciously implemented by doctors on both sides. Patients also learned by observation – fellow patients who got well got discharged home, or to garrison duty – and thus, as long as the prevailing medical model (shell-shocked soldiers were constitutionally weak, but could be helped by a class of highly educated doctors) went unchallenged, this escape route remained open. Many patients rewarded their doctors with often stunning treatment successes, for which the doctors could take credit in their publications, and thus did their best to make sure that they would not change their opinion about shell shock; however, patients who did not abide by these rules often had to face negative consequences.

In Chapter 12, we encountered Binswanger's patient who failed to recover his voice, and was duly sent back to the front line. Similar attitudes prevailed amongst the Queen Square doctors, as can be gleaned from the case of Private John P. of the 6th Black Watch:[23] born and bred in Glasgow, John had left school at 14 to become a grocer; he had always been in good health and was keen to serve his country. John enlisted in May 1916 (when he turned 18) – and soon, he was sent to the Western Front. On 27 April 1917, John's regiment was advancing at Arras, and 'going into a shell hole he was struck in the head. He fell, was not unconscious, but was unable to get up. His head was dressed, and a few minutes later he lost complete use of the right side. [He] was left in the shell hole all night, then taken to C.C. Station'. Afterwards, he was transferred to Frevent Hospital (40 miles west of Arras), where he remained for three days. He soon regained control of his right leg, but his right arm remained paralysed; John was sent to the National Hospital straight away – arriving at Queen Square five days after his injury. Apart from a 'slight superficial scar' on his scalp, the Queen Square doctors could not find any organic signs. The 'short and stout' Scotsman could not move his right shoulder and arm, and he complained of numbness in his right arm and leg, and the right side of his neck. John was told that he would be treated and cured, which was part of the general procedure of suggestive treatment preparation; yet, two days after admission – before Yealland could even start to apply his treatment – power and feeling in John's right arm fully returned; he was

---

23 QSA: Queen Square Records, Dr Wilson, 1917, male and female L-Z: case record Private John P.

completely cured. John was discharged from hospital on 13 June 1917, and – unlike the vast majority of his successfully treated comrades – was sent back to his regiment after a short period of furlough. John P. was killed in action on 30 September 1917; he was only 19 years old. His 'non-compliance' with the rules of the medical establishment ultimately cost him his life.

Quest for organic explanation

The doctors of the First World War still do not seem to have been entirely comfortable with their psychological illness models: even late into the war, they still had a tendency to come up with organic labels wherever possible (Chapter 13);[24] this may have been partly motivated by the benevolent attempt to spare their patients the stigma of a mental illness. The general public's attitude towards mental illness, which Smith and Pear described as 'a mixture of ignorant superstition and exaggerated fear',[25] and the 'taunt of having nothing to show' encouraged soldiers without obvious wounds to express their trauma through physical symptoms;[26] however, this does not explain the intense search for organic causes of functional disorders through dissection of the brains of deceased soldiers, and through animal experiments intended to prove brain damage after distant shell explosions. Why were doctors so keen to find an organic cause when, clearly, many soldiers with shell shock symptoms had not been exposed to shell explosions, or other potential physical causes, other than the general hardship of the war they shared with millions of others? In fact, as we saw in Chapter 11, shell shock even occurred in those who had not been to the front line at all, or after minor injuries on the Berlin Tramway. One explanation might be that doctors were afraid to overlook conditions that might be amenable to more specific treatments (for example, bleeds that required brain surgery); however, in the absence of obvious injuries, this was an unlikely scenario. It is more likely that the quest for organic models can be explained by a general reluctance to accept psychological explanations of disease, which are, by their very nature, less mechanistic and more controversial than purely biological explanations. Questions of an individual's character, morality and upbringing just come up much less – if at all – if an illness has a biological root, and it may be easier to argue for compensation and pension payments. For doctors, organic models may be more comfortable as well: successful treatment is then clearly owed to their professional competence and clinical acumen, rather than the interaction between doctor and patient and their mutual expectations, which would devalue the role of the doctor and limit his or her power. These motives may explain why doctors, patients and veteran organisations have often been keen to find organic causes for traumatic war syndromes; even the methods have been remarkably static over time.

24 Hargreaves, 'Psychiatric Organisation in the Services', pp.169-170.
25 Smith and Pear, *Shell Shock and its Lessons*, p.78.
26 Smith and Pear, *Shell Shock and its Lessons*, p.14.

Although magnetic resonance imaging has been added to the arsenal of neurologists, present-day examinations of post-mortem brains for effects of mTBI in soldiers exposed to IEDs are not miles away from Mott's search for micro-haemorrhages in cases of shell shock – and Rusca's rabbits, rats and fish (Chapter 4) and Carver and Dinsley's fish, mice and rats (Chapter 13) were subject to very similar blast experiments as the pigs recently used by the UK Ministry of Defence to test body armour.[27]

Organic models today: is PTSD a brain disorder after all?

The hypothesis that behavioural anomalies and cognitive impairments may be secondary to organic changes in the brain of military personnel after blast exposure (rather than being a primary psychological consequence) is on the agenda again. Modern PTSD researchers are looking for molecular and physiological correlates of brain damage with the aim of preventing further 'cell death' and developing effective treatments;[28] why, then, do today's researchers hope to find the organic solution to the conundrum Major Mott faced a century ago? Some argue that Mott lost his vision and creative spirit somewhere on his path to the organic origin of shell shock: had he pursued his mission, and also possessed the right instruments, he might have succeeded (so they believe).[29] 'Visibility' is a relative term; to the proponents of an organic illness model, it merely depends on our eyesight and the powers of our microscopes and scanners[30] – thus the search for an organic lesion continues, only on a greater scale and with more sophisticated measures than were available to Mott 100 years ago. The idea that psychological trauma can leave psychological scars that are beyond visualisation is too hard to accept for medicine and the individual sufferer.

The similarities between 2016 and 1916 are not confined to the proponents of organic models; even sceptical voices today sound very much like their counterparts from the shell shock era. Some experts on PTSD caution against attributing symptoms to 'mild traumatic brain injury, because associated PTSD and depression may be the primary problem'; they warn that the incorrect belief that symptoms are the result of brain injury, rather than psychological distress, jeopardises recovery.[31] This is the same argument Charles Samuel Myers – consultant psychologist to the BEF in France

---

27 <http://www.mirror.co.uk/news/uk-news/ministry-defence-kills-28000-animals-2951774)> 'Horrific toll on helpless creatures: 28,000 each year are killed by the Ministry of Defense: Pigs are blown up to test body armour…' – accessed 24 January 2016.
28 See (e.g. <www.usuhs.mil/cnrm/>) – accessed 20 April 2015.
29 Shively, Sharon B. and Perl, Daniel P., 'Traumatic Brain Injury, Shell Shock, and Posttraumatic Stress Disorder in the Military – Past, Present, and Future' – *Journal of Head Trauma Rehabilitation*, 27: 3 (2012), pp.234-239.
30 Bury, 'Remarks on the Pathology of War Neuroses', pp.97-99.
31 Bryant, Richard A., 'Disentangling Mild Traumatic Brain Injury and Stress Reactions' – *The New England Journal of Medicine*, 358:5 (2008), pp.525-527.

and editor of the *British Journal of Psychology* – made in his *Lancet* article in December 1919 (see Chapter 13): misattributing psychological symptoms to brain injury could take away a person's hopes of recovery; if the medical profession fails to cure the symptoms, the patient is left with an organic disorder – bereft of any hope of a cure.

Since the First World War, the face of so-called 'medically unexplained symptoms' has changed and new diagnostic techniques have rendered certain psychosomatic illnesses obsolete, but therapeutic approaches and discussions on illness models, and the origins of symptoms, have remained the same – thus, what did the medical profession learn from the Great War (the first large-scale study on the effects of physical and psychological stress on body and mind)?

The – medical – lessons of the First World War

The First World War marked a turning point in the history of neurological treatment, because clinicians were provided with the opportunity and resources to treat and evaluate large numbers of patients with similar symptoms;[32] the challenge posed by thousands of traumatised soldiers awakened the creativity und pioneering spirit of a profession that had, previously, largely resigned to therapeutic nihilism. Psychiatric and neurological journals and conferences became a forum for discussion of psychopathology, aetiological concepts, treatments and treatment outcomes – including the first systematic therapeutic trials in the history of psychiatry.

Therapies developed for shell shock were diverse and covered a wide range of complexity and invasiveness: treatments for paralysis ranged from simple encouragement, rest and mild exercises, to the application of strong electric currents, or the plastering of parts of the body. Many treatments worked through the systematic reinforcement of 'healthy' behaviour and aimed to transform the traumatised soldier into a valuable labourer (but not necessarily to return him to active duty). As we have learned in Chapter 12, psychiatrists of the First World War were not only familiar with concepts of reinforcement, model learning and gradual exposure, but also with schedules of reinforcement (or punishment) for small learning steps – similar to what was later called 'shaping' in operant conditioning. It was not until after the Second World War, however, that behaviour therapy – or behaviour modification – were deployed on a greater scale (initially, in the USA and later, in Europe).

Although many of the specific treatments were forgotten after the armistice, or superseded by the increasing influence of psychoanalysis,[33] they experienced a revival in the 1970s and 1980s when small case series of isolation treatment and faradic stimulation were published in psychiatric and rehabilitation journals.[34] Furthermore,

---

32 Linden and Jones, 'German Battle Casualties'.
33 Shorter, *A History of Psychiatry*, pp.145-189.
34 Dickes, Richard A., 'Brief therapy of conversion reactions: an in-hospital technique' – *American Journal of Psychiatry*, 131:5 (1974), pp.584-586; Khalil, T.M., Abdel-Moty, E.,

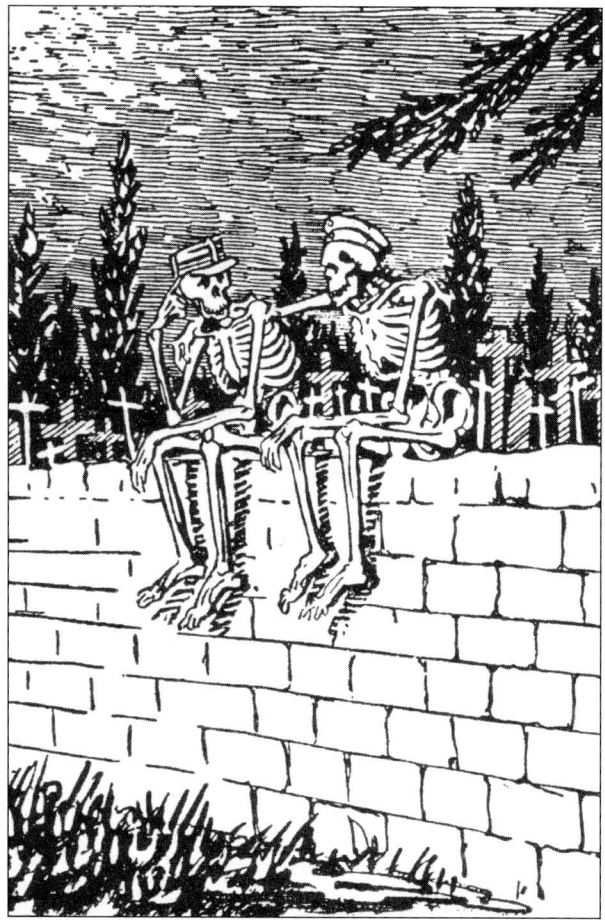

'On the cemetery in Ypres: "Remind me, why did we actually kill each other?"'; from Hirschfeld, M. and Gaspar, A., Sittengeschichte des ersten Weltkrieges. (Hanau: Müller & Kiepenheuer, 1929; reprint of the 2nd revised edition, 1980, p.569)

the psychological and physiological approaches to functional disorders established by Yealland and his contemporaries are conceptually similar to some modern treatments, although they are rarely acknowledged as precursors; for example, a group of researchers in Florida developed a biofeedback procedure with electromyography (EMG) (a technique that picks up electrical signals from muscles) for patients with paralysed legs:[35] a biofeedback apparatus played the signals from their own muscles

    Asfour, S.S., Fishbain, D.A., Rosomoff, R.S. and Rosomoff, H.L., 'Functional electric stimulation in the reversal of conversion disorder paralysis' – *Archives of Physical Medicine and Rehabilitation*, 69:7 (1988), pp.545-547.
35 Fishbain, D.A., Goldberg, M., Khalil, T.M., Asfour, S.S., Abdel-Moty, E., Meagher, B.R., Santana, R., Rosomoff, R.S. and Rosomoff, H.L., 'The utility of electro-myographic

back to the patients through a visual display on a television screen. In the first training session, the non-paralysed counterpart muscle in the normal leg was used to demonstrate how voluntary muscle contraction translates into movements on the screen; in the next session, electrodes were placed on the 'paralysed' muscle, and the patient was asked to try to contract this muscle just like the normal one. This generated a noticeable, but small, signal on the screen – indicating to the patient that although the leg did not move, the muscles and nerves in their paralysed legs were undamaged and functioning normally. This procedure, like Yealland's interventions, incorporated the communication of a somatic illness model: patients participating in this trial were told that their brains had lost the ability to communicate with their peripheral nerves – thereby losing the ability to control the muscles in their legs; they were also reassured before the treatment that biofeedback would ultimately cure them. The Florida patients received up to 70 training sessions, with the whole treatment lasting several months – and furthermore, they also received other treatments in addition to EMG biofeedback, which included physical and occupational therapy, behaviour modification, vocational counselling and electrical stimulation. Although the four patients of the study eventually regained their lower limb function, it took them much longer to recover than the average patient treated by Yealland.

Modern versions of electrotherapy also include transcranial magnetic stimulation (TMS) and transcranial direct current stimulation (tDCS):[36] TMS applies brief, strong magnetic pulses to the head, which induce electrical field changes in the brain; for example, a single pulse over the left motor cortex can lead to a twitch of the right thumb. Reports in stroke patients show that excitatory (high-frequency) repeated magnetic stimulation of the affected brain hemisphere and inhibitory (low-frequency) stimulation of the unaffected hemisphere can improve motor function. A team of researchers from Rouen treated 70 patients with functional paralysis with repetitive transcranial magnetic stimulation (rTMS) to the contralateral primary motor cortex, with high success rates[37] and the authors argued that demonstration of function was an essential part of their treatment. Similarly, Yealland had argued that the patient's experience of preserved motor function was crucial for the recovery of movement.

Transcranial direct current stimulation (tDCS), which uses low currents delivered directly to the scalp via small electrodes, also seems to be a promising approach in the

---

biofeedback in the treatment of conversion paralysis' – *American Journal of Psychiatry*, 145:12 (1988), pp.1,572-1,575.
36   Wassermann, Eric M. and Zimmermann, Trelawny, 'Transcranial Magnetic Brain Stimulation: Therapeutic Promises and Scientific Gaps' – *Pharmacology and Therapeutics*, 133:1 (2012), pp.98-107.
37   Chastan, Nathalie and Parain, Dominique, 'Psychogenic paralysis and recovery after motor cortex transcranial magnetic stimulation' – *Movement Disorders*, 25:10 (2010), pp.1,501-1,504.

rehabilitation of stroke patients;[38] it has also been suggested that TMS is a powerful add-on therapy in the rehabilitation of patients who lose awareness of one side of their body after a lesion to the other side of the brain.[39] One might suspect that suggestion played a substantial part in these treatment approaches – past and present – as already foreseen by Yealland and his contemporaries.

Suggestion, deception and coercive treatments

Yealland's attitude to the ethics of coercive treatments was one-dimensional: '… the only merits that can be assigned to such methods of treatment are to be found in the result.'[40] His paternalistic attitude – justification by results and disregard for patient autonomy – has been superseded by present, more patient-centred approaches; however, faced with the challenge of treating functional movement disorders, some authors have advocated a revival of suggestive methods and the associated ethical concept of 'asymmetric paternalism'.[41] This approach aims to guide patients towards a particular outcome (when it is judged that they might otherwise act against their best interests) without subverting the principle of autonomy.

Even the use of deception in medicine – standard practice amongst doctors of the First World War, but later censored by medical ethics – has become a matter of significant interest and debate again. Philosophers Shlomo Cohen and Haim Shapiro have recently proffered an argument in favour of placebo treatment: moving away from the rigorous stance of the German 18th century philosopher Immanuel Kant, who considered deception to be morally wrong under all circumstances (even when it was employed to save innocent lives), they argue that placebo treatment can be defended on paternalistic grounds – and, in certain circumstances, even preserve patient autonomy.[42] In their view, placebo treatment can be considered morally legitimate because it fulfils the two most important criteria for the rightness of an action: good intention and good result; paradoxically, 'placebo treatment is a 'lie'

---

38 Higgins, Johanne, Koski, Lisa, Xie, Haiqun, 'Combining rTMS and Task-Oriented Training in the Rehabilitation of the Arm after Stroke: A Pilot Randomized Controlled Trial' – *Stroke Research and Treatment*, 2013:539146; Khedr, Eman M., Ahmed, Mohamed A., Fathy, Nehal and Rothwell John C., 'Therapeutic trial of repetitive transcranial magnetic stimulation after acute ischemic stroke' – *Neurology*, 65:3 (2005), pp.466-468.
39 Müri, René Martin, Cazzoli, Dario, Nef, Tobias, Mosimann, Urs P., Hopfner, Simone and Nyffeler, Thomas, 'Non-invasive brain stimulation in neglect rehabilitation: an update' – *Frontiers in Human Neuroscience*, 7 (2013), p.348.
40 Yealland, *Hysterical Disorders of Warfare*, p.57.
41 Hallett, Mark, Lang, Anthony, Jankovic, Joseph, Fahn, Stanley, Halligan, Peter, Voon, Valerie and Cloninger, Robert (eds), *Psychogenic Movement Disorders and other Conversion Disorders* (Cambridge: Cambridge University Press, 2012), p.298.
42 Cohen, Shlomo and Shapiro, Haim, '"Comparable Placebo Treatment" and the Ethics of Deception' – *Journal of Medicine and Philosophy*, 38:6 (2013), pp.696-709.

that (ideally) becomes true once believed'[43] – thus, one could argue that it is administered without the intention to deceive. Furthermore, although placebos are classically defined as 'inert' agents – without the properties of the 'real drug' – recent research has produced growing evidence that objective parameters of the mechanisms of action of the placebo can be virtually indistinguishable from those of the 'real' drugs they are supposed to simulate: neuroimaging studies with positron emission tomography (PET) use radioactively-labelled markers of drug receptors and can show how a placebo drug affects the brain. It appears that placebo analgesia, where patients received a mere starch pill – but believed it to be a pain-altering medication – can mimic the actions of opiates on the opioidergic system, which is the most potent pain-reducing system of the body.[44]

Another potential way of justifying deceptive treatments is based on the assumption that the patient would give his retrospective approval after a successful outcome; indeed, many patients welcome 'a local or temporary suspension of knowledge' and are eager to be guided through the momentous decision about the best treatment. Placebo treatment generally has fewer side effects than an active drug, which is another reason why many patients would probably prefer to receive a placebo and, retrospectively, approve of it. Despite all the arguments in favour of placebos, doctors might find it emotionally difficult to 'manipulate' the patient and violate the principle of honesty that governs doctor-patient relationships. Cohen and Shapiro suggest that the individual practitioner would be relieved of this burden by a public discussion on the benefits and moral justification of placebos because they consider a broad agreement regarding its permissibility to be more than likely; this 'global pact' between patients and therapists would make it easier for the individual therapist to temporarily 'deceive' his patient.

Today, up to a third of patients who see their family physicians complain of medically unexplained symptoms – and these functional syndromes constitute one of the major public health and socio-economic challenges of our time: the debate on covert placebo treatment of such conditions was foreshadowed in the letter on 'the justifiability of therapeutic lying' that Myers sent to *The Lancet* shortly after the publication of Yealland's *Hysterical Disorders of Warfare*.[45]

This book has traced the history of shell shock, from the lecture theatres of *fin de siècle* Paris, to the trenches of the Great War; the hospitals set up all around the world to treat its victims; and the streets of London and Berlin, where the impact of trauma transformed everyday life. Shell shock was one of the defining medical and cultural phenomena of the early part of the 20th century and has revolutionised our

---

43   Cohen and Shapiro, '"Comparable Placebo Treatment"', pp. 696-709.
44   Price, Donald D., Finniss, Damien G. and Benedetti, Fabrizio, 'A comprehensive review of the placebo effect: recent advances and current thought' – *Annual Review of Psychology*, 59 (2008), pp.565-590.
45   Myers, 'The justifiability of therapeutic lying', pp.1,213-1,214.

views of the human psyche – and few would have predicted that psychological reactions to combat stress could reach such an epidemic scale. This book has described the constellation of medical knowledge, scientific theories, and cultural and social factors that produced the particular symptoms that were described as 'shell shock'; it has also offered an explanation why, during subsequent conflicts, psychological breakdown has manifested itself in other ways. Although symptoms have changed over the last century, the basic psychological mechanisms of traumatic reactions have remained the same; however, now – as then – doctors and patients remain uneasy about purely psychological explanations of physical suffering, and the search for organic causes goes on. Although it was officially abandoned mid-way into the war, the term 'shell shock' never lost its attraction and continues to symbolise the ambiguity of the relationship between body and mind that was exposed by the Great War.

Bibliography

Medical Case Records

Historisches Psychiatriearchiv Charité: Krankenakten.
Universitätsarchiv Jena, Bestand S/III Abt. IX, Kriegsarchiv.
Queen Square Archives, Queen Square Records.

Books

Bandura, Albert, *Self-efficacy: The exercise of control* (New York: Freeman, 1997).
Barham, Peter, *Forgotten Lunatics of the Great War* (New Haven, London: Yale University Press, 2004).
Barker, Pat, *Regeneration* (London: Penguin, 2008).
Berger, Hans, *Trauma und Psychose: mit besonderer Berücksichtigung der Unfallbegutachtung* (Berlin: Springer, 1915).
Binneveld, Hans, *From Shell Shock to Combat Stress: a Comparative History of Military Psychiatry* (Amsterdam: Amsterdam University Press, 1997).
Binswanger, Otto, *Die Pathologie und Therapie der Neurasthenie: Vorlesungen für Studierende und Aerzte* (Jena: Verlag von Gustav Fischer, 1896).
—— *Der deutsche Krieg. Die seelischen Wirkungen des Krieges. Politische Flugschriften, zwölftes Heft* (Stuttgart, Berlin: Deutsche Verlags-Anstalt, 1914).
Breuer, Josef and Freud, Sigmund, *Studien über Hysterie* (Leipzig, Wien: Franz Deuticke, 1895).
Bridger, Geoff, *The Battle of Neuve Chapelle* (Barnsley: Leo Cooper, Pen & Sword Books Ltd., 2000).
Cannon, Walter B., *Bodily Changes in Pain, Hunger, Fear and Rage: An Account of Recent Researches into the Function of Emotional Excitement* (New York, London: Appleton and Company, 1915).
Clarke, David, *The Angel of Mons: Phantom Soldiers and Ghostly Guardians* (Chichester: John Wiley & Sons, 2004).
Dejerine, Joseph J. and Gauckler, E., *The Psychoneuroses and Their Treatment by Psychotherapy* (Philadelphia and London: J.B. Lippincott Company, 1913).
Dubois, Paul, *Die Psychoneurosen und ihre psychische Behandlung* (Bern, Verlag von A. Francke, 1905).

Eder, Montague D., *War-Shock, the Psycho-Neuroses in War* (London: William Heinemann, 1917).
Ferguson, Niall, *The Pity of War* (London: Penguin Books, 1999).
Flatau, Georg, *Kursus der Psychotherapie und des Hypnotismus* (Berlin: S. Karger, 1920).
Gray, Peter and Oliver, Kendrick (eds), *The Memory of Catastrophe* (Manchester: Manchester University Press, 2004).
Gröbe, Benjamin, *Desertion im deutschen Weltkriegsheer 1914-1918* (Norderstedt: GRIN Verlag, 2005).
Hallett, Mark, Lang, Anthony, Jankovic, Joseph, Fahn, Stanley, Halligan, Peter, Voon, Valerie and Cloninger, Robert (eds), *Psychogenic Movement Disorders and other Conversion Disorders* (Cambridge: Cambridge University Press, 2012).
Hawes, James, *Englanders and Huns: How five decades of enmity led to the First World War* (London: Simon & Schuster, 2014).
Healy, David, *Images of Trauma* (London: Faber and Faber, 1993).
Hirschfeld, M. and Gaspar, A., *Sittengeschichte des ersten Weltkrieges* (Hanau: Müller & Kiepenheuer, 1929; re-print of the 2nd revised edition, 1980).
Holmes, Gordon, *The National Hospital, Queen Square, 1860–1948* (Edinburgh: E. & S. Livingstone, 1954).
Hurst, Arthur F., *Medical Diseases of the War* (London: Edward Arnold, 1918).
Jahr, Christoph, *Gewöhnliche Soldaten: Desertion und Deserteure im deutschen und britischen Heer 1914-1918* (Göttingen: Vandenhoek & Rupprecht, 1998).
Janet, Pierre, *L'automatisme psychologique: Essai de psychologie expérimentale sur les formes inférieures de l'activité humaine* (Paris: L'Harmattan, 1889).
—— *The Major Symptoms of Hysteria*, 2nd edition (New York: The Macmillan Company, 1924).
Jaspers, Karl, *Allgemeine Psychopathologie*, 9th edn (Berlin: Springer, 1973; 1st edn 1913).
Jones, Edgar and Wessely, Simon, *Shell Shock to PTSD: Military Psychiatry from 1900 to the Gulf War* (Hove, New York: Psychology Press, 2005).
Kahlbaum, Karl L., *Klinische Abhandlungen über Psychische Krankheiten, I. Heft: Die Katatonie* (Berlin: August Hirschwald, 1874).
Killen, Andreas, *Berlin Electropolis: Shock, Nerves, and German Modernity* (Berkeley, Los Angeles, London: University of California Press, 2006).
Leed, Eric J., *No Man's Land: Combat & Identity in World War I* (Cambridge: Cambridge University Press, 1981).
Leese, Peter, *Shell Shock: Traumatic Neurosis and the British Soldiers of the First World War* (New York: Palgrave, 2002).
Lerner, Paul, *Hysterical Men: War, Psychiatry and the Politics of Trauma in Germany, 1890-1930* (Ithaca, London: Cornell University Press, 2003).
MacCurdy, John T., *War Neuroses* (Cambridge: Cambridge University Press, 1918).
Marneros, Andreas and Pillmann, Frank, *Acute and Transient Psychoses* (Cambridge: Cambridge University Press, 2004).

Micale, Mark S. and Lerner, Paul F., *Traumatic Pasts: History, Psychiatry, and Trauma in the Modern Age, 1870-1930* (Cambridge: Cambridge University Press, 2001).

Miller, Emanuel, *The Neuroses in War* (London: Macmillan & Co., 1940).

Mott, Frederick W., *War Neuroses and Shell Shock* (London: Oxford University Press, 1919).

Myers, Charles S., *Shell Shock in France, 1914-1918* (Cambridge: Cambridge University Press, 1940).

Neuner, Stephanie, *Politik und Psychiatrie: Die Staatliche Versorgung Psychisch Kriegsbeschädigter in Deutschland 1920-1939* (Göttingen: Vandenhoeck & Ruprecht, 2011).

Nonne, Max, *Anfang und Ziel meines Lebens: Erinnerungen* (Hamburg: Hans Christians Verlag, 1971).

Porter, Roy, *The Greatest Benefit to Mankind: A Medical History of Humanity from Antiquity to the Present* (London: Fontana Press, 1999).

Reid, Fiona, *Broken Men: Shell Shock, Treatment and Recovery in Britain 1914-1930* (London: Continuum International Publishing Group, 2010).

Sassoon, Siegfried, *Sherston's Progress* (London: Faber and Faber, 1936).

Scull, Andrew, *Hysteria* (Oxford: Oxford University Press, 2009).

Shephard, Ben, *A War of Nerves: Soldiers and Psychiatrists 1914-1994* (Cambridge, MA: Harvard University Press, 2001).

Shorter, Edward, *From Paralysis to Fatigue: A History of Psychosomatic Illness in the Modern Era* (New York: The Free Press, 1992).

——*A History of Psychiatry: From the Era of the Asylum to the Age of Prozac* (New York: Wiley, 1997).

Showalter, Elaine, *The Female Malady: Women, Madness and English Culture 1830–1980* (London: Virago, 1987).

Smith, Grafton E. and Pear, Tom H., *Shell Shock and its Lessons*, 2nd edn (Manchester: Manchester University Press, 1917).

Temkin, Owsei, *The Falling Sickness: The History of Epilepsy from the Greeks to the Beginnings of Modern Neurology* (Baltimore, London: Johns Hopkins University Press, 1945).

Thorndike, Edward L., *The Elements of Psychology* (New York: A.G. Seiler, 1912).

White, Jerry, *Zeppelin Nights: London in the First World War* (London: Vintage Books, 2014).

Winter, Jay and Robert, Jean-Louis, *Capital Cities at War: Paris, London, Berlin 1914-1919* (Cambridge: Cambridge University Press, 1999).

Yealland, Lewis R., *Hysterical Disorders of Warfare* (London: MacMillan and Co., 1918).

Journal Articles

Adams, Barfield J., 'Attempted Suicide among Soldiers ['*Il Tentato Suicidio nei Militari*'] – *British Journal of Psychiatry*, 66:273 (1920), pp.164-165.

'An epitome of current medical literature. "Big belly" in soldiers' – *British Medical Journal*, 2:2961 (1917), p.9.

Bar-El, Yair, Durst, Rimona, Katz, Gregory, Zislin, Josef, Strauss, Ziva and Knobler, Haim Y., 'Jerusalem syndrome' – *British Journal of Psychiatry*, 176:1 (2000), pp.86-90.

Bartsch, Andreas J., Neumärker, Klaus-J., Franzek, Ernst and Beckmann, Helmut, 'Karl Kleist (1879-1960)' – *American Journal of Psychiatry*, 157:5 (2000), p.703.

Bayliss, William M., 'On the Origin of Electric Currents led off from the Human Body, especially in Relation to "Nerve-Leaks"' – *British Medical Journal*, 1:2934 (1917), pp.387-388.

Beveridge, Allan W. and Renvoize, Edward B., 'Electricity: a history of its use in the treatment of mental illness in Britain during the second half of the 19th century' – *British Journal of Psychiatry*, 153:2 (1988), pp.157-162.

Beyer, E., 'Die Heilung des Zitterns und anderer nervöser Bewegungsstörungen' – *Psychiatrisch-Neurologische Wochenschrift*, 35/36 (1917-1918), pp.225-228

Boycott, A.E., Damant, G.C.C. and Haldane, J.S., 'The Prevention of Compressed-Air Illness' – *Journal of Hygiene*, 8:3 (1908), pp.342-443.

Bresler, J., 'Das Kaufmann-Verfahren bei funktionellen Nervenstörungen' – *Psychiatrisch-Neurologische Wochenschrift*, 17/18 (1917-1918), pp.101-105.

Brown, William, 'The treatment of cases of shell shock in an advanced neurological centre' – *The Lancet*, 192:4955 (1918), pp.197-200.

Bruce, Ninian, 'The treatment of functional blindness and functional loss of voice' – *Review of Neurology and Psychiatry*, 14 (1916), pp.195-198.

Brunner, José, 'Psychiatry, Psychoanalysis, and Politics during the First World War' – *Journal of the History of the Behavioral Sciences*, 27:4 (1991), pp.352-365.

Bryant, Richard A., 'Disentangling Mild Traumatic Brain Injury and Stress Reactions' – *The New England Journal of Medicine*, 358:5 (2008), pp.525-527.

Burton-Fanning, F.W., 'Neurasthenia in soldiers of the home forces' – *The Lancet*, 189:4894 (1917), p.907.

Bury, Judson S., 'Remarks on the Pathology of War Neuroses: An Address given to the Officers at the Lord Derby War Hospital, Warrington', *The Lancet*, 192:4952 (1918), pp.97-99.

By a Correspondent, 'Medical Aspects of Severe Trauma in War. Insanity and Psychic Trauma – *British Medical Journal*, 2:2815 (1914), pp.1,038-1,039.

Carmalt-Jones, Dudley W., 'War-Neurasthenia, Acute and Chronic' – *Brain*, 42:3 (1919), pp.171-213.

Chambers, W.D., 'Mental Wards with the British Expeditionary Force: A Review of Ten Months' Experience – *British Journal of Psychiatry*, 65:270 (1919), pp.152-180.

Chastan, Nathalie and Parain, Dominique, 'Psychogenic paralysis and recovery after motor cortex transcranial magnetic stimulation' – *Movement Disorders*, 25:10 (2010), pp.1,501-1,504.

Cohen, Shlomo and Shapiro, Haim, '"Comparable Placebo Treatment" and the Ethics of Deception' – *Journal of Medicine and Philosophy*, 38:6 (2013), pp.696-709.

Dahl, A.A., 'The DSM-III classification of the functional psychoses and the Norwegian tradition' – *Acta Psychiatrica Scandinavica Supplement,* 328 (1986): pp. 45-53.
Dickes, R.A., 'Brief therapy of conversion reactions: an in-hospital technique' – *American Journal of Psychiatry,* 131:5 (1974), pp.584-586.
Dub, D., 'Heilung psychogener Taubheit, Stummheit (Taubstummheit)' – *Deutsche Medizinische Wochenschrift,* 42:52 (1916), pp.1,601-1,602.
Duffy, Dennis, 'The Strange Second Death of Lewis Yealland' – *Ontario History,* 103:2 (2011), pp.127-149.
Dunnill, Michael S., 'Victor Horsley (1857-1916) in World War I' – *Journal of Medical Biography,* 18:4 (2010), pp.186-193.
Eager, R., 'A Record of Admissions to the Mental Section of the Lord Derby War Hospital, Warrington, from June 17th, 1916, to June 16th, 1917' – *Journal of Mental Science,* 64:266 (1918), pp.272-295.
Eder, Montague E., 'The Psycho-Pathology of the War Neuroses' – *The Lancet,* 188:4850 (1916), pp.264-268.
Elliott, T.R., 'Transient paraplegia from shell explosions' – *British Medical Journal,* 2:2815 (1914), p.1,006.
Fauser, A., 'Kriegspsychiatrische und -neurologische Erfahrungen und Betrachtungen' – *Archiv für Psychiatrie und Nervenkrankheiten,* 59:1 (1918), pp.260-280.
Fishbain, D.A., Goldberg, M., Khalil, T.M., Asfour, S.S., Abdel-Moty, E., Meagher, B.R., Santana, R., Rosomoff, R.S. and Rosomoff, H.L., 'The utility of electromyographic biofeedback in the treatment of conversion paralysis' – *American Journal of Psychiatry,* 145:12 (1988), pp.1,572-1,575.
Fraser, Francis and Wilson, R.M., 'The sympathetic nervous system and the "Irritable heart of soldiers."' – *British Medical Journal,* 2:3002 (1918), pp.27-29.
Freeman, Hugh and Berrios, German E., *150 Years of British Psychiatry* (London, Atlantic Highlands, NJ: Athlone, 1996).
Friedman, Bruce H., 'Feelings and the body: the Jamesian perspective on autonomic specificity of emotion' – *Biological Psychology,* 84:3 (2010), pp.383-393.
From a Special Correspondent in Northern France, 'Medical arrangements of the British Expeditionary Force' – *British Medical Journal,* 2:2815 (1914), pp.1,037-1,038.
Gamgee, Arthur, 'An account of a demonstration on the phenomena of hystero-epilepsy and on the modification they undergo under the influence of magnets and solenoids; given by Professor Charcot at the Salpêtrière' – *British Medical Journal,* 2:928 (1878), pp.545-548.
Ganser, Sigbert J.M., 'Über einen eigenartigen hysterischen Dämmerzustand, Vortrag, gehalten am 23. October 1897 in der Versammlung der mitteldeutschen Psychiater und Neurologen zu Halle' – *Archiv für Psychiatrie und Nervenkrankheiten,* 30:2 (1898), pp.633-640.
Geddes, Jennian F., 'The Women's Hospital Corps: forgotten surgeons of the First World War' – *Journal of Medical Biography,* 14:2 (2006), pp.109-117.

Gersons, Berthold P. and Carlier, Ingrid V., 'Post-traumatic stress disorder: the history of a recent concept' – *British Journal of Psychiatry*, 161:6 (1992), pp.742-748.
Gijswijt-Hofstra, Marijke and Porter, Roy, *Cultures of Neurasthenia. From Beard to the First World War* (New York, Amsterdam: Rodopi, 2001).
Gottstein, A., 'Die Sterblichkeit in Berlin während des ersten Kriegshalbjahres' – *Deutsche Medizinische Wochenschrift*, 41:25 (1915), p.740.
Green, Edith M.N., 'Blood pressure and surface temperature in 110 cases of shell shock' – *The Lancet*, 190:4908 (1917), pp.456-457.
Grzybowski, Andrzej and Pietrzak, Krzysztof, 'Napoleon Cybulski (1854-1919)' – *Journal of Neurology*, 260:11 (2013), pp.2,942-2,943.
Harford, Charles F., 'Visual neuroses of miners in their relation to military service' – *British Medical Journal*, 1:2879 (1916), pp.340-342.
Hart, Ernest, 'Special Correspondence: Medical Paris of today. Letter from Mr. Ernest Hart' – *British Medical Journal*, 1:1466 (1889), pp.266-268.
——'Medical Paris of today. Notes made in December, 1888' – *British Medical Journal*, 1:1467 (1889), pp.322-324.
Harzbecker, O., 'Über die Ätiologie der Granatkontusionsverletzungen' – *Deutsche Medizinische Wochenschrift*, 40:47 (1914), p.1,985.
Henderson, D.K., 'War Psychoses: An Analysis of 202 Cases of Mental Disorder occurring in Home Troops' – *Journal of Mental Science*, 64:265 (1918), pp.165-189.
Higgins, Johanne, Koski, Lisa and Xie, Haiqun, 'Combining rTMS and Task-Oriented Training in the Rehabilitation of the Arm after Stroke: A Pilot Randomized Controlled Trial' – *Stroke Research and Treatment*, 2013:539146.
Hirschfeld, R., 'Zur Behandlung im Kriege erworbener hysterischer Zustände, insbesondere von Sprachstörungen' – *Zeitschrift für die gesamte Neurologie und Psychiatrie*, 34:1 (1916), pp.195-205.
Hollender, Marc H. and Hirsch, Steven J., 'Hysterical Psychosis' – *American Journal of Psychiatry*, 120:11 (1964), pp.1,066-1,074.
'Home Hospitals and the War: Brighton, Second Eastern General Hospital: Complete Loss of Memory' – *British Medical Journal*, 2:2814 (1914), p.992.
Hotchkis, Robert D., 'Renfrew District Asylum as a War Hospital for Mental Invalids: Some Contrasts in Administration. With an Analysis of Cases admitted during the First Year' –*Journal of Mental Science*, 63:261 (1917), pp.238-249.
Hübner, A.H., 'Über Kriegs- und Unfallpsychosen' – *Archiv für Psychiatrie und Nervenkrankheiten*, 58:1 (1917), pp.324-400.
Hunt, Elizabeth J.F., Wessely, Simon, Jones, Norman, Rona, Roberto J. and Greenberg, Neil, 'The mental health of the UK Armed Forces: where facts meet fiction' – *European Journal of Psychotraumatology*, 5 (2014), 23617.
Hurst, Arthur F., 'Observations on the etiology and treatment of war neuroses' – *British Medical Journal*, 2:2961 (1917), pp.409-414.
'Insanity and the War' – *The Lancet*, 186:4801 (1915), pp.553-554.
James, William, 'What is an emotion?' – *Mind*, 9:1884, pp.188-205.
Johnson, W., 'Hysterical tremor', *British Medical Journal*, 2:3023 (1918), pp. 627-628.

Jones, Edgar, 'Historical approaches to post-combat disorders' – *Philosophical Transactions of the Royal Society B: Biological Sciences*, 361:1468 (2006), pp.533-542.

—— 'Shell Shock at Maghull and the Maudsley: Models of Psychological Medicine in the UK' – *Journal of the History of Medicine and Allied Sciences*, 65:3 (2010), pp.368-395.

—— 'War Neuroses and Arthur Hurst: A Pioneering Medical Film about the Treatment of Psychiatric Battle Casualties' – *Journal of the History of Medicine and Allied Sciences*, 67:3 (2012), pp.345-373.

Jones, Edgar, Everitt, Brian, Ironside, Stephen, Palmer, Ian and Wessely, Simon, 'Psychological Effects of Chemical Weapons: A Follow-up Study of First World War Veterans' – *Psychological Medicine*, 38:10 (2008), pp.1,419-1,426.

Jones, Edgar, Hodgins Vermaas, Robert, McCartney, Helen, Beech, Charlotte, Palmer, Ian, Hyams, Kenneth and Wessely, Simon, 'Flashbacks and post-traumatic stress disorder: the genesis of a 20th-century diagnosis' – *British Journal of Psychiatry*, 182:2 (2003), pp.158-163.

Jones, Edgar and Wessely, Simon, 'War Syndromes: The Impact of Culture on Medically Unexplained Symptoms' – *Medical History*, 49:1 (2005), pp.55-78.

—— 'British prisoners-of-war: from resilience to psychological vulnerability: reality or perception' – *Twentieth Century British History*, 21:2 (2010), pp.163-183.

—— 'Battle for the mind: World War 1 and the birth of military psychiatry' – *The Lancet*, 384:9955 (2014), pp.1,708-1,714.

Kehrer, Ferdinand, 'Zur Frage der Behandlung der Kriegsneurosen' – *Zeitschrift für die gesamte Neurologie und Psychiatrie*, 36:1 (1917), pp.1-22.

Khalil, T.M., Abdel-Moty, E., Asfour, S.S., Fishbain, D.A., Rosomoff, R.S. and Rosomoff, H.L., 'Functional electric stimulation in the reversal of conversion disorder paralysis' – *Archives of Physical Medicine and Rehabilitation*, 69:7 (1988), pp.545-547.

Khedr, Eman M., Ahmed, Mohamed A., Fathy, Nehal and Rothwell, John C., 'Therapeutic trial of repetitive transcranial magnetic stimulation after acute ischemic stroke' – *Neurology*, 65:3 (2005), pp.466-468.

Kleist, Karl, 'Schreckpsychosen' – *Allgemeine Zeitschrift für Psychiatrie und psychisch-gerichtliche Medizin*, 74 (1918), pp.432-510.

Leva, J., 'Epilepsie im Kriege' – *Archiv für Psychiatrie und Nervenheilkunde*, 65 (1922), pp.386-410.

Liebermeister, G. and Siegerist, 'Über eine Neurosenepidemie in einem Kriegsgefangenenlager' – *Zeitschrift für die gesamte Neurologie und Psychiatrie*, 37:1 (1917), pp.350-355.

Linden, Stefanie, Harris, Margaret and Healy, David, 'Religion & Psychosis: The effects of the Welsh Religious Revival in 1904/5' – *Psychological Medicine*, 40:8 (2010), pp.1,317-1,323.

Linden, Stefanie C., Hess, Volker and Jones, Edgar, 'The Neurological Manifestations of Trauma: Lessons from World War I' – *European Archives of Psychiatry and Clinical Neuroscience*, 262:3 (2012), pp.253-264.

Linden, Stefanie C. and Jones, Edgar, 'German Battle Casualties: The Treatment of functional Somatic Disorders during World War I' – *Journal of the History of Medicine and Allied Sciences*, 68:4 (2013), pp.627-658.

—— '"Shell Shock" Revisited: An Examination of the Case Records of the National Hospital in London' – *Medical History*, 58:4 (2014), pp.519-545.

Linden, Stefanie C., Jones, Edgar and Lees, Andrew J., 'Shell Shock at Queen Square: Lewis Yealland 100 years on' – *Brain*, 136:6 (2013), pp.1,976-1,988.

Maclean, W.C., 'Diseases of the heart in the British Army, the cause and the remedy' – *British Medical Journal*, 1:320 (1867), pp.161-164.

McDowall, Colin, 'Mutism in the Soldier and its Treatment' – *Journal of Mental Science*, 64:264 (1918), pp.54-64.

Maloney, W.J.M.A., 'Obituary: "The National" and Dr. F.E. Batten' – *Journal of Nervous and Mental Disease*, 49:1 (1919), pp.91-94.

Mammis, Antonios, Eloy, Jean A. and Liu, James K., 'Early descriptions of acromegaly and gigantism and their historical evolution as clinical entities: Historical vignette'– *Journal of Neurosurgery*, 29:4 (2010), p.E1.

Mann, G., 'Zur Frage der traumatischen Neurose' – *Wiener Klinische Wochenschrift*, 52 (1916), pp.257-261.

Medical Society of London, 'Surgical experiences of the present war. Functional blindness' – *British Medical Journal*, 2:2813 (1914), pp.938-942.

Meyer, Semi, 'Die nervösen Krankheitsbilder nach Explosionsschock' – *Zeitschrift für die gesamte Neurologie und Psychiatrie*, 33:1 (1916), pp.353-370.

Milligan, E.T.C., 'A method of treatment of "shell shock"' – *British Medical Journal*, 2:2898 (1916), p.73.

Mörchen, Friedrich, 'Der vorläufige Abschluß der Auseinandersetzung über das Wesen der nervösen Kriegsschädigungen' – *Psychiatrisch-Neurologische Wochenschrift*, 39/40 (1916-1917), pp.301-305.

Mott, Frederick W., 'The psychic mechanism of the voice in relation to the emotions' – *British Medical Journal*, 2 (1915), pp.845-847.

—— 'The microscopic examination of the brains of two men dead of commotio cerebri (shell shock) without visible external injury' – *British Medical Journal*, 2:2967 (1917), pp.612-615.

—— 'The Chadwick Lecture on Mental Hygiene and Shell Shock during and after the War' – *British Medical Journal*, 2:2950 (1917), pp.39-42.

Muck, Otto, 'Psychologische Betrachtungen bei Heilungen funktionell stimmgestörter Soldaten' – *Münchner Medizinische Wochenschrift*, Feldärztliche Beilage, 63 (1916), p.441.

Müri, René M., Cazzoli, Dario, Nef, Tobias, Mosimann, Urs P., Hopfner, Simone and Nyffeler, Thomas, 'Non-invasive brain stimulation in neglect rehabilitation: an update' – *Frontiers in Human Neuroscience*, 7 (2013), p.348.

Myers, Charles S., 'The justifiability of therapeutic lying: Correspondence' – *The Lancet*, 194:5026 (1919), pp.1,213-1,214.

'Nerves and War: The Mental Treatment Bill' – *The Lancet*, 185:4783 (1915), pp.919-920.

Nonne, Max, 'Über erfolgreiche Suggestivbehandlung der hysteriformen Störungen bei Kriegsneurosen' – *Zeitschrift für die gesamte Neurologie und Psychiatrie*, 37:1 (1917), pp.191-218.

Norman, Hubert J., 'Treatment of Insanity: Treatment by Suggestion' – *Journal of Mental Science*, 63:260 (1917), pp.122-123.

Opjordsmoen, Stein, 'Reactive psychosis and other brief psychotic episodes' – *Current Psychiatry Reports*, 3:4 (2001), pp.338-341.

Oppenheimer, B.S. and Rothschild, M.A., 'The psychoneurotic factor in the "irritable heart" of soldiers' – *British Medical Journal*, 2:3002 (1918), pp.29-31.

Oram, Gerard, '"The administration of discipline by the English is very rigid": British Military Law and the Death Penalty (1868 – 1918)' – *Crime, Histoire et Sociétés/ Crime, History and Societies*, 5:1 (2001), pp.93-110.

Pedersen, Susan, 'Gender, welfare, and citizenship in Britain during the Great War' – *The American Historical Review*, 95:4 (1990), p.999.

Playfair, William S., 'Notes on the systematic treatment of nerve prostration and hysteria connected with uterine disease' – *The Lancet*, 117:3013 (1881), pp.857-859.

Powell, Michael, 'Sir Victor Horsley – an inspiration' – *British Medical Journal*, 333:7582 (2006), pp.1,317-1,319.

Price, Donald D., Finniss, Damien G. and Benedetti, Fabrizio, 'A comprehensive review of the placebo effect: recent advances and current thought' – *Annual Review of Psychology*, 59 (2008), pp.565-590.

Raether, M., 'Neurosen-Heilungen nach der Kaufmann-Methode' – *Deutsche Medizinische Wochenschrift*, 43:11 (1917), pp.321-323.

Rafferty, Anne Marie and Solano, Diana, 'The Rise and Demise of the Colonial Nursing Service: British Nurses in the Colonies, 1896-1966' – *Nursing History Review*, 15:1 (2007), pp.147-154.

'Reviews and Notices: Leçons du Mardi à la Salpêtrière. Par Professeur Charcot' – *British Medical Journal*, 2:1015 (1890), pp.1,015-1,016.

Reynolds, Edward H., 'Jackson, Todd, and the Concept of "Discharge" in Epilepsy' – *Epilepsia*, 48:11 (2007), pp.2,016-2,022.

Rivers, W.H.R., 'Freud's Psychology of the Unconscious' – *The Lancet*, 189:4894 (1917), pp.912-991.

Rohde, Max, 'Neurologische Betrachtungen eines Truppenarztes im Felde' – *Zeitschrift für die gesamte Neurologie und Psychiatrie*, 29 (1915), pp.379-415.

Rothmann, M., 'Zur Beseitigung psychogener Bewegungsstörungen bei Soldaten in einer Sitzung' – *Münchner Medizinische Wochenschrift*, 63 (1916), pp.1,277-1,278.

Rusca, F., 'Experimentelle Untersuchungen über die traumatische Druckwirkung der Explosionen' – *Deutsche Zeitschrift für Chirurgie*, 132:3-4 (1914), pp.315-374.

Schioldann, Johan, 'Classic Text No. 87: "Psychogenic Psychoses" by August Wimmer (1936): Part I' – *History of Psychiatry*, 22:3 (2011), pp.347-367.

Schneider, Kurt, 'Schizophrene Kriegspsychosen' – *Zeitschrift für die gesamte Neurologie und Psychiatrie*, 43:1 (1918), pp.420-429.
Shively, Sharon B. and Perl, Daniel P., 'Traumatic Brain Injury, Shell Shock, and Posttraumatic Stress Disorder in the Military – Past, Present, and Future' – *Journal of Head Trauma Rehabilitation*, 27: 3 (2012), pp.234-239.
Shorter, Edward, 'Paralysis: The Rise and Fall of a "Hysterical" Symptom' – *Journal of Social History*, 19:4 (1986), pp.549-582.
Shorvon, Simon, 'Fashion and cult in neuroscience – the case of hysteria' – *Brain*, 130:12 (2007), pp.3,342-3,348.
Sichel, Max, 'Der Selbstmord im Felde' – *Zeitschrift für die gesamte Neurologie und Psychiatrie*, 49:1 (1919), pp.385-392.
Smith, Grafton E., 'Shock and the soldier' – *The Lancet*, 187:4834 (1916), pp.853-857.
Smyly, Cecil P., 'Treatment by Suggestion' – *Dublin Journal of Medical Science*, 139:4 (1915), pp.252-268.
Sommer, Robert, 'Beseitigung funktioneller Taubheit, besonders bei Soldaten, durch eine experimental-psychologische Methode' – *Archiv für Psychiatrie und Nervenkrankheiten*, 57:2 (1917), pp.574-575.
Stone, Jon, Carson, A., Duncan, R., Coleman, R., Roberts, R., Warlow, C., Hibberd, C., Murray, G., Cull, R., Pelosi, A., Cavanagh, J., Matthews, K., Goldbeck, R., Smyth, R., Walker, J., Macmahon, A.D. and Sharpe, M., 'Symptoms "unexplained by organic disease" in 1144 new neurology out-patients: how often does the diagnosis change at follow-up?' – *Brain*, 132:10 (2009), pp.2,878-2,888.
Stoney, Florence A., 'On the connexion between "soldier's heart" and hyperthyroidism' – *The Lancet*, 187:4832 (1916), pp.777-780.
Storch, Alfred, 'Beiträge zur Psychopathologie der uncrlaubten Entfernung und Fahnenflucht im Felde' – *Zeitschrift für die gesamte Neurologie und Psychiatrie*, 46:1 (1919), pp.348-367.
'The death-rate in Berlin during the first six months of the War' – *British Medical Journal*, 2:2851 (1915), pp.302-303.
'The War: Notes from German and Austrian Medical Journals. Disciplinary Treatment of Shell Shock' – *British Medical Journal*, 2:2921 (1916), p.882.
Tombleson, J. Bennett, 'A series of military cases treated by hypnotic suggestion' – *The Lancet*, 188:4860 (1916), pp.707-710.
Turner, William A., 'Remarks on Cases of Nervous and Mental Shock' – *British Medical Journal*, 1:2837 (1915), pp.833-835.
——'Nervous and Mental Shock' – *British Medical Journal*, 1:2893 (1916), pp.830-832.
'Vital statistics of England and Wales' – *British Medical Journal*, 2:3107 (1920), pp.79-80.
Vuilleumier, Patrik, 'Hysterical conversion and brain function' – *Progress in Brain Research*, 150 (2005), pp.309-329.
Wassermann, Eric M. and Zimmermann, Trelawny, 'Transcranial Magnetic Brain Stimulation: Therapeutic Promises and Scientific Gaps' – *Pharmacology and Therapeutics*, 133:1 (2012), pp.98-107.

Wells, S. Russell, 'A collective investigation of ten thousand recruits with doubtful heart conditions' – *British Medical Journal*, 2:3010 (1918), pp.248-251.

Wetzel, A., 'Über Schockpsychosen. Ergebnisse von Untersuchungen an ganz frischen Fällen' – *Zeitschrift für die gesamte Neurologie und Psychiatrie*, 65:1 (1921), pp.288-330.

Yealland, Lewis R. and Adrian, Edgar D., 'The treatment of some common war neuroses' – *The Lancet*, 189:4893 (1917), pp.867-872.

Ziegler, Walther and Hegerl, Ulrich, 'Der Werther-Effekt: Bedeutung, Mechanismen, Konsequenzen' – *Nervenarzt*, 73:1 (2002), pp.41-49.

Index

INDEX OF PEOPLE

Adrian, Edgar D. 195-198, 227
Alexander, Rachel F. 53, 55
Alexander, William Cleverly 53
Alzheimer, Alois 204
Anderson, Louisa Garrett 57-58
Ashby, Elizabeth 57, 111

Babinski, Joseph Jules François Félix 33, 226
Back, Reverend John 110
Barker, Pat 39, 194-195
Batten, Frederick Eustace 54, 56
Beauchamp, Lord 51
Berger, Hans 127, 236
Bernard, Claude 210
Binswanger, Otto 153, 201-202, 205-206, 211, 236, 241
Bird, Golding 197
Blandy, Majorie A. 57-59
Bonhoeffer, Karl 77, 131-132, 149-150, 164-166, 169, 174-176, 189
Breuer, Josef 214
Briquet, Paul 22
Bruce, Ninian 205
Bury, Judson S. 223, 231
Buzzard, S. Farquhar 52, 204

Cannon, Walter 76
Carmalt-Jones, Dudley William 32, 219, 225
Carver, Captain Alfred 230-231, 233, 243
Chambers, Captain W.D. 155-157
Charcot, Jean-Martin 19-22, 25-27, 30, 32-33, 37, 72, 120, 203, 206, 213

Clarke, Robert Henry 51
Cohen, Shlomo 247-248
Collier, James 52
Critchley, Macdonald 137-138
Cushing, Harvey 108
Cybulski, Napoleon 237

Dejerine, Joseph Jules 33, 80, 213
Dinsley, Lieutenant A. 230-231, 233, 243
Dubois, Paul 213
Duchenne, Guillaume-Benjamin-Amand 197

Eager, R. 218
Eder, David Montague 78-79, 207, 218-219
Ehrlich, Paul 51
Elliot Smith, Grafton 43-44, 76, 151-152, 216, 242
Elliott, T.R. 42-43

Farranridge, Clive 107-108, 110-119, 182
Ferguson, Niall 39
Forster, Edmund 150
Freud, Sigmund 20, 143, 214-215
Friedreich, Nikolaus 108
Froment, Jules 226

Ganser, Sigbert 126-129, 165, 169
Gauckler, Ernest 213
Goethe, Johann Wolfgang von 156
Gottstein, Adolf 153
Green, Edith 75, 220

Hadfield, J.A. 206-207, 218
Haldane, John Scott 74
Hart, Ernest Abraham 20-21, 26
Hata, Sahachiro 51
Henson, Hensley 138-139
Hitler, Adolf 150
Horsley, Colonel Sir Victor 49-50, 60, 62-63, 66
Hotchkis, Robert D. 219
Hurst, Arthur 27, 33, 80, 123, 205, 217, 224, 226

James, William 76
Janet, Pierre 32, 72, 114, 120, 238
Jaspers, Karl 127, 133, 143, 238
Jelenska-Macieszyna, Sabina 237
Jolowicz, Ernst 31
Jones, Edgar 234-235, 239

Kahlbaum, Karl Ludwig 129
Kaufmann, Fritz 200-201
Kehrer, Ferdinand 204-205, 209
Kempster, Frederick 108-110
Killen, Andreas 236
Klein, Josua 187
Kleist, Karl 120, 122-123, 125, 130, 133-134, 164, 238-239
Knutsford, Lord 52-53
Korsakoff, Sergei 150

Lange, Carl 76
Leese, Peter 94-95

MacCurdy, John Thomson 181, 204, 208
Machen, Arthur 139
Maclean, W.C. 224
Mann, Thomas 69
McDowall, Colin 208
Mesmer, Franz 20
Mott, Major Frederick Walker 69, 73-78, 88-89, 94, 134, 181, 197, 209-210, 212, 220, 223, 226, 231, 233, 243
Muck, Otto 207
Murray, Flora 57, 59
Myers, Charles Samuel 68-69, 76, 94, 142, 222, 243, 248

Nietzsche, Friedrich 153
Nonne, Max 25, 33, 82, 193, 206, 209, 217-218, 234

Oppenheim, Hermann 72-73, 77, 223
Owen, Wilfred 99, 101

Pear, Tom Hatherley 43-44, 76, 123, 151, 216, 242
Playfair, William Smout 210
Purdon Martin, James 58

Richer, Paul Marie Louis Pierre 23-24
Rivers, William H.R. 39, 95, 114, 174, 181, 194-195, 214
Rivington, Eveleen B. 57
Rows, Lieutenant Colonel R.G. 49
Rusca, F. 73, 243
Russell, Bertrand 174
Russell, Charles Taze 174

Sassoon, Siegfried 95, 142, 173-174, 176, 194, 214
Schneider, Kurt 141
Schroeder van der Kolk, Jacobus 236
Shapiro, Haim 247-248
Showalter, Elaine 39, 194
Sommer, Robert 208
Steward, Grainger 227
Stokes, Captain A. 73
Stoney, Florence A. 224-225
Stoney, G. Johnstone 225
Storch, Alfred 164-165, 169

Thorndike, Edward 208, 241
Tibbits, Herbert 197
Todd, Robert Bentley 236-237
Tombleson, J. Bennett 207
Tooth, Howard Henry 56, 101
Turner, Violet 57
Turner, William Aldren 52, 56, 120

Walshe, Francis 28, 96, 97, 101
Weir Mitchell, Silas 210-211

Wernicke, Carl 134
Wessely, Simon 235
Westphal, Carl 199
Wilhelm II of Germany (Kaiser) 100, 148
Winter, Jay 152
Wire, David 114-115

Yealland, Lewis Ralph 80-81, 90, 112, 117-119, 124, 180, 191-199, 201, 217, 220-223, 227, 230, 235, 241, 245-248

Zuckmayer, Carl 167

INDEX OF CASE STUDIES

Adolf S. (Belgian soldier) 52, 54-55
Adolf S. (German soldier) 166-170, 175
Albert W. (Dragoon Guards) 27-29
Albert W. (Northamptons) 173
Alfred K. 227-228
Alfred P. 143-144
Arthur T. 140-141

Benno B. 187

Charles A. 207-208
Charles S. 116
Cornelius B. 179-180, 182

Daniel T. 171
Devitt O. 78, 177-179, 182

Edward C. 111, 182-183
Edward E. 131-132
Ernst R. 123
Eugen B. 31

Frank D. 66-67
Franz B. 25, 34
Frederick C. 117
Frederick J. 117
Frederick J.W. 124-125
Frederick O. 191-192
Frederick R. 103-104
Friedrich S. 202

George B. 112
George C. 60, 62-63
George D. 89-90
George H. (Argyll and Sutherland Highlanders) 194-195

George H. (2nd Coldstream Guards) 115-116
George H. (RAMC) 183
Gustav B. 30

Hans K. 185-187
Harry D. 128-129
Harry M. 101-102
Henry M. 67-69
Herbert M. 90-91, 96
Hermann G. 127, 165

Jakob B. 127
James E. 111
James H. 112-113
James John S. 34-36, 118
James T. 192-193
John L. 183-185
John N. 129
John P. 118-119, 198, 241-242
John T. 110-111
John W. 86-87
Joseph B. 102-103
Joseph M. 199-200, 207

Karl E. 174-176

Max K. 146-151, 153, 155, 157

Nikolaus K. 125-126
Norman H. 98

Otto K. 189

Patrick D. 116-117
Patrick R. 79-80

Percy W. 198
Peter R. 87-89
Philip P. 81

Randolph S. 228-230
Richard N. 31
Ronald C. 96-97

Samuel D. 130-131
Stanley S. 115
Steward, B. 54, 56, 140-141

Walter E. 54, 56
Walter L. 187-188
Walter S. (German Musketeer) 125
Walter S. (ex-soldier) 196
Wilhelm B. 158-163, 166-167, 169-170, 175
Wilhelm H. 132
William B. 113-114William Charles L. 29-30
William Henry W. 115-116
William S. 84, 86

INDEX OF PLACES INCLUDING INSTITUTIONS

1 Canadian General Hospital, Étaples 98, 112
1 London General Hospital, Camberwell 49, 52, 54, 62
1 Southern General Hospital, Birmingham 91
2 Canadian General Hospital, Le Tréport 227
4 London General Hospital 35, 48, 73, 117, 179-180, 209
4 Stationary Hospital, Arques 32, 219
6 Stationary Hospital, Frevent 241
8 General Hospital, Rouen 107
8 Stationary Hospital, Wimereux 155
9 General Hospital, Rouen 177
12 General Hospital, Rouen 67, 129
13 General Hospital, Boulogne 79-80
21 General Hospital, Alexandria 60, 62

Aarshot 52
Aberdeen 137
Albert 198
Aldershot 27, 49, 107
Alexandria 47, 60, 62-63
Alsace-Lorraine 166
Amara 63, 66
ANZAC Cove 60, 63
Armentières 83, 89, 130, 171, 173, 177
Arras, 79, 131, 241
Ashurst War Hospital, Oxford 206, 218
Aubers Ridge 83

Aubrey House, Kensington 53-54
Aumerval 88
Australia 35, 47, 62-63

Belfast 129
Belgrade 147-149
Bloomsbury 49, 227
Bois Grenier sector 95, 98
Bologna 184
Bonn 162, 166
Boulogne 54, 80, 89, 91, 101, 155
Brest-Litovsk 131
British General Hospital, Amara 63
Bruges 146

Cairo 185
Calais 98, 155
Cambridge 49, 142, 174
Cambridge Military Hospital, Aldershot 107
Canada 195
Cape Helles 63
Champagne region 131, 158
Charité University Hospital, Berlin 25, 30-31, 37,, 69, 77, 127, 131, 143, 146, 149-150, 157, 163, 165-166, 168-169, 175, 181, 185-189, 199-200, 235-236
Claybury Asylum, Woodford, Essex 45-46
Cleve 160
Coblenz 159, 161

Cologne 146, 159, 168
Craiglockhart 60, 95, 114, 142, 174, 181, 194, 214, 216
Crimea 224, 234

The Dardanelles 64-65
Denmark 35, 162, 167,
Diksmuide 185
Dinant 161-162
Dublin 49, 206, 224
Durham 117, 130, 138
Düsseldorf 161, 165
Dutch border 160, 162
Dykebar War Hospital 219

Eastern Front 25, 83, 125, 131, 146, 150, 166, 188
Edinburgh 49, 60, 74, 174, 205
Egypt 47, 60, 62, 183, 228
Endell Street Military Hospital 58
Essen 207
Étaples 98, 112

Frankfurt 122, 131
Fulda 158
Fulham Military Hospital 36, 49, 224

Gallipoli 47, 60, 63, 65
Galway 116
Geneva 146
Giessen 164
Givenchy 87
Golders Green, London 60
Greifswald 150, 189
Grove House, Ewell 54

Hamburg 33, 37, 82, 146, 164, 167, 206, 217
Hampshire 48, 107
Hill 60 (battle of) 83, 99-104, 195
Hotel Claridge ('Hôpital Anglo-Belge') 58-59

India 47, 117

Jena 74, 123-128, 132, 153, 201-202, 205, 216
Jena Military Hospital 123-125, 132, 202, 205

Kaldenkirchen 160-161
Karlsruhe 124
King George V Hospital, Dublin 49
King George Hospital, London 227
King's College Hospital xvii, 56, 90-91, 118, 179, 194, 210, 236
Kinmel Park 179

La Bassée 87-88
Le Cateau 165
Le Havre 87
Lemnos 60
Lille 83, 122, 194
London School of Medicine for Women (LSMW) 57-58
Loos 194-195
Lord Derby War Hospital, Warrington 218
Lorduterre 88

Malta 111, 207, 219
Manchester Royal Infirmary 223
Manchester University 223
Maudsley Neurological Clearing Hospital 28, 48-49, 73, 75, 197, 209, 220
Mesopotamia 47, 63, 81
Mönchengladbach 160-161
Mons 35, 136-139, 143-144, 195
Munich 77, 148-149, 158, 204

Napsbury Asylum 80
National Hospital, Queen's Square London 27-30, 36-37, , 49-60, 62-63, 66-69, 79-81, 83 86-87, 89-91, 96-98, 101-118, 120, 124-125, 128-131, 140-141, 149, 171-173, 179-180, 182-183, 185, 191-196, 198, 201, 203-204, 208, 215-216, 226-228, 230, 235, 241
Netherlands 160, 162-163, 236
Neuss 158, 161
Neuve Chapelle, 83-94, 96, 98, 104, 195

Newcastle 128
Newham, London Borough of 111, 182
Nieuwpoort, Flanders 146
North Wales 144, 179
Nottingham 90

Osnabrück 132
Oxford 69, 179, 196, 207, 218

Palace Green 53
Paris 19-26, 32-34, 58, 206, 210, 236, 248
Philadelphia 80, 178
Ploegsteert ("Plug Street") 171
Poperinghe 191
Port Said 184
Posen 31, 146

Red Cross Military Hospital, Maghull 48-49, 181, 204, 215-216
Redlands War Hospital, Reading 35
Rhineland 158, 167
Rostock 122
Rouen 67, 86, 101, 107, 115, 129, 177-178, 198, 246
Royal Victoria Hospital, Edinburgh 49, 205
Royal Victoria Hospital, Netley 33, 48-49, 173, 205, 224
Russia 123, 131, 146

Saargemuend 166
Salonica 113, 195
Salpêtrière Hospital 19-21, 25-26, 33, 213

Santomischel, Posen 146
Schleswig 167
Sedan 25
Silvertown explosion 111, 182
The Somme 34-35, 111, 115, 117, 158, 172, 220
Souchez 98
Southampton 56, 62, 173, 183
Springfield War Hospital, London 35, 48
St. George's Hospital, London 130
St. John's Ambulance Association 116
St. Julien 192
St. Mary's Hospital, London 81
St. Quentin 131
Sulva Bay 63
Switzerland 146, 162, 164, 187
Sydney 107

Tübingen 164

United States of America 76, 156, 177-178, 233, 237-238, 244

Venlo 160-161
Verdun 143
Victoria Hospital, Bombay 81
Vietnam 70, 134, 232-234, 239

Warsaw 167
Wimereux 58, 155

Ypres 83, 100-101, 171, 173, 185, 191-192, 195, 245

INDEX OF GENERAL & MISCELLANEOUS TERMS

Acromegaly 108
American Civil War 223-224
Amyotrophic lateral sclerosis 19, 107
Angels of Mons 136-139, 143, 144
Anglican Church 138-139
ANZACs 60-61, 63
Arc de cercle 21, 22, 27, 37
Army Pay Corps 185
Army Service Corps 191
Australian Infantry 60

Behavioural models 198, 208-209, 211, 215, 240
Belgian soldiers 53-54, 58, 60
Boer War 86
British Expeditionary Force (BEF), 44, 83, 86-87, 100, 112, 136-138, 222, 243
British Psychological Society 142

Catatonia 129
Compagnie Internationale des Wagons-Lits 146
Conditioning 198, 208-209, 240, 244
Crimean War 47

Desertion 158-176
Disordered Action of the Heart (DAH) 32, 63, 223-224
Dissociation 113-114, 133-135, 141-142, 175, 188, 238
Electroencephalogram (EEG) 236
Electromyography (EMG) 245
Electrotherapy 37, 39, 63, 67, 80, 101, 104, 117, 118, 124-125, 146, 180, 192-193, 195-202, 205, 209, 210, 215, 216, 218, 221-222, 235, 246
Epilepsy 107, 110, 112-113, 227-228, 236

Friedreich's ataxia 108

Ganser syndrome 126-129, 165, 169
Gas attacks 83, 100-104,194
General Paralysis of the Insane (GPI) 47, 51-52, 155, 216

Glengorm Castle (hospital ship) 62
Gorlice-Tarnów offensive 146
Grande hystérie 22, 25, 27, 30

Hoechst (company) 51
Homosexuality 188
Huntington's chorea 108
Hypnosis 20, 33, 76, 199, 204, 206-207, 214-215, 217, 218, 219

Illegitimate children 154, 183
Infanticide 183
Isolation treatment 36, 201-202, 216, 235

Jerusalem Syndrome 144

'Kaufmann cure' 200-201, 218
Korean War 70, 233
Korsakoff syndrome 150

Lafayette Squadron 177-178
Landsturm 187

Marital infidelity 154, 183-185
Medical Research Committee (today Medical Research Council) 75, 220
Medical Society of London 41, 75
Mediterranean Expeditionary Force 62
Mental Treatment Bill 44, 134
Mild traumatic brain injury (mTBI) 231, 233, 237, 243
Military Formations/Units:
British
  Argyll & Sutherland Highlanders 194
  Bedford Regiment 103
  East Lancashire Regiment 171, 228
  Machine Gun Corps 81
  North Staffordshire Regiment 102
  Nottinghamshire and Derbyshire Regiment (Sherwood Foresters) 98, 113
  Queen's Royal West Surrey Regiment 118
  Royal Garrison Artillery 73, 198

Royal North Lancashire Regiment 88
Suffolk Regiment 96
Welsh Pioneers 111
6th Black Watch 241
2nd Coldstream Guards 115
5th Dragoon Guards 27, 29
2nd Durham Light Infantry 117
20th Durham Light Infantry 130
8th Gloucestershire Regiment 107
18th Hussars 67-68
2nd Irish Guards 129
5th King's Own Yorkshire Light Infantry 117
2nd Leinster Regiment 79
14th London Regiment (London Scottish) 54, 141, 207
20th London Regiment (County of London) 111, 227
1st Monmouthshire Regiment 66
5th Northamptonshire Regiment 173
1st Rifle Brigade 140
2nd Royal Berkshires 84
1st Royal Dragoons 54
9th Royal Fusiliers 34, 36, 118
10th Royal Sussex Regiment 27
1st Seaforth Highlanders 87
2nd Seaforth Highlanders 101
5th Seaforth Highlanders 110
4th Suffolk Regiment 90
2nd Yorkshire Regiment 86
German
   6th Bavarian Reserve Division 86
   161st Infantry Regiment 158
   166th Infantry Regiment 166
   8th Leib-Grenadier Regiment 146
   203rd Reserve Infantry Regiment 167
   207th Reserve Infantry Regiment 146
   208th Reserve Infantry Regiment 146
Miner's nystagmus 63
Ministry of Pensions 56-57
MStGB (German military penal code) 169-170
Multiple sclerosis 19, 108

Neurasthenia 47-48, 59, 71, 94, 110, 115-116, 153, 174, 199, 211, 225

Neurosurgery 49-50

Officers 53, 60, 63, 78, 94-97, 104, 114, 115-116, 161, 175, 214

Parkinson's disease 19, 116
Persuasion therapy 37, 76, 104, 198, 213, 216
Placebo 220, 248
Poliomyelitis 107
Positron emission tomography (PET) 248
Post-traumatic stress disorder (PTSD) 70, 122, 134, 152, 224, 232-234, 237, 239, 243
Prisoners of War (POW) 77, 92
Psychoanalysis 39, 114, 143, 207, 214-215, 219
Psychopathic constitution 37, 69, 131, 152, 162, 164-166, 169, 186, 187, 188, 189, 200, 232
Psychosis 143-144, 165, 238-239

Railway spine 71, 180
Reflex nervous disorder 226
Religious Revival 144, 174
Royal Air Force 178
Royal Army Medical Corps 56, 58, 73, 107, 155, 228, 230
Royal Army Ordnance Corps 230
Royal Engineers 230
Royal Field Artillery 115, 124
Royal Flying Corps 86
Royal Society 73-74
Salvarsan 51
Second World War 137, 234-235, 244
Serbian campaign 147
Siemens 236-237
Simulation 69, 97-98, 152, 188
Stigma of mental illness 151-153, 154, 220, 226, 242
Suggestion 80, 114, 156, 197, 200-207, 213-216, 217-219, 221-223, 235
Suicide 146-151, 153-157, 189
Surprise attack 207-208

Terror psychosis (*Schreckpsychose*) 120-135, 164, 238-239

Transcranial direct current stimulation (tDCS) 246-247
Transcranial magnetic stimulation (TMS) 196, 246-247
Traumatic neurosis 38, 72, 86, 152-153
Twilight states 123-129, 133, 141, 164-165, 175

War Ministry 162-163, 209
War Office 51-53, 56, 58, 105, 224
Wellcome Chemical Works 52
Women's Hospital Corps (WHC) 57-59

Zeppelin raids 105-106, 227-229

Wolverhampton Military Studies

www.helion.co.uk/wolverhamptonmilitarystudies

Editorial board

Professor Stephen Badsey
Wolverhampton University

Professor Michael Bechthold
Wilfred Laurier University

Professor John Buckley
Wolverhampton University

Major General (Retired) John Drewienkiewicz

Ashley Ekins
Australian War Memorial

Dr Howard Fuller
Wolverhampton University

Dr Spencer Jones
Wolverhampton University

Nigel de Lee
Norwegian War Academy

Major General (Retired) Mungo Melvin President of the British Commission for Military History

Dr Michael Neiberg
US Army War College

Dr Eamonn O'Kane
Wolverhampton University

Professor Fransjohan Pretorius
University of Pretoria

Dr Simon Robbins
Imperial War Museum

Professor Gary Sheffield
Wolverhampton University

Commander Steve Tatham PhD
Royal Navy
The Influence Advisory Panel

Professor Malcolm Wanklyn
Wolverhampton University

Professor Andrew Wiest
University of Southern Mississippi

Submissions

The publishers would be pleased to receive submissions for this series. Please contact us via email (info@helion.co.uk), or in writing to Helion & Company Limited, 26 Willow Road, Solihull, West Midlands, B91 1UE.

Titles

No.1 *Stemming the Tide. Officers and Leadership in the British Expeditionary Force 1914* Edited by Spencer Jones (ISBN 978-1-909384-45-3)

No.2 *'Theirs Not To Reason Why'. Horsing the British Army 1875–1925* Graham Winton (ISBN 978-1-909384-48-4)

No.3 *A Military Transformed? Adaptation and Innovation in the British Military, 1792–1945* Edited by Michael LoCicero, Ross Mahoney and Stuart Mitchell (ISBN 978-1-909384-46-0)

No.4 *Get Tough Stay Tough. Shaping the Canadian Corps, 1914–1918* Kenneth Radley (ISBN 978-1-909982-86-4)

No.5 *A Moonlight Massacre: The Night Operation on the Passchendaele Ridge, 2 December 1917. The Forgotten Last Act of the Third Battle of Ypres* Michael LoCicero (ISBN 978-1-909982-92-5)

No.6 *Shellshocked Prophets. Former Anglican Army Chaplains in Interwar Britain* Linda Parker (ISBN 978-1-909982-25-3)

No.7 *Flight Plan Africa: Portuguese Airpower in Counterinsurgency, 1961–1974* John P. Cann (ISBN 978-1-909982-06-2)

No.8 *Mud, Blood and Determination. The History of the 46th (North Midland) Division in the Great War* Simon Peaple (ISBN 978 1 910294 66 6)

No.9 *Commanding Far Eastern Skies. A Critical Analysis of the Royal Air Force Superiority Campaign in India, Burma and Malaya 1941–1945* Peter Preston-Hough (ISBN 978 1 910294 44 4)

No.10 *Courage Without Glory. The British Army on the Western Front 1915* Edited by Spencer Jones (ISBN 978 1 910777 18 3)

No.11 *The Airborne Forces Experimental Establishment: The Development of British Airborne Technology 1940–1950* Tim Jenkins (ISBN 978-1-910777-06-0)

No.12 *'Allies are a Tiresome Lot' – The British Army in Italy in the First World War* John Dillon (ISBN 978 1 910777 32 9)

No.13 *Monty's Functional Doctrine: Combined Arms Doctrine in British 21st Army Group in Northwest Europe, 1944–45* Charles Forrester (ISBN 978-1-910777-26-8)

No.14 *Early Modern Systems of Command: Queen Anne's Generals, Staff Officers and the Direction of Allied Warfare in the Low Countries and Germany, 1702–11* Stewart Stansfield (ISBN 978 1 910294 47 5)

No.15 *They Didn't Want To Die Virgins: Sex and Morale in the British Army on the Western Front 1914–1918* Bruce Cherry (ISBN 978-1-910777-70-1)

No.16 *From Tobruk to Tunis: The Impact of Terrain on British Operations and Doctrine in North Africa, 1940–1943* Neal Dando (ISBN 978-1-910294-00-0)

No.17 *Crossing No Man's Land: Experience and Learning with the Northumberland Fusiliers in the Great War* Tony Ball (ISBN 978-1-910777-73-2)

No.18 *"Everything worked like clockwork": The Mechanization of the British Cavalry between the Two World Wars* Roger E Salmon (ISBN 978-1-910777-96-1)

No.19 *Attack on the Somme: 1st Anzac Corps and the Battle of Pozières Ridge, 1916* Meleah Hampton (ISBN 978-1-910777-65-7)

No.20 *Operation Market Garden: The Campaign for the Low Countries, Autumn 1944: Seventy Years On* Edited by John Buckley & Peter Preston Hough (ISBN 978 1 910777 15 2)

No.21 *Enduring the Whirlwind: The German Army and the Russo-German War 1941-1943* Gregory Liedtke (ISBN 978-1-910777-75-6)

No.22 *'Glum Heroes': Hardship, fear and death – Resilience and Coping in the British Army on the Western Front 1914-1918* Peter E. Hodgkinson (ISBN 978-1-910777-78-7)

No.23 *Much Embarrassed: Civil War Intelligence and the Gettysburg Campaign* George Donne (ISBN 978-1-910777-86-2)

No.24 *They Called It Shell Shock: Combat Stress in the First World War* Stefanie Linden (ISBN 978-1-911096-35-1)